Ambulatory Anorectal Surgery

Springer
New York
Berlin
Heidelberg
Barcelona
Hong Kong
London
Milan
Paris
Singapore
Tokyo

H. Randolph Bailey, M.D.   Michael J. Snyder, M.D.

Editors
University of Texas Medical School at Houston, Division of Colon and Rectal Surgery

Ambulatory Anorectal Surgery

With 118 Illustrations

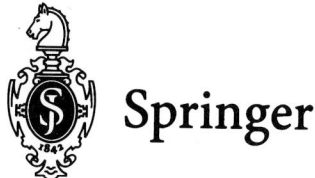

Springer

H. Randolph Bailey, M.D.
University of Texas Medical School at Houston
Division of Colon and Rectal Surgery
6550 Fannin
Smith Tower, Suite 2307
Houston, TX 77030

Michael J. Snyder, M.D.
University of Texas Medical School at Houston
Division of Colon and Rectal Surgery
6550 Fannin
Smith Tower, Suite 2307
Houston, TX 77030

Library of Congress Cataloging-in-Publication Data

Ambulatory anorectal surgery / [edited by] H. Randolph Bailey, Michael
    J. Snyder.
        p.   cm.
    Includes bibliographical references and index.
    ISBN 0-387-98603-0 (hardcover)
    1. Anus—Surgery.   2. Rectum—Surgery.   3. Ambulatory surgery.
    I. Bailey, H. Randolph.   II. Snyder, Michael J.
    [DNLM: 1. Anus Diseases—surgery.   2. Rectal Diseases—surgery.
    3. Ambulatory Surgical Procedures—methods.   WI 650 A497 1999]
    RD544.A53   1999
    617.5′55—dc21
    DNLM/DLC
    for Library of Congress   98-52782

Printed on acid-free paper.

Production coordinated by Impressions Book and Journal Services, Inc. and managed by Terry Kornak; manufacturing supervised by Joe Quatela.
Typeset by Impressions Book and Journal Services, Inc., Madison, WI.
Printed and bound by Maple-Vail Book Manufacturing Group, York, PA.
Printed in the United States of America.

9 8 7 6 5 4 3 2 1

ISBN 0-387-98603-0   Springer-Verlag   New York   Berlin   Heidelberg   SPIN 10689513

Preface

In the 25 years since the beginning of my residency in colon and rectal surgery, both the specialty of colon and rectal surgery and the entire face of medical practice have changed dramatically. Technology has exploded with such advances as the use of surgical staplers and imaging systems (CT and MRI). Colonoscopy, in its infancy in 1973, is now widely used (perhaps overused) for its potential for reducing the incidence of colorectal cancer. Surgical techniques, such as the ileal pouch-anal anastomosis, and colo-anal anastomosis, have moved from the theoretical to the mainstream in the treatment of inflammatory bowel disease and rectal cancer. Local treatment for rectal cancers, many of which in 1973 would have been treated by abdominoperineal resection, has now become widely accepted and practiced. Widespread use of adjuvant radiation and chemotherapy has improved survival in patients with colorectal cancer and has made some rectal tumors resectable or amenable to sphincter-saving procedures.

One of the most dramatic changes that has occurred during the past 25 years has been the shift in the performance of surgical procedures requiring lengthy inpatient hospital stays to ambulatory settings. A striking example of this change is seen with excisional hemorrhoidectomy. In 1973, at the Ferguson Hospital, Grand Rapids, Michigan, patients undergoing hemorrhoidectomy were admitted to the hospital the evening before surgery and stayed an average of 7 days postoperatively. In our practice today, virtually all operations for hemorrhoids, as well as most other anorectal surgical procedures, are performed on an ambulatory basis with a postoperative stay of less than 4 hours.

I was first made aware of the concept of "outpatient" anorectal surgery by the work of William G. Friend and Stephen Medwell of Seattle, Washington.[1] Their writings and lectures about their experience performing anorectal operations on an ambulatory basis showed benefits for the surgeon, the patient, and those who pay for medical care. For example, benefits for the surgeons included elimination of postoperative rounds and reduction in the number and frequency of postoperative telephone calls. Their patients had an improved sense of well-being when they were allowed to return home to familiar surroundings, food, and family. Finally, the elimination of an extended postoperative hospital stay saved the payers a considerable sum of money.

Our clinic embraced the concept of ambulatory anorectal surgery early in its development and soon realized that Friend and Medwell were correct in their assessment of its benefits. One unexpected benefit of ambulatory surgery that we noted was a significant decrease in the incidence of postoperative urinary retention. A paper from our institution by Stuart Hoff[2] touting ambulatory surgery as a solution to postoperative urinary retention probably led to the development of this book. When Laura Gillan, an editor with Springer-Verlag Publishers, was looking for someone to edit a book on ambulatory colon and rectal surgery, she found Dr. Hoff's paper and contacted us.

Crucial to the decision to begin this project was the fact that Mike Snyder, my new partner, agreed, while he was still a Fellow, to help edit the book. With his assistance, as well as that of the publisher, a group of enthusiastic and experienced contributors, and our excellent medical illustrator, Scott Barrows, we have put together in a relatively short period of time a collection of material that we hope will be helpful to both the colon and rectal surgeon and the general surgeon.

We have tried to include a wide range of topics including the facility, technical aspects of the surgery, and coding and other economic issues in ambulatory surgery. The chapters on positioning the patient for surgery and those on techniques of hemorrhoidectomy are controversial enough to justify the point–counterpoint approach. Other areas where the editors disagree with the approaches of the chapter authors are covered by a series of "Editor's notes."

This book was our first undertaking of this magnitude. A project such as this is always more time-consuming than one predicts. The time commitment necessary to finish the manuscript has meant less time for our families and friends. Mike and I are grateful for the understanding of our wives, Elizabeth and Kelly, as well as of our partners, as we have worked to complete the project. We are also appreciative of the editorial assistance from my friend and editorial adviser Carolyn Gurklis Huff.

H. Randolph Bailey

Bibliography

1. Medwell SJ, Friend WG. Outpatient anorectal surgery. Dis Colon Rectum 1979;22:480–482.
2. Hoff SD, Bailey HR, Butts DR, Max E, Smith KW, Zamora LF, et al. Ambulatory surgical hemorrhoidectomy—a solution to postoperative urinary retention? Dis Colon Rectum 1994; 37:1242–1244.

Contents

Contributors

H. Randolph Bailey, M.D., F.A.C.S., Clinical Professor of Surgery, The University of Texas Medical School at Houston, Houston, Texas

Richard P. Billingham, M.D., F.A.C.S., Clinical Associate Professor, Department of Surgery, University of Washington, Seattle, Washington

Scott M. Browning, M.D., Staff Colorectal Surgeon, Wilford Hall Medical Center, Lackland AFB, Texas, Assistant Professor of Surgery, Uniformed Services University of the Health Sciences, Bethesda, Maryland

Ian G. Faragher, M.B., B.S., F.R.A.C.S., F.R.C.S.(Ed.), Senior Lecturer, Department of Surgery—Western Hospital, University of Melbourne, Victoria, Australia

Andrea Ferrara, M.D., F.A.C.S., Colon and Rectal Clinic of Orlando, Clinical Assistant Professor of Surgery, University of Florida College of Medicine, Gainesville, Florida

Charles O. Finne III, M.D., F.A.C.S., Clinical Associate Professor, Division of Colon and Rectal Surgery, University of Minnesota, Minneapolis, Minnesota

Debra Holly Ford, M.D., F.A.C.S., Assistant Professor and Chief, Division of General Surgery, Head, Section of Colon and Rectal Surgery, Howard University College of Medicine, Washington, D.C.

Joseph Gallagher, M.D., Colorectal Fellow, University of Florida College of Medicine, Gainesville, Florida, Orlando Regional Healthcare System Fellowship Program, Colon & Rectal Clinic of Orlando, Orlando, Florida

Julio Garcia-Aguilar, M.D., Ph.D., Clinical Associate Professor, Division of Colon and Rectal Surgery, University of Minnesota Cancer Center, Minneapolis, Minnesota

J. Byron Gathright Jr., M.D., F.A.C.S., Chairman Emeritus, Department of Colon and Rectal Surgery, Ochsner Clinic, New Orleans, Louisiana

Stanley M. Goldberg, M.D., F.A.C.S., Hon.F.R.A.C.S., Hon.F.R.C.S.(Eng), Hon.A.F.C.(Fr), Hon.G.R.C.P.S.(Glasg), Hon.F.R.S.M.(Lond), Division of Colon and Rectal Surgery, Department of Surgery, University of Minnesota, Minneapolis, Minnesota

Ernest D. Graves III, M.D., F.A.C.S., Associate Professor of Surgery, University of South Alabama College of Medicine, Mobile, Alabama

Stuart D. Hoff, M.D., F.A.C.S., Private Practice, Colon and Rectal Surgery, Tulsa, Oklahoma

Susanna Hudson, R.N., Director of Nursing, Medical Center Endoscopy, The University of Texas Medical School at Houston, Houston, Texas

John T. Isler, M.D., F.A.C.S., Clinical Instructor, Department of Surgery, University of Washington, Attending Surgeon, Northwest Hospital, Swedish Hospital Medical Center, and Providence Medical Center, Seattle, Washington

Richard E. Karulf, M.D., F.A.C.S., Division of Colon and Rectal Surgery, Department of Surgery, University of Minnesota, Minneapolis, Minnesota

Sergio W. Larach, M.D., F.A.C.S., Clinical Associate Professor of Surgery, University of Florida, College of Medicine, Gainesville, Florida

Michael Lavan, R.N., Director of Surgical Services, HealthSouth Hospital for Specialized Services, Houston, Texas

Ann C. Lowry, M.D., F.A.C.S., Division of Colon and Rectal Surgery, Department of Surgery, University of Minnesota, Minneapolis, Minnesota

Martin A. Luchtefeld, M.D., F.A.C.S., Program Director for Residency Training, The Ferguson-Blodgett Digestive Disease Institute, Associate Professor of Surgery, Michigan State University College of Human Medicine, Grand Rapids, Michigan

John M. MacKeigan, M.D., F.R.C.S.(C.), F.A.C.S., Ferguson Clinic, Grand Rapids, Michigan

Fatima A. Mawji, M.D., M.B.A., Chief of Anesthesia and Medical Director, HealthSouth Hospital for Specialized Surgery, Houston, Texas

Ernest Max, M.D., F.A.C.S., Clinical Associate Professor, Department of Surgery, Baylor College of Medicine, Houston, Texas

Frank G. Opelka, M.D., F.A.C.S., Colorectal Surgeon, Department of Colon and Rectal Surgery, Ochsner Clinic, New Orleans, Louisiana

M. Parker Roberts, M.D., F.A.C.S., Clinical Instructor, The University of Texas Medical School at Houston, Houston, Texas

Andrew A. Shelton, M.D., Division of Colon and Rectal Surgery, Department of Surgery, University of Minnesota, Minneapolis, Minnesota

Michael J. Snyder, M.D., Clinical Instructor, The University of Texas Medical School at Houston, Houston, Texas

Judy Swanson, R.N., Director of Perioperative Services, The Methodist Hospital, Houston, Texas

1

Facilities for Ambulatory Surgery

Part A: The Freestanding Ambulatory Surgery Center

Michael Lavan, R.N.

The ambulatory surgery center (ASC) differs from the general hospital (GH) in several respects. First and foremost, the ASC is a facility for the exclusive treatment of patients through surgery. Second, the purpose of the ASC is to perform only surgical procedures that can be expected to be managed with a short postoperative stay at the facility.

The ASC has many advantages over the GH facility, some of which are financial and others related to patient flow and satisfaction. Clearly, a facility that has a limited purpose and scope can eliminate many services and costs that are necessary in the GH. As many hospital administrators will attest, the management of medical problems within the hospital is frequently a drain on the resources of the facility, balanced only by the more profitable surgical services. Examples of expensive cost centers in the GH include the intensive care units, emergency room, and many full-time ancillary services. A freestanding ASC may also provide a more satisfactory experience for the patient and family. Examples of this include parking near the facility (often at no additional cost), streamlined flow of the patient through the registration and preoperative process, and the ability for the family to be with the patient most of the time while at the facility (except in the operating room). In some facilities, the patient may also encounter the

same personnel both preoperatively and postoperatively. From the standpoint of the surgeon, the ASC may function more efficiently than the GH for many of the reasons already mentioned. In addition, the efficiencies of time that are possible in a small unit with regard to turnover time between cases and working with the same personnel on a daily basis may allow the surgeon to complete his or her operative schedule in less time than would be required in a GH. The mindset and efficiency of the anesthesia personnel may also play a large role in making the ASC a more time- and cost-effective working environment for the surgeon.

Issues that must be faced by the freestanding ASC that are taken for granted by the GH include standard hospital services such as laboratory, electrocardiography, radiology, pathology, and pharmacy. Another critical issue is what to do with the occasional patient in whom something unexpected occurs requiring more intensive medical care than is possible in the ASC.

The Facility

The only nonsurgical procedures performed in our facility are endoscopic procedures. The ASC provides an ideal environment for such procedures as well. Patients who experience complications of their endoscopic procedure such as perforation or bleeding can be promptly transferred, as mentioned below, to a tertiary facility for treatment. Fortunately, such a situation is rare, and no endoscopy patient has required transfer for such reasons in the 4 years since our facility opened.

To be eligible for contracting with Medicare as well as most other third-party payers, the facility must be accredited by the Joint Commission on Accreditation of Healthcare Organizations (JCAHO). This involves a rigorous inspection of the facility as well as its medical staff organization and policies and procedures. One of the requirements for the ASC to be accredited by the JCAHO is proper credentialing and re-credentialing of the medical staff members. Our Medical Executive Committee is made up of the chiefs of the various specialties represented in the facility as well as administration and pharmacy. The Medical Executive Committee fulfills the JCAHO requirement for staff meetings, and the minutes of these meetings are distributed to the other members of the medical staff.

Planning and Resource Utilization

One of the greatest challenges in operating an ASC efficiently (and a major difference from a hospital setting) is the necessity of effective planning. Unlike a hospital that has seemingly unlimited resources, the ASC is self-contained and has to rely on careful preparedness in order to function effectively. General hospitals typically have several supply areas from which to draw, much larger inventory of equipment and instruments, and an extensive support staff. In an ASC, the instruments and equipment may be limited to those needed to perform specific procedures. Because of limited storage areas and budgetary restraints, supplies are ordered on an "as needed" basis, making advance planning extremely important.

Because of limited equipment, supplies, and instruments, it is imperative that the ASC maintain a network of external support with other facilities and resources. By developing reciprocal relationships with other facilities, the ASC is able to borrow instruments and equipment when needed. It is also extremely important to maintain close contact and open communication with the surgeons to ensure that all of the necessary equipment, instruments, and other supplies that will be needed for each procedure can be provided and will be available.

The issue of how to deal with patients in whom something unexpected occurs that cannot be handled with the facilities available at the ASC is crucial in planning and establishing the facility. A signed agreement with a nearby full-service general hospital that allows the transfer of patients requiring services unavailable at the ASC is mandatory. Although most hospitals may not be enthusiastic about being what they envision as the "dumping ground" for the competing ASC, such an arrangement may be sweetened by combining it with an agreement to use their laboratory and/or radiology facilities. Transfer of patients can be accomplished by ambulance, with critically ill patients accompanied by a physician (usually an anesthesiologist) from the ASC. Fortunately, the need for transfer of patients is quite rare, especially if patients are properly selected for their procedures in the ASC.

Patient Flow within the Facility

An issue crucial to the efficiency of the ASC is patient flow. Our facility has two levels. The patients enter on the first level, where they are promptly registered and their insurance information is verified. Patients and their families are then escorted to the second-floor preoperative area, where the patient is prepared for surgery. A brief anesthesia interview takes place and intravenous access is established. Laboratory information is checked and informed consent documents are signed. Once the surgeon arrives and the history and physical examination are completed, the patient is sedated and transported to the operating room.

After completion of the operative procedure, the patient is taken to the postanesthesia care unit (PACU), which is immediately adjacent to the operating suites. A family member is allowed into the PACU as soon as the patient is stable and semi-alert. As the patient awakens, he or she is either kept in the PACU or moved to the progressive recovery area until discharge. Distances are quite short between all areas in the facility, a factor in increasing the efficiency of patient flow. In addition to the regular PACU, our facility also has a separate pediatric area for recovery after anesthesia. When the patient is stable and ready for discharge, he or she is transported downstairs by wheelchair to his or her transportation home.

Nursing and Staffing Issues

To handle the day-to-day surgical schedule, which averages 16 cases a day, our center has six operating rooms, two endoscopy rooms, and one cystoscopy room. The types of procedures we perform include general surgical, colon and rectal, gastroenterologic, gynecologic, orthopedic, genitourinary, plastic, ophthalmologic, and otorhinolaryngologic. To handle the staffing of the operating room (OR), the preoperative area, and the recovery room, the facility maintains a mix of full-time, part-time, and per-diem nurses. The operating room has five full-time registered nurses (RNs), five full-time operating room technicians, and several part-time and per-diem nurses and technicians to help accommodate fluctuations in the OR schedule and to help cover vacations and requested time off. To keep costs down, nurses must be flexible, leaving early at times when cases are completed and staying late to finish cases when necessary. The preoperative area has one full-time RN, one licensed vocational nurse (LVN), and one nurse technician. We also use one part-time RN to help when the schedule is busy. Our preoperative nurses are cross-trained to PACU and endoscopy and are all advanced cardiac life support (ACLS) certified. The PACU has two full-time RNs and several per-diem and part-time nurses. All of these nurses are also cross-trained to preoperative, endoscopy, and patient care rooms and must also be ACLS certified. We have several RNs and LVNs to cover patient care rooms on a 24-hour basis. In the event that we do not have any overnight patients, the facility is still staffed on a 24-hour basis, but it is staffed with either an LVN or a paramedic to cover the emergency room. We are not required to staff with an RN in this instance.

Ancillary Services

Laboratory

An area that requires careful planning is the laboratory in the ASC. Our center is able to provide only limited laboratory services, which include measuring serum electrolytes, hemoglobin and hematocrit,

blood urea nitrogen, glucose, and bleeding time; analyzing urine pregnancy tests; performing urinalysis; and measuring arterial blood gases. We also have the capability of performing frozen section examination of tissue specimens. We have a contract with a neighboring hospital that provides services for any other laboratory studies that are needed. A taxi company, with which we contract, transports specimens to the hospital. Tests are completed, and results are transmitted via telephone lines and modem to our computer and printer, which are interfaced with the contracted hospital's laboratory computer. The total turnaround time for this process is approximately 2 hours. Physicians are made aware of the limitations of our laboratory capabilities when they join our medical staff. They are strongly encouraged to carefully assess the needs for preoperative testing and to send patients for their preoperative visit at least 2 to 3 days before surgery. We contract with a group of pathologists for histologic evaluation of all tissue specimens. The pathologists also come to the ASC to perform frozen section tissue examinations, both planned and unplanned. The pathologists are also responsible for maintaining our laboratory policies and procedures, performing laboratory quality control, and preparing for JCAHO and Clinical Laboratory Improvement Act (CLIA) surveys. A member of this group also sits on our Medical Executive Committee to ensure adequate representation for laboratory/pathology.

Radiology

Our facility has only limited radiographic capabilities. These capabilities include obtaining chest radiographs, obtaining x-ray films during cystoscopic procedures, and performing radiographic studies (cholangiograms, C-arm studies, etc.) in the operating rooms using portable equipment. A nearby facility, with which we contract, has full-service radiology capabilities, including fluoroscopy, computed tomographic (CT) scanning and magnetic resonance imaging (MRI). The radiologists in the contract facility also interpret studies performed in our ASC.

Pharmacy

For obvious reasons, our facility does not have a full-time staff pharmacist. Instead, a part-time/contract pharmacist assists us in organizing and maintaining our pharmacy. The pharmacist is responsible for ordering all drugs, including controlled substances; maintaining and updating the formulary as needed; assisting with policies and procedures; and completing all paperwork required for state pharmacy license and JCAHO accreditation. Another role of the contract pharmacist is assisting with cost-containment issues by ensuring limited but adequate inventory of drugs, using generics when feasible, returning outdated medications for credit in a timely manner, and so forth. He is used as a resource person and also sits on the Medical Executive Committee to ensure that standards are met and that the pharmacy is represented. Drugs are removed from the pharmacy and signed out with the patient's name, date, and other information in a log book so the pharmacist is able to keep proper records of drug usage. Our pharmacy does not dispense medications for take-home prescriptions. A nearby retail pharmacy will deliver take-home medications to the facility as a convenience to our patients

A major difference between a GH and an ASC is that a hospital generally provides services such as food and nutrition, blood bank, anesthesia, electrocardiography, housekeeping, laundry, interpretation, and medical transcription. Our ASC must contract for these services as well as those listed above.

Dietary

Although we function as an ASC, we are licensed as a hospital (see Hospital License, below) and therefore must have a registered dietitian to oversee and plan our patients' diets. We do not have a kitchen on the premises. We contract with a neighboring hospital, which provides us with a registered dietitian who visits our facility at least twice weekly and as needed to review patient charts. The contract hospital also supplies us with food trays for our patients. We have a nutrition room that is utilized to hold the patient trays as well as to prepare snacks and light meals for patients.

Blood Bank

Our center contracts with the regional blood center to provide blood and blood products as needed. Blood products should ideally be cross-matched and ordered in advance of the procedure so that

they can be available in the "blood bank refrigerator" in the facility during the surgical procedure. In emergency situations, the clot is transported to the blood center by taxi or ASC personnel and blood products are returned to the facility by the blood center.

Anesthesia

We contract with a group of anesthesiologists to provide anesthesia for our surgical patients. Under this contract the anesthesiologists provide the anesthesia machines, but our facility provides the maintenance on the machines and all drugs and supplies used by anesthesia. The anesthesiologists are responsible for their own professional liability insurance as well as that for any certified registered nurse anesthetists who work with them. One of the anesthesiologists also serves as the medical director of the facility and sits on the Medical Executive Committee.

Electrocardiography

The facility has a contract with a company that provides us with electrocardiography (ECG) capabilities. Under this contract the ECG company provides us with ECG equipment and a transmitter. The ECG is recorded from the patient and is immediately transmitted to the ECG company via telephone. A copy of the computer-interpreted ECG is then faxed to us, usually within 10 to 20 minutes. The anesthesiologist evaluates the ECG and makes the immediate decision as to the patient's suitability for undergoing anesthesia. Each ECG is subsequently read and interpreted by a cardiologist, and the original copy is then mailed to our facility.

Housekeeping

Housekeeping services are provided through an agency that is contracted to maintain and clean our facility in accordance with hospital policy and JCAHO standards. The housekeeping company is responsible for ongoing training of their employees, including orienting them to job safety techniques and universal precautions. They also maintain all records for these employees. This company is also responsible for maintaining and updating our Material Safety Data Sheets (MSDS) manual for all cleaning chemicals and agents used within the facility.

Linen

The facility also has a contract with a linen company that provides and maintains all linens within the center. We are billed according the usage of linens only. Our facility purchases operating room attire (scrub clothing) and patient gowns, and the linen service launders them for us.

Other Ancillary Services

We also have contracts with an interpreter service and a medical transcription service. The interpreter service is utilized on an as-needed basis only and is available 24 hours a day. The medical transcription service provides transcription of all operative reports, patient histories and physical examinations, and other information. Dictation is done via telephone and the reports are transcribed and sent via modem to our facility, usually within 24 to 48 hours. A short-form, handwritten history and physical examination report is used for a majority of our patients undergoing surgery. This form meets all requirements of the JCAHO. Patient charts are maintained in the facility's medical records department, and the same policies found in hospitals also apply in the ASC.

It is readily apparent that our facility relies heavily on contracted services. It is essential to the operation of the facility that such services are coordinated and that all employees become knowledgeable regarding how or where to obtain these services as needed.

Patient Satisfaction

There are several major differences between a hospital and an ASC. Perhaps the most notable difference is the potential for patients to experience greater overall satisfaction in their experience with the surgical procedure. There can be much more personal attention and less "hassle factor" in an ASC than in a hospital. It may begin with parking close to the front door of the facility, often for free. Patients are greeted at the door, begin their registration process immediately upon arrival, and then are sent promptly to the preoperative area. Because of short distances between different areas as well as efficiency of personnel, the time needed from arrival at the ASC to the start of the surgical procedure may be considerably shorter than in the GH. Family members may be allowed and even encouraged to stay with the patient throughout much of the process. The preoperative area, the surgical suites, and the recovery areas are all in close proximity, a factor that facilitates efficient flow of patients from one area to the other. Family members may be allowed into the recovery area once the patient is awake and stable. The friendly, relaxed atmosphere as well as the presence of family members may help to reduce the stress of the surgical process. Our facility frequently hears comments and compliments from patients and their families regarding the personal attention they receive and how this made their surgery a much more positive experience.

Hospital License

Whereas our center is basically structured and functions as an ambulatory surgery center, it is somewhat unique in that it is formally licensed as a hospital and accredited as such by the JCAHO. Although we are licensed as a hospital we do not admit patients for nonsurgical problems. We function to serve patients having only elective surgical procedures. To be licensed as a hospital, we must be staffed 24 hours a day. State law also mandates that we maintain a fully equipped emergency room. This is the reason behind our need for 24-hour staffing regardless of our census (or absence thereof). We see an average of only 2 or 3 patients a year through our emergency room. If a patient presents to our emergency facility with a life-threatening condition or injuries, our goal is to stabilize and transfer the patient immediately to a tertiary care facility with which we have a contract. This is similar to our transfer contract as mentioned for other seriously ill patients. Being licensed as a hospital may at times be burdensome. However, the advantage that it affords us is in allowing our patients the possibility of staying beyond the 23-hour time constraint that is usually present with ambulatory surgery centers. This also allows our surgeons to perform surgical procedures in our facility that they might not consider in a more limited ASC. Our hospital has a total of seven patient care rooms, and on average three to four of these rooms are occupied daily.

Conclusions

The freestanding ASC is a facility that may serve the needs of both patients and surgeons. It allows a patient-friendly and hassle-free experience for the patient that may be less costly and stressful for all involved. For the surgeon, a facility in which surgical procedures may be promptly and efficiently completed while at the same time providing a safe environment that is acceptable to patients is clearly a win-win situation. The freestanding ASC can provide the environment for efficient performance of a majority of the surgical procedures carried out in the United States today.

Part B: The Hospital Ambulatory Surgery Center

Judy Swanson, R.N.

During the late 1970s and early 1980s there was a dramatic shift in how patients were cared for when surgical intervention was identified as their course of treatment. Before that time, all surgical patients were admitted to the hospital the night before surgery for the customary workup. This workup involved extensive blood tests, radiographs, and an electrocardiogram and provided the physicians with clinical data that allowed them to proceed comfortably with the surgery. Little thought was given to the cost of those diagnostic tests or whether those tests were even necessary before anesthesia or the surgical procedure. As hospitals filled with patients, it became necessary to build additional facilities to accommodate the surgical volumes.

As hospital occupancy rose, procedures were then identified that could be done on a same-day surgery or ambulatory basis. The development of short-acting anesthetic agents allowed the patients to recover quickly and to go home the same day. With further refinements of anesthetic agents, the same-day surgery process became a reality. The advent of ambulatory surgery led many hospitals to identify areas in close proximity to the main campus where outpatient surgical facilities could be constructed. The concept of separate sites for ambulatory procedures grew rapidly. Some systems aligned ambulatory facilities directly to the main campus, whereas many others located them on a freestanding site in a remote location.

The popularity of ambulatory or same-day surgery facilities continues to increase with both surgeons and patients. Convenience for both physicians and patients has been a key factor in the rapid growth of these facilities nationwide. The growth and expansion of outpatient surgical facilities ultimately resulted in hospitals with vacant inpatient operating rooms. Underutilization of these operating rooms became a major focus of attention for hospital administrators as they watched their revenue base slip away to freestanding surgery centers. The length of stay for inpatients decreased as same-day admissions and "23-hour observation status" became common practice. This entire phenomenon created an excess of inpatient capacity. Nursing units were, of necessity, consolidated and closed, leaving valuable real estate unoccupied. Empty wards became support space for new categories of administrative functions such as case management and utilization review.

The Hospital-Based Ambulatory Unit

The technology explosion has created easier ways to perform what were once considered very complex surgical procedures. Advanced technology and minimally invasive surgery have given the surgeon opportunities to drastically decrease the morbidity of some surgical procedures. These advances allow patients to return to normal activities in days rather than weeks or months. However, many of these procedures are very complex and may require extensive postoperative intervention. Freestanding centers typically do not have the ability to keep patients overnight if their condition requires additional care and observation. Hospitals are able to use prime real estate to develop programs to care for these patients. Inpatient facilities that can provide cost-efficient, quality outpatient surgical procedures can compete extremely well for these patients. Establishing an outpatient environment in the inpatient setting serves the purposes of convenience, cost containment, and comprehensive care.

Preoperative Assessment

Since the higher-risk patient may require more extensive preoperative assessment, the time involved for this can also be significant. The patient's physical status may require intervention earlier than the day of surgery. Diagnostic testing and clearance from an internist may be required before the patient can be accepted for surgery and anesthesia. Areas devoted to this evaluation will facilitate the patient's care. An assessment center is best located in close proximity to the outpatient laboratory, patient registration area, and radiology department. The ideal assessment center will provide for a single stop by the patient. The patient will have a nurse assessment, anesthesia evaluation, and all required diagnostic testing in one location. This encounter provides the patient and family a nonthreatening introduction to the hospital personnel and services while establishing a relationship with the health care team.

Preoperative teaching, emotional support, and discharge planning are important interactions that require time for open dialogue with the patient and family. These activities should begin during the preoperative assessment.

The medical record is initiated at the assessment center, and documentation is completed at the initial visit. This time-consuming process is a priority to ensure that important information is gathered and not overlooked until the day of the surgery. Neither the age nor the physical status of the patient provides absolute contraindications to outpatient surgery. The preoperative assessment center should meet the needs of all ages.

The preoperative assessment process by nursing and anesthesia personnel successfully completes the reconciliation of the chart. All the data and documentation are reviewed, the physical assessment is evaluated, and the anesthesiologist concludes whether or not this patient can undergo anesthesia

and proceed with the scheduled procedure. This advance detection of the need for additional physician intervention is critical to the successful management of surgical schedules. When this process is followed, patient confidence and satisfaction will be high, and costly interruptions of operating room schedules will be minimal.

Minimizing the length of stay has increased the intensity of the visit for the patient and family. The patient who has been assessed before the day of surgery and who had properly directed preoperative teaching will enter the unit with confidence. The medical record has been completed and reconciled. This advance chart review promotes staff awareness of the need for further actions and allows most corrections or additional requirements to be rectified in the time allotted before surgery.

Outpatient Admission Unit

When designing the outpatient admission area, the following requirements should be considered. Proximity to the operating room is desirable for the convenience of the surgeon, patient, and family. Contiguous space gives all the disciplines easy access to the patient. An admission unit where patients and their families come to be prepared for the surgery is preferred over the ward-like preoperative "holding" areas often found in ambulatory facilities. The area is designed to promote ease of processing the patient through the system. A unit must contain all the support space that is needed to support nursing care. The nursing station should be located so that patients and their families are greeted as they arrive. An inpatient unit converted to outpatient space may require redesign of the desk where patients report. The secretarial functions in this unit are more extensive than in an inpatient unit and may thus require additional space in which to assemble and consolidate charts. A small dietary area is used to provide nourishment to the patients in the postoperative phase. Rooms equipped with bathrooms and televisions are desirable because they may make the waiting time more pleasant for patients and their families. The rooms can be both private and semiprivate, and assignment to the space can be based on the patient's physical status and needs. Since the ultimate postoperative status is not determined in many patients until after the recovery phase, all patients are assessed preoperatively as completely as for an inpatient admission. During patient assessment, maintenance of privacy is nicely accomplished in these converted nursing units. Preoperative teaching is accomplished in this setting and early discharge teaching is initiated.

Timing of arrival is a very important aspect of outpatient surgery. A minimum of 1 hour is required if patients have completed their preoperative assessment. If advance preoperative evaluation has not been completed, a minimum of 2 hours is needed. Even with a 2-hour window, it is difficult to guarantee that all the necessary information can be retrieved and evaluated for its relevancy and the patient can be cleared for surgery. This time frame becomes even more complicated with patients who are scheduled for early start times in the operating room. Many cancellations and delays result when patients who are scheduled for early surgery do not have their preoperative evaluation in advance of the day of surgery. The requirement for immediate laboratory work when the patient arrives on the unit may be easily managed by the patient's arriving 30 minutes early. Again, this need for additional testing must have been identified as a result of the preoperative assessment.

Point-of-care testing (the performance of studies such as measurement of glucose and potassium levels at the bedside) for screening purposes has become very popular with outpatients. However, these urgent laboratory studies should be minimized in frequency and limited to patients who require evaluation based on current illness and medications. In the preoperative evaluation of complex patients, the comprehensive laboratory facility located in the hospital can provide information quickly and accurately, thus giving the hospital outpatient facility an edge over the freestanding unit. In summary, early patient arrival and preoperative assessment before the day of surgery are crucial to the success of a well-managed surgery schedule for both inpatients and outpatients.

Hospital Services

The technical aspects of the operation can be carried out equally well in either a freestanding or a hospital ASC. Advantages of performing outpa-

tient surgery in the hospital setting are the hospital's extensive support services and their ready availability. Such resources and technology may be too costly to purchase in a freestanding surgery site based on the frequency with which they may be used. Examples include the full-service laboratory, blood bank, pharmacy, and cardiology services that may not be readily available in a freestanding center. The extensive food and nutrition services in the hospital setting offer a distinct advantage to patients having special dietary requirements. Education about food and drug interactions is necessary in more complicated patients and is easily accomplished when pharmacists and clinical nutritionists are on site. If for some reason a scheduled surgical case is canceled or delayed, it is more likely in the hospital unit that another patient can easily be moved into the slot and the schedule can proceed.

Many patients' surgical plan must be altered based on the unexpected findings noted during the procedure. The patient may need a more extensive procedure than planned and may therefore require inpatient postoperative services. Such adjustments can easily be made when the surgery is being performed in the hospital setting.

Postanesthesia Care Unit

While in the postanesthesia care unit (PACU), patients receive pharmacologic agents to control their pain as well as assessment of their status for determination of postoperative care. The patient must meet certain criteria for discharge from the PACU. These criteria do not, however, always determine that the patient will be discharged to home. It may be concluded instead that the proper care requires observation status. The hospital outpatient setting again provides the options and the flexibility to respond to this type of situation. The decision to use the PACU may be optional depending on the extent and nature of the surgery and the patient's response to anesthesia. Patients may instead be returned to the discharge unit for reasonable observation time before discharge to home. Bypassing the PACU altogether will eliminate additional costs. PACU policies, which are agreed on by both nursing and anesthesia personnel, may be formulated to address the issue of which patients may avoid the PACU.

Discharge Unit

The discharge unit is usually the last stop for the outpatient. The admission unit where the patient originated is easily converted to the discharge area later in the day. This area, by serving a dual function, provides great continuity of care and continued relationships with the nursing personnel for the patients and their families.

As mentioned, patient teaching should occur both before surgery and on admission the day of the procedure. The patient must know what to expect and be mentally prepared to go home the day of surgery. To be discharged the same day, the patient must (1) be able to take oral pain medications without nausea, (2) be able to walk with assistance, and (3) be able to void and take fluids without nausea. (*Editor's note:* Patients undergoing ambulatory anorectal surgery should not be required to void prior to discharge. As discussed in Chapter 7, fluid restriction during and following surgery may postpone bladder fullness for 12 to 18 hours after surgery, and thus voiding may be delayed for many hours. Urinary retention in the fluid-restricted patient is quite rare and does not justify keeping the patient in the ASC until voiding occurs.) In addition to the general discharge requirements, each procedure may have specific criteria that must be met if the patient is to be discharged. The discussion of discharge goals with the patient and family before the procedure is critical to their successful attainment. The patient must also have a ride home and someone must be designated to stay with him or her at home overnight. If not arranged before the procedure, these deficiencies can be a major setback in discharging the patient.

A postprocedure instruction sheet is a tool that is widely used and should be given to the patient be-fore the procedure. The information on the sheet can be reinforced throughout the experience with the patient, and the patient's awareness of the material can be documented at discharge. The surgeon's office initiates this teaching with the patient. The preoperative nurse then reinforces the teaching that began in the office. Patients who are prepared and know what to expect have a higher degree of satisfaction with the entire experience and are more likely to go home the day of surgery.

Patient Flow

Patient flow is most easily accomplished when the various units are contiguous within the facility. The patient reports to the admission/discharge unit and is prepared for surgery. The patient is then moved to the preoperative area to be assessed and prepared by the anesthesiologist. When the patient is fully prepared and the surgeon has identified the patient, he or she is transported to the operating room. When the operation is completed, the patient is then transferred to the PACU. The final phase is completed in the admission/discharge unit, where the patient was admitted earlier in the day. The discharge to home is facilitated in that unit. The contiguous space makes this a pleasant experience for all concerned.

Relative Advantages

Table 1.1 summarizes the advantages and disadvantages of hospital ambulatory surgery. Technology acquisitions and duplication of instrumentation are among the most costly capital outlays made by surgical services. If instruments and equipment are

TABLE 1.1. Advantages and disadvantages of the hospital-based ambulatory surgery center.

Advantages	Disadvantages
Technology availability	Difficulty in accessing the facility
Comprehensive hospital services	High fixed costs
Maximization of underutilized space	Overutilization of resources
Flexibility	
Lower variable costs	
Increased utilization of personnel	
Physician convenience	
Patient convenience and satisfaction	

available for both inpatients and outpatients, an economy is realized with volume of use as well as the availability of additional equipment when repairs are needed. Standardization of equipment is desired but is very difficult to achieve when many surgeons are involved. Such standardization may be better achieved with a smaller group in a freestanding setting.

Discussed earlier is the distinct advantage of having the diverse services typically available in a large hospital. Higher-risk outpatients can be cared for in this setting with a great deal of security. The physician often chooses a hospital-based outpatient facility when a patient presents with comorbid conditions that could require more comprehensive services. Many patients, especially elderly patients, may require overnight stays under observation status. Patients can be accommodated in an observation unit or any acute-care bed. The ability of the hospital unit to provide observation beds or hospitalization, when needed, provides flexibility to the surgeon in caring for all types of patients and their individual needs. This flexibility allows the hospital to maximize available resources. It is very important, and a JCAHO requirement, that the same standard of care be delivered for both outpatients and inpatients.

A hospital-based ambulatory surgery center can be set up in space previously used by inpatients. Approximately 50% of surgical procedures being performed in hospitals today have been converted to outpatient procedures.

The transformation of currently available underutilized space into ambulatory surgery units assists hospitals in spreading their fixed costs. However, there are disadvantages to this scenario as well. Due to the nature of inpatient services, fixed costs are higher in the hospital setting than in a freestanding surgery center. These costs are increased because of the departments that must be available for inpatients, staff, and visitors 24 hours a day. Assessing high fixed costs to outpatients may make the procedures appear unprofitable. There is no easy way to distinguish fixed costs for inpatients and outpatients in a cost accounting system. However, all activity contributes to the fixed costs and may increase overall facility profitability. Since surgery has shifted to so many outpatient procedures, there is contribution to the bottom line and some contribution to the fixed costs. In a freestand-

ing center, all activity must contribute and shoulder the entire fixed costs associated with a successful program. The reimbursement rates for certain procedures based on their location should be evaluated before any decision is made. (*Editor's note:* The subject of cost accounting is quite complex and may require several semesters of study for its mastery. Detailed explanation of these issues is beyond the scope of this book.)

Other costs are more manageable when patient populations are mixed. An economy of scale is realized when supplies are purchased in volume. Large hospital systems have purchasing agreements that may make them more cost effective. Other variable, indirect costs are spread over a larger patient base, thus decreasing the cost per unit.

Employee costs are lower when the degree of utilization can be consistently predicted. This is achievable when inpatient and outpatient surgery are performed in the same setting. Many of the fixed labor costs can be spread over a larger base. Often the number of personnel needed to perform certain tasks will be the same whether caring for 5 or 10 patients (not exponential with volume). Personnel management techniques such as cross training and "floating" of employees may increase the job security of staff and allow employers less dependence on small groups of employees.

Physicians whose practice is based near the hospital may utilize their time more productively in a hospital-based unit. Operating on both the inpatient and ambulatory populations in the same setting may eliminate travel time to other sites. Downtime or turnover time can be made productive for the surgeon if he or she can make rounds on inpatients or attend to administrative functions in nearby areas.

A disadvantage of a hospital-based ambulatory surgery center is that patients may experience more difficult access. Since the center is located in the hospital, patients may get lost trying to find the admission unit (especially in units that were converted from acute care beds). Depending on its location, the hospital may be difficult to reach by car because of traffic and parking problems. Many hospital facilities have added amenities, such as valet parking, for outpatients to make the experience more convenient.

Overutilization of resources for the ambulatory patient may be a significant problem in a hospital unit. When services and supplies are readily available, utilization and costs may increase. Care must be exercised to keep this to a minimum. Continuing evaluation of costs by all the disciplines involved in caring for the ambulatory patient population helps keep the program viable.

Summary

The benefits of ambulatory services in a hospital setting far outweigh the disadvantages. As the population ages, it becomes essential for us to care for complicated elderly patients in the safest environment available. That environment is and will remain the hospital ambulatory setting. Surgeon needs and procedural costs will adjust to the fluctuations in activity. Increased utilization of existing hospital facilities will continue to rise. More procedures will be done on an outpatient basis if surgeons, anesthesia personnel, and hospital employees are committed to goal-oriented care. As minimally invasive surgery increases, the opportunities exist to move more procedures to the outpatient environment while still providing quality, cost-effective care in the hospital ambulatory setting.

Part C: The Physician-Owned Ambulatory Surgery Center for Colon and Rectal Surgery

Andrea Ferrara, M.D.
and
Joseph Gallagher, M.D.

Freestanding outpatient surgery centers have become substantial contributors to the delivery of modern health care. During the early 1970s, surgery centers were unable to thrive because of insufficient reimbursement.[1] As a result of these failures, the efficacy of the surgery center was tested in an experimental paradigm. In the next few years, studies showed that ASCs could be considered successful because they were responsible for reducing hospital charges by 25% to 30%. In the early 1980s, additional financial incentives were implemented with the introduction of the prospective payment system (PPS), a reimbursement method that encouraged a decreased hospital stay.

Overall, study results showed that inpatient and outpatient surgery had similar clinical outcomes, with the addition of several benefits for the outpatient.[2-4] Unquestionably, outpatient surgery allows patients the benefits of home recovery and the avoidance of potential inpatient hazards. Additionally, physicians are able to implement better management of their time. As a result of these benefits, ambulatory surgery has grown exponentially and accounts for 50% of all surgical procedures performed in the United States today. In particular, ASCs are compatible with the vast majority of the anorectal surgical procedures performed by the colon and rectal surgeon.

This subchapter focuses on a unique surgery center that is physician owned and devoted to colon and rectal surgery. We explore some of the economic considerations in establishing such a center and its benefits for both surgeon and patient. Some aspects of the operation of the center, as well as a review of the surgical results, are presented.

It has been reported that more than 90% of anorectal problems requiring surgical correction can be treated in an outpatient surgery center.[5] Also, physician-owned ASCs can provide unique opportunities and benefits for the colon and rectal surgeon. The benefits of the unit include greater control of the operative schedule by the surgeon, the ability to work in a unit that is specifically dedicated to the performance of colorectal procedures, and improved patient satisfaction. Based on these factors, we began the planning for an independent physician-owned colorectal ambulatory center in July 1994.

Before beginning construction, feasibility studies to evaluate the financial viability of the center are essential. Overall, the financial success of the surgical center relies primarily on reimbursement per procedure and the number of procedures performed. When our surgery center was contemplated during the early 1990s, third-party payers did not present as much difficulty with reimbursement as they do today. An increasing number of managed-care programs are now limiting out-of-network benefits for ambulatory surgery, thus reducing the number of patients who are allowed to utilize our center. In addition, per-case reimbursement has dropped, in some cases, as much as 40% in the last 2 years alone. Although these developments are in general quite unfavorable, in our experience, with careful planning, the ASC remains financially viable. In addition, the colorectal specialty ASC has some cost advantages over the general outpatient unit. The initial equipment costs are relatively low because the instrumentation is limited and high-cost technology such as lasers and laparoscopic equipment is not needed. Also, the technology that is needed is not rapidly outdated. Reimbursement per case can still be relatively favorable, especially with minimal variable costs such as laboratory studies, drugs, and sutures. Finally, the surgical complications after anorectal surgical procedures are minimal.

Our facility was constructed in approximately 8 months. The ambulatory care facility is licensed by the state, meets all safety guidelines for a surgical facility, and is certified by Medicare. JCAHO certification was not pursued because of the significant cost involved and because such certification did not provide additional benefits for the center beyond certification by the State of Florida and Medicare. We are currently working toward American Association of Ambulatory Health Care (AAAHC) accreditation, which is specifically directed toward the ASC.

Our building is free standing and is located next to our surgical clinic (office) building. The outpatient unit covers 3000 square feet and consists of one complete operating room, an anorectal physiology laboratory, an endoscopy suite, and a preoperative/recovery area. The full-time staff includes an office manager who coordinates activity in the facility, an endoscopy nurse, a surgical scrub technician, two registered nurses, and a receptionist. The staff members deal specifically with colorectal diseases and therefore develop a great deal of expertise with these problems. Staff members also assist with preoperative testing and preparation (including intravenous access) and postoperative recovery. In addition, there is a physician on call for the unit 24 hours a day. A certified risk manager is also employed to help with the implementation and oversight of the facility's risk management program. Issues associated with risk management are discussed at quarterly meetings, with particular emphasis on postoperative complications, patient complaints, and compliance with accepted standards of care. In addition, a pharmacy consultant is used to maintain and monitor medications used within the ASC.

We have developed several strategies designed to improve the efficiency of the surgery center. First, the operative schedule alternates with endoscopic procedures to expedite the schedule and optimize the time spent during room turnover. All patients who will receive monitored anesthesia care (MAC) or general anesthesia are seen before surgery by the nurses in the center. Appropriate preoperative testing can be arranged. The nursing staff helps to clarify patient medications and arrange medical or cardiac clearance in advance to prevent cancellations on the day of surgery. Furthermore, all necessary supplies are readily available for the specialty procedures that we perform.

Currently, all of our patients follow a standardized preoperative and postoperative protocol. Before the day of surgery, the patients visit the center and become familiarized with the center and the staff. All patients are given detailed instructions for preoperative and postoperative care according to their diagnosis and proposed surgical treatment. The patients also receive a facility and staff evaluation form to complete at home after their initial visit. Following their indicated procedure, patients are discharged from the ambulatory unit within 2 to 4 hours after surgery. Patients are called the following day by the center's nursing staff for an assessment of their status. Also, patients return to the clinic 1 week after surgery for postoperative follow-up.

All patients undergo preoperative bowel preparation using enemas the night before and the morning of surgery. The majority of patients are sedated and monitored by the anesthesia personnel (MAC). A perianal block of bupivacaine (Marcaine, Sterling Winthrop Pharmaceutical, New York, NY) 0.25% with epinephrine 1:200,000 in combination with two ampules (150 U/amp) of hyaluronidase (Wydase, Wyeth-Ayerst Laboratories, Philadelphia, PA). Approximately 30 mL of the anesthetic solution is used to infiltrate the perianal skin, anal canal mucosa, and intramuscular plane. The local anesthetic is beneficial in achieving hemostasis, intraoperative and postoperative analgesia, and relaxation of the anal sphincters. According to surgeon preference, some patients receive ketorolac tromethamine (Toradol, Syntex International, Palo Alto, CA). Sixty mg of ketorolac is injected into the anal sphincter muscles at the end of the procedure.[6-7] Other patients receive a postoperative subcutaneous morphine pump.[8] Intraoperative fluid administration is limited to approximately 100 mL. (*Editor's note:* It is probably easier to achieve this low volume of intravenous fluids in a specialized unit. In the general ASC, the surgeon must work with a variety of anesthesia personnel and remind them frequently of the goal of fluid restriction.)

TABLE 1.2. Age distribution of patients.

Age, yr	Patients	
	No.	%
<30	53	13.2
30–39	112	27.9
40–49	85	21.2
50–59	51	12.7
60–69	41	10.2
>70	59	14.7
Total	401	100

TABLE 1.3. Postoperative complications.

Complications	Patients	
	No.	%
None	369	92.0
Infection	12	3.0
Urinary retention	10	2.5
Fecal impaction	7	1.7
Bleeding	3	0.7
Total complications	32	7.9

Between July 1994 and April 1997, 961 consecutive patients underwent surgical treatment for anal conditions at our center. In addition, 1470 colonoscopic examinations, 202 anal manometric studies, and 295 invasive electromyographic studies were performed during the same time period. The mean age of all patients was 45.9 (SD ± 14.8) years. Of these patients, 787 were male (54%). More recently, we have obtained more detailed data from 401 patients. Currently, all patients are entered into a computer database. The ages of patients are shown in Table 1.2. The indications for operation in our group of patients were similar to the distribution found in the literature.[9,10] The diagnoses of the patients were as follows: 192 hemorrhoids, 47 anal fissures, 50 anal fistulae, 16 condylomata acuminata, 23 pilonidal cysts, 17 abscesses, 31 hemorrhoids associated with anal fissure, and 4 anal fissures with concomitant anal fistula and other pathologies (anal adenoma, anal carcinoma, hidradenitis suppurativa, etc.).

Between 1994 and 1997, the American Society of Anesthesiologists (ASA) classifications of our patients included 67% ASA I, 28% ASA II, and 5% ASA III. (See Table 2.1 for details of this classification.) No ASA IV or ASA V patients underwent ambulatory treatment in our center. The anesthesiologist performed a preoperative evaluation in all patients to determine if they were appropriate candidates for surgery in our outpatient center.

The responses of our patients to a mailed self-report questionnaire were extremely positive for the center. Patients gave a rating of excellent to the following areas: courtesy of staff (85%), professionalism of staff (85%), efficiency (80%), preoperative instructions (88%), and personal interest (92%). In addition, 96% of patients stated that they would again utilize the colorectal surgery center and 100% would recommend it to friends. Also, patients perceived the center as having a supportive atmosphere that encouraged discussion with other individuals who have similar complaints and symptoms.

The most common operation performed in the center was hemorrhoidectomy (one- to three-column resection; 57.8%); the second most common was lateral sphincterotomy for anal fissure (11.5%). The mean time to the first postoperative visit was 9.3 days, and for the last visits 40.8 days. The majority of patients required only two visits in the postoperative period. Thirty-two of our patients (7.9%) had postoperative complications. Twenty-five were considered minor complications and were managed on an outpatient basis, whereas seven patients (1.7%) had major complications requiring admission to the hospital. The complications are listed in Table 1.3.

Infection, the most frequently noted postoperative complication, occurred in 3% of patients (8 after hemorrhoidectomy and 4 after operations for anal fistula. The next most frequent complication was urinary retention, which had an incidence of 2.5% (10 cases following hemorrhoidectomy). The third most common complication was fecal impaction, which occurred in 1.7% of patients. The incidence of these complications compared favorably to those reported in historical literature from previous inpatient series. These studies indicated that urinary retention occurred in 10% to 20% of patients, fecal impaction in 1%, and infection in 1%.[11,12]

All cases of urinary retention was treated by insertion of a Foley catheter. The catheter was left in place for a mean of 2 days. Fecal impaction was treated with manual extraction in the office. Four patients required admission to the hospital for infections, which were treated with incision and drainage and administration of antibiotics. Three patients were admitted for observation after experiencing bleeding from the surgical site, but none required a blood transfusion.

Overall, our experience with the physician-owned colorectal surgical center has been extremely positive. During the last 4 years, we have found that most anorectal surgical procedures can be successfully performed in an ambulatory setting when a dedicated colorectal surgery unit is utilized. In addition, continued investment into preoperative and postoperative care at our ambulatory center continues to produce optimal surgical outcomes and high levels of patient satisfaction.

References

1. Medical World News 1971;12:58.
2. Detmer DE, Gelijins AC. Ambulatory surgery, a more cost-effective strategy? Arch Surg 1994;129:123–127.
3. Davis JE, Detmer DE. The ambulatory surgical unit. Ann Surg 1972;175:856–862.
4. Stephenson SV. Ambulatory surgical centers. JAMA 1985;253:342–343.
5. Smith LE. Ambulatory surgery for anorectal diseases: an update. South Med J 1986;79:163–166.
6. Reichmann IM. Use of Toradol in anorectal surgery. Dis Colon Rectum 1993;36:295–296.
7. O'Donovan S, Ferrara A, Larach SW, et al. Intraoperative use of Toradol facilitates outpatient hemorrhoidectomy. Dis Colon Rectum 1994;37:793–799.
8. Goldstein ET, Williamson PR, Larach SW. Subcutaneous morphine pump for postoperative hemorrhoidectomy pain management. Dis Colon Rectum 1993;36:439–446.
9. Changyul O, Celia M, Randolph M. Anal fissure 20-year experience. Dis Colon Rectum 1995;4:378–382.
10. Leong A, Husain M, Seow-Choen F, et al. Performing internal sphincterotomy with other anorectal procedures. Dis Colon Rectum 1994;11:1130–1132.
11. Hoff S, Bailey R, Butts D, et al. Ambulatory surgical hemorrhoidectomy—a solution to postoperative urinary retention. Dis Colon Rectum 1994;37:1242–1244.
12. Bleday R, Pena JP, Rothenberger DA, et al. Symptomatic hemorrhoids: current incidence and complications of operative therapy. Dis Colon Rectum 1992;35:477–481.

Part D: The Colonoscopy Suite in the Ambulatory Surgery Center

Susanna Hudson, R.N.

In choosing procedures suitable for performance in the ambulatory surgery center (ASC), consideration should be given to the length and complexity of the procedure, the risk of significant complications, the extent of anesthesia or sedation required for the procedure, and the amount of care required by the patient after the procedure. Among the procedures that lend themselves well to being performed on an ambulatory basis are endoscopic procedures, both diagnostic and therapeutic.

When flexible endoscopy was in its infancy 25 years ago, many patients undergoing colonoscopy were hospitalized. Today, the vast majority of these procedures are performed on an ambulatory basis. In 1998, colonoscopic procedures are among the most commonly performed diagnostic studies in the United States. It is widely believed that examination of the entire colon in patients at risk for colorectal cancer and removal of premalignant polyps, if found, will result in a significant reduction in the number of deaths from colon and rectal cancer. In addition, patients with chronic inflammatory bowel can be monitored for disease surveillance with this relatively simple procedure.

Flexible endoscopic evaluation of the large bowel is performed in a variety of different settings. Flexible sigmoidoscopy examinations, which evaluate the distal 60 cm of the colon and rectum, require little or no sedation and are commonly performed in an office or clinic setting. Hospital-based endoscopy suites located in general hospitals are the most common sites for performance of endoscopic procedures on both the inpatient and the outpatient population. Newest on the healthcare scene is the ASC. Since the endoscopist typically has little need for many of the ancillary services found in the traditional hospital setting, the credentialed ASC is an appropriate practice setting. This subchapter provides a discussion of colonoscopy as it pertains to the ambulatory setting.

Colonoscopy

Colonoscopy is the visualization of the large bowel from the rectum to the cecum, and, in many cases, the terminal ileum, using a long, flexible endoscope. Direct visualization of the colon with a flexible instrument is a relatively safe technique. Each colonoscope is a flexible tube with angulation knobs to control the distal tip as it travels through the colon. The scope also has a channel inside that allows the endoscopist to apply suction to remove liquid that may obscure visibility as well as to pass various working accessories to perform tasks, such as biopsy of colonic mucosa or polypectomy. Air and water channels in the scope help keep the distal lens clear of debris and aid in insufflation of air into the colon to enhance visualization of the lumen.

Regulation

According to the Federal Ambulatory Surgery Association, ASCs are among the most highly regulated providers of ambulatory medical care, with

17

most being regulated at the federal, state, and peer levels. The federal government has determined that safe, high-quality medical care can be achieved in both ambulatory surgery centers and hospital outpatient departments.

All outpatient surgery centers wishing to be approved for Medicare reimbursement must submit to rigorous inspections by the federal government. Nearly 90% of ASCs are Medicare approved. Forty-one states require licensure for ambulatory surgery centers. The Joint Commission on Accreditation of Healthcare Organizations (JCAHO) and the Accreditation Association for Ambulatory Health Care (AAAHC) are voluntary peer-based accreditation organizations that certify processes that mandate a safe environment in which patients can receive quality medical care.

There are several organizations available to the gastroenterology endoscopy professional. These organizations to provide educational support and information regarding the setup of an endoscopy practice. The American Society for Gastrointestinal Endoscopy (ASGE) and the Society of Gastroenterology Nurses and Associates (SGNA) are two organizations that provide written guidelines for the scope of professional endoscopy practice. The American Nurses Association (ANA) provides guidelines to direct the behavior of the professional nurse.

Technical standards are often developed from the individual endoscopy units' guidelines. Such guidelines are referenced in order to maintain a safe and effective endoscopy practice. An example of such referencing would be the recommended guidelines for infection control written by the SGNA.

Federal regulations play a major part in the operations of an ASC. The foremost focus of most federal regulations is infection control. Several government agencies have developed guidelines and regulations that have an impact on disinfection and sterilization practice in the ASC and the endoscopy suite. Such agencies include the Centers for Disease Control and Prevention (CDC), the Environmental Protection Agency (EPA), the Food and Drug Administration (FDA), and the Occupational Safety and Health Administration (OSHA). Of these, the most important to the ASC are the CDC and OSHA.

Centers for Disease Control and Prevention

The CDC has formulated guidelines for the prevention and control of nosocomial infections. They cover handwashing; cleaning, disinfecting, and sterilization of patient care equipment; microbiological sampling; management of infectious waste; housekeeping; and laundry. The CDC guidelines are not regulation or law but are respected as a representation of the best information available on practical and solid infection control practices. Some of these recommendations are based on documented epidemiological studies. More often, the guidelines are based on reasonable theoretical rationale.

Occupational Safety and Health Administration

The Occupational Safety and Health Administration is the federal agency responsible for enforcing safety and health regulations in the workplace. OSHA's primary function is to protect the healthcare worker by ensuring that employers comply with health and safety issues under federal law. OSHA has issued compliance directives that are used by enforcement officers during inspections. Such directives address issues such as occupational exposure to blood-borne pathogens.

Architectural Environment

Because of the flow of personnel and the activities involved in performing a colonoscopic procedure, the architectural setting becomes a very important issue. If one is fortunate enough to be involved in the design of an endoscopy suite, attention to even the smallest of details becomes important. Examples include such aspects as the lighting scheme, sink location and size, door swing direction, and location of the telephone. Errors made in planning these seemingly inconsequential things can place a definite strain on the environment.

Figure 1.1 is an example of an endoscopy room floor plan. The concept of an "ideal" procedure

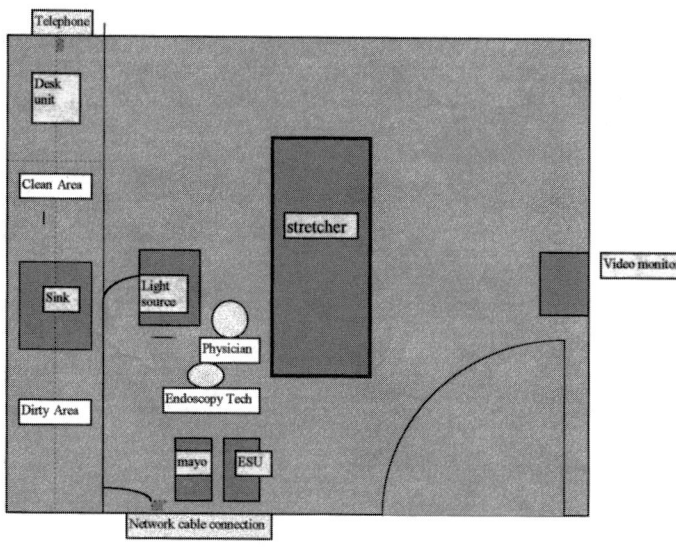

FIGURE 1.1. Sample layout of an endoscopy procedure room.

room must take into account many different factors, some of which cannot be controlled. Often, one must try to make the best of circumstances. This is especially true when utilizing an existing space. If you are involved in the design of a new facility, then more options are available to you and your architect. Common sense and experience become important attributes as the design reaches its completion.

For example, room lighting should be controlled to allow for various light levels and without the light shining directly into the face of the patient, who may be lying on his or her back. Also, the location and size of the sink are important issues. When specifying your needs to your architect, stipulate the inside dimensions of the sink such that it can easily accommodate your flexible endoscope when it is immersed for leak testing. An improperly sized sink can cause expensive damage to the fiberoptic components of your scope should it be forced into too tight a coil.

In the initial discussions with the architectural/engineering company that will design your new facility, be sure to request extensive input into the plans before they are finalized and sent to the construction companies for bids. Allow yourself time to "walk through" all the plans and ask questions of your architect before final decisions are made. This will help avoid costly change orders and delays during the construction phase. Ask about such

things as electrical outlets, nurse call systems, narcotic box placement, emergency electrical outlets (connected to uninterruptible power supplies), and direction of door swings relevant to how you, the user, envision the space being utilized. Think about how you plan on getting through each door and what you might be carrying in your hands, as well as the activities being conducted on the other side of the door. Do you perceive any traffic snarls? Inquire about placement of computer workstations, data cable outlets, and telephone line outlets. In this age of technology, many systems use some type of computer device. These systems may require their own "mechanical room" for this type of hardware. This mechanical room or closet should have electricity and lighting as well as some sort of mounting board. Inquire of your utility vendors exactly what they will require for the installation of their system. One may be surprised at the complexity of these requirements.

If your architect has done other healthcare facility projects, he or she should be knowledgeable on the rules and regulations governing architectural designs to accommodate the Americans with Disabilities Act (ADA). This legislation can affect such areas as sink access and turning radius in your restrooms and soiled utility room. The Texas Department of Health has an Architecture Division that approves all building plans before local construction permits can be obtained. Similar requirements may be present in your state. The medical person responsible for the facility should maintain rapport with the architect as well as the construction company and be available to check on construction on a regular basis

Interior design may or may not be included in the architectural agreement. This issue should be clarified during the negotiation phase. If it is not part of the architect's agreement, then interior design must be included in the final budget for the facility. Interior design will usually include a graphics component covering appropriate signage throughout the facility. ADA regulations may again be a factor; therefore, someone who is knowledgeable is very valuable to your endeavor.

Artwork is another factor that can do much to add the proper atmosphere to your facility. Someone who can guide you in this matter is another valuable asset. An interior designer can also guide you in the selection of furnishings for each area of your facility. There is much to consider to achieve the appearance you desire, and each member of the team will work together to help you achieve this overall goal. This will require many hours and meetings to set the groundwork in place. However, when your efforts come to fruition, the facility will be one of which you can truly be proud.

Staffing

The accredited endoscopy unit should have adequate staffing that is trained in gastrointestinal endoscopy. The endoscopy team consists of the endoscopist (surgeon, gastroenterologist, or other qualified practitioner), a registered nurse (RN), and a trained technician, who can be a certified scrub technician, a patient care associate, or a licensed vocational nurse.

Each member of the team is necessary to achieve the goal of a pleasant, efficient, and uncomplicated experience for the patient. The endoscopist brings an expertise of the actual procedure to complement his or her medical management of the patient's condition.

The RN is a professional whose role during the procedure is to continually assess and support the patient's response to the procedure and the medications given. The RN also uses general nursing knowledge combined with his or her endoscopy experience to complement the endoscopist's skills to provide the best possible outcome for the patient.

The endoscopy technician provides care and expertise related to the equipment itself and assists the endoscopist with such tasks as biopsy and polypectomy. A good technician learns to anticipate the endoscopist's needs in a given situation and acts as a valued extra hand during the procedure itself.

The SGNA has developed a standard regarding minimal staffing during an endoscopy procedure to ensure that the patient's safety is maintained throughout the endoscopy experience. The standard states that two persons per room will staff any routine endoscopy procedure such as colonoscopy. At least one staff member must be an RN whose sole duty is to monitor the patient's condition throughout the procedure. The nurse will use his or her endoscopy knowledge to allay the patient's fears and anxieties as well as to support his or her responses throughout the procedure.

During the preoperative phase, one nurse obtains a general medical history of the patient. Areas of particular concern are the surgical history, brief medical history to include any respiratory and cardiac problems, a review of current medications and medication allergies, and any information relevant to the current complaint.

Before the procedure can be performed, the nursing staff must verify that the patient has given informed consent for the procedure. The patient should be asked if he or she has a thorough understanding of the planned procedure. The patient may have questions that might seem trivial or even embarrassing to ask of the physician. A nurse who is sensitive to the patient's vulnerability can do much to calm anxious patients by treating their anxiety and questions with respect and knowledge. Many patients fear the unknown procedure that lies ahead.

In addition, it is important to verify that the procedure preparation was adequate. In the case of a colonoscopy, it is imperative that a bowel preparation be verified for the procedure to take place. Endoscopists use several different bowel preparations, and these are discussed later in the chapter.

Staffing during the recovery phase should consist of an RN skilled in assessing the patient's return to his or her preprocedure baseline without untoward events. A patient care technician or licensed vocational nurse can supplement this RN when multiple patients are cared for in the same unit.

Equipment

Colonoscopy is accomplished with a flexible endoscope approximately 120 to 180 cm in length. Older flexible endoscopes transmit images via a fiberoptic bundle back to a lens system that focuses the image at the eyepiece. This system allows only the endoscopist to view the colon. The modern colonoscope is a video endoscope that transmits the image from a camera chip on its tip to a video monitor. The monitor allows the entire endoscopy team to participate in the examination. Video endoscopes still use fiberoptic technology for light transmission from the light source to the colon.

In addition to the viewing capabilities of the flexible endoscope, there is an air–water system inside the scope allowing for controlled insufflation of room air into the colon. Water is available primarily to keep the viewing lens at the distal tip washed clean of debris and to minimize fogging. A larger working channel is built in for suctioning liquid effluent and introducing accessories. The working channel is of varying size depending on the type of scope selected. Different devices are available to perform a variety of tasks that may be necessary during even a routine examination. Accessories for biopsy, polypectomy, electrocoagulation, and brush cytology, as well as laser fibers, can be passed through the colonoscope. Because of variation in channel size, not all scopes will accommodate every accessory.

Some of these tasks will require additional equipment. Hot biopsy and polypectomy require an electrosurgical unit. The minimum equipment needed for any endoscopy unit is based on the range of procedures to be performed in the center, but an electrosurgical unit with coagulation capabilities is an essential item.

JCAHO and SGNA standards require that the patient's heart rate and rhythm, blood pressure, and pulse oximetry readings be monitored continually during the examination and recorded every 5 minutes. Monitoring instruments are available that measure these parameters and provide a written record for the chart. Respiratory rate must also be monitored, but this parameter can be recorded manually. Similar monitors can be used in the preoperative and recovery phase of the patient's stay. The unit must be prepared for unforeseen emergencies with a defibrillator and a crash cart for cardiopulmonary support.

Conscious Sedation

Conscious sedation has received considerable attention in recent years because of its classification as a form of anesthesia and the lack of specific formal training available. Most persons performing conscious sedation are not anesthesiologists or certified registered nurse anesthetists but have attained certain performance standards. If conscious sedation is performed correctly, anesthesia personnel are not necessary. Most regulating agencies agree on the definition of conscious sedation as providing a minimally reduced level of consciousness in which the patient retains the ability to maintain an airway independently and to respond appropriately to physical stimulation and/or verbal command. The goals of conscious sedation are to decrease the patient's anxiety and elevate the pain threshold to ensure cooperation from the patient while providing some degree of amnesia.

The agents used in conscious sedation are commonly a benzodiazapine (usually midazolam or diazepam) in combination with a narcotic agent (such as fentanyl or meperidine) administered intravenously (by the physician or by the RN under the direction of the physician) and titrated to achieve the desired response from the patient. Some patients may benefit from a dose of gastrointestinal anticholinergic (such as hyoscyamine sulfate) when there is spasm and discomfort. Of course, the medical history of the patient must be reviewed by the medical professionals for them to be aware of conditions, such as narrow-angle glaucoma, myasthenia gravis, or prostatic hypertrophy, that might contraindicate the use of anticholinergics. Glucagon can also be given to decrease gastrointestinal motility and relax the colon. In many instances, the timely use of one of these agents may markedly improve the patient's tolerance of the procedure. The nurse must know each of these drugs and their potential benefit.

It is the responsibility of the RN to administer and maintain conscious sedation during endoscopic procedures under the auspices of the physician. This supervision does not absolve the nurse of all responsibility should adverse effects occur. As a professional, the RN should know the scope of his or her practice. The nurse should know the agents used in conscious sedation and their desired as well as adverse effects. It is very important to be aware of the drugs' onset of action and half-life so that the patient's response to medication can be monitored and documented. Reversal agents such as flumazenil and naloxone should be available for use if necessary. These reversal agents should not be used routinely because of the short duration of the recovery phase and possible complications, such as resedation, that may occur after the patient has been discharged.

Conscious sedation, when properly administered and with the correct goals in mind, may allow the patient to tolerate a difficult examination. A balance must be achieved among the medications given, the patient's anxiety, and stimulation from the scope for the procedure to be considered a success by the most sensitive of critics: the patient. Proper sedation is one factor that allows the reluctant patient to come back for follow-up examinations and is thus a good public relations tool for endoscopy.

Colonoscopy

Preparation

The colonoscopic examination is performed with minimal disruption when team members do their parts. Once the need for the procedure has been established and the examination scheduled, the patient is provided with instructions from the physician's office regarding the bowel preparation regimen that has been selected. Each physician has a favorite preparation for general use, and this can be altered depending on the specific needs of the patient. The most widely used bowel preparations are polyethylene glycol (Golyteley, Braintree Laboratories, Braintree, MA) and sodium phosphate (Fleet Phospho-Soda, C.B. Fleet Co., Lynchburg, VA). Both of these preparations will adequately cleanse the colon of fecal material. Each preparation has its own advantages and disadvantages.

Setup and Procedure

It is the responsibility of the endoscopy technician or assistant to prepare the room for the procedure. The patient's privacy can be maintained by simply turning the operative part away from the door. An occupied/unoccupied sign on the outside of the door will further deter unwanted traffic into the room during the procedure.

As the technician arranges the room, he or she must allow enough space to assist the physician and still get to the supplies that might be needed during the examination. The RN can be an extra hand from time to time, but the technician should have everything prepared and within reach for the routine examination.

The monitor should be on the opposite side of the stretcher from the endoscopist, and the light source/processor should be behind him or her. The arrangement should be checked to avoid any trailing electrical cords that might pose a safety hazard. Work spaces should be planned to provide for a dirty area for the endoscopy technician to place contaminated articles during the procedure. A clean space for the RN and endoscopist to use for paperwork is very helpful in avoiding the unwanted spread of potentially infectious material.

Once the general layout of the room is determined, the endoscopy team must assemble the needed equipment and accessories. A list of necessary equipment is shown in Table 1.4. In addition to these items, the RN will need to have available the required pharmacology items preferred by the endoscopist as previously discussed.

TABLE 1.4. Equipment needed for colonoscopic examination.

An appropriate colonoscope
Appropriate biopsy forceps
Polypectomy snare
Electrosurgical unit
Sterile water bottle filled with sterile water
Bowl or emesis basin filled with tap water
Simethicone drops
Nonsterile 4 × 4 gauze sponges
Water-soluble lubricating jelly
60-ml syringe with metal introducer or Luer slip tip for
  irrigation
Paper or cloth absorbent pad under buttocks
Personal protection to include eye protection, gown, and gloves

After the preoperative assessment is completed and the consent signed, intravenous access is established with an intravenous line running at a slow rate. There are two main advantages of a running intravenous line compared to a saline lock. First, there is a decreased incidence of phlebitis from medications used during the procedure with a running intravenous line. Second, some patients complain of a headache presumably related to hypoglycemia from decreased oral intake during preparation. The headache is often relieved with a bolus of intravenous fluid with even a minimal amount of dextrose in the bag (e.g., D_5W, D_5LR, or D_5NS). Also, should any fluids need to be given during the procedure, an intravenous line is readily available. The cost of the intravenous catheter plus the bag of intravenous fluid is comparable to the multiple small vials of normal saline used for flushing the medications into the vein. After any premedications, such as intravenous antibiotics, have been given, the patient is transported to the procedure room.

A sturdy cloth pad or draw sheet on the stretcher may be useful for repositioning a sleepy patient during the procedure. The endoscopy technician should be sure that the colonoscope and any requested equipment are in working order before the examination starts and should remain in the room ready to be of assistance while the patient is being medicated.

Once the endoscopist has greeted the patient, conscious sedation commences with the initial medications given by either the endoscopist or the RN and the dose adjusted slowly to achieve the desired effects. Additional medication can be given as the procedure progresses based on the needs of the patient. Individual responses to medications will vary based on the patient's age, physical status, and current medication regimens. Vital signs are monitored continuously and are recorded every 5 minutes according to JCAHO standards. In addition to electrocardiogram, heart rate, blood pressure, and pulse oximetry, the nurse should be aware of the patient's level of consciousness, warmth and dryness of skin, facial expressions as an indicator of pain tolerance, respiratory rhythm, and abdominal distention. Such assessments can provide many clues to the patient's tolerance of the procedure.

During the procedure, the endoscopy technician may be called upon to do more than assist the endoscopist with the equipment. He or she may be asked to assist with the advancement of the endoscope itself. This requires a thorough knowledge of how the colonoscope behaves after it is introduced into the rectum as well as verbal communication with the endoscopist regarding how the scope "feels." Often, gentle pressure on the abdomen will assist the advancement of the scope and may be accompanied by well-timed deep breaths on the part of the patient. It may be necessary to turn the patient on his or her back or even on the right side to facilitate passage of the scope beyond a particularly difficult segment of the colon.

Therapeutic Colonoscopy

In the case of a diagnostic colonoscopy, the activities described above may be all that is required, but many times a diagnostic colonoscopy will identify polyps or other abnormalities that require intervention. Such pathological findings as colon polyps, arteriovenous malformations, colitis, stricture, or even apparently normal tissue in view of a history of chronic colitis may be indications for the endoscopist to perform biopsies, polypectomy, or even coagulation therapy during the course of a therapeutic colonoscopy.

Therapeutic colonoscopy can be as simple as taking biopsies or as complicated as the coagulation of an arteriovenous malformation. Each procedure requires that the endoscopy technician and the RN be knowledgeable regarding the indications for the appropriate accessory and how that accessory functions. Biopsies require additional items to process the specimen. In addition to the items needed for a diagnostic colonoscopy, the handling of specimens may require the following items:

- Appropriate biopsy forceps
- Toothpick or fine-tipped tweezers
- Labels
- Pathology laboratory slip or requisition
- Formalin-filled containers
- Biohazard-labeled specimen bag

Biopsy and Polypectomy

Biopsy forceps come in different styles. The style used will be primarily dependent on the endoscopist's preferences. Large cup forceps, sometimes known as "big bites," can be used for most situations. Caution should be used with colitis, however, as the mucosa can be more fragile. A change to the regular or small-bite forceps is not necessary if the endoscopist is made aware of the equipment he or she is given. A slight change in the pressure used when obtaining the tissue is helpful in avoiding unnecessary trauma to the mucosa. The biopsy forceps should be sharpened and in good repair at all times to avoid unnecessary trauma for the patient.

Proper management of the tissue samples is the primary responsibility of the endoscopy technician. The RN can support this responsibility by recording the number of polyps removed and the location of each sample taken. This requires communication among all members of the endoscopy team. A tissue sample incorrectly labeled or placed in the wrong specimen container can have serious consequences for the patient.

Colon polyps can be removed using several different techniques based on the shape, size, and length of any stalk. Small sessile polyps, less than 8 mm, can be completely removed using either cold biopsy forceps or hot biopsy forceps. (*Editor's note:* Although the removal of small polyps using "cold biopsy" technique is widely practiced by gastroenterologists, it is my opinion that this is inappropriate. There is little if any risk from properly used electrocautery to ablate the base of the polyp and achieve hemostasis. More importantly, the residual neoplastic tissue present at the base of the biopsy site typically regrows and presents as another polyp at the time of the next colonoscopic examination.) Either technique allows for easy recovery of the polyp tissue for pathologic examination. In the case of hot biopsy forceps, an electrocautery unit is used with specially insulated forceps to capture and ablate the polyp when the coagulation current is applied. A grounding pad is applied to the patient and connected to the electrosurgical unit (ESU). The preferred placement of the grounding pad is lengthwise on the patient's thighs, avoiding any bony prominence. The endoscopy technician adjusts the ESU to the endoscopist's preferred settings and provides the endoscopist with access to the foot pedal. After handing the hot biopsy forceps to the endoscopist for passage through the scope, the technician awaits instructions to open and close the forceps to capture the polyp.

Polypectomy can be performed on pedunculated polyps or those larger than 8 mm using a snare (a sheathed wire loop). Using a snare, the base of the polyp is encircled and the snare is attached to the ESU. The electrical current (coagulation, cutting, or blended) is applied by the endoscopist in brief pulses until the polyp is transected. The technician may have control of the snare during the actual polypectomy or the snare may be manipulated by the endoscopist. A trap can be attached to the suction line to retrieve the polyp tissue. For large polyps that cannot be brought back through the scope, a basket or tripod grabber may be used. Polyp retrieval accessories allow the endoscopist to securely hold the polyp while still allowing visualization of the colon.

Polyps with a broad base or that appear to be an active or potential source of bleeding can be injected at their base before polypectomy to minimize bleeding and protect the underlying wall of the colon. A sclerotherapy needle is inserted into the submucosa and the tissue is injected with normal saline or a 1:10,000 mixture of epinephrine and saline. The endoscopist will instruct the RN when to insert or withdraw the needle and when to inject. The RN should communicate how much fluid is being injected at 0.5-mL intervals and if any undue pressure is incurred during injection. Snare polypectomy assisted by the technician follows as usual. Hemostasis of a biopsy or polypectomy site can occasionally also be achieved using this technique.

Cytology and Cell Culture

In cases where the presence of an infection is suspected, a specimen of the tissue can be obtained and cultured for fungi, bacteria, and other organisms. These specimens can be obtained by direct biopsy techniques, by aspiration of fecal material, or by cytologic brushing. Brush cytology can obtain whole cells for examination. The sheathed brush is introduced through the scope, as are other endoscopic accessories, and the endoscopist instructs the endoscopy technician to put the brush out to brush the area of concern. After gathering cells from the suspected area, the brush is pulled back into the sheath for removal of the accessory from the endoscope. In cases of cytology, the cells are then smeared on a glass microscope slide, which is labeled and sprayed with a fixative before being placing in a slide holder or a container of alcohol for transport to the laboratory.

If cell culture is requested, the tip of the brush can be cut off, moistened with a few drops of bacteriostatic saline, and placed in a sterile container. The specimen is labeled and the correct requisition slip is attached before transport to the laboratory. Any specimen collection process should be confirmed with the appropriate laboratory before any specimen is collected to minimize collection errors that might invalidate the tissue specimen.

Coagulation Techniques

Coagulation techniques can be performed using a specialized wand accessory and a standard ESU or may require an entire specialized setup using monopolar or bipolar electrocoagulation. With bipolar electrocoagulation a grounding pad is not required, since the current travels back to the generator through the bipolar electrode. Electrical energy is converted into thermal energy on contact with the tissue. Bipolar electrocoagulation produces a predictable depth of injury to the tissue, which reduces the risk of perforation and thermal burn of the colonic tissue. In addition to its use in hemostasis of actively bleeding lesions, bipolar probes can also be used to destroy neoplastic cells (tumor ablation) and thereby relieve symptoms of obstruction, and even to destroy hemorrhoidal tissue. It is important that the patient be cooperative and that direct visualization of the bleeding site be maintained throughout the procedure.

It is very important that all persons using ESUs be thoroughly trained in their use and be able to troubleshoot problems that might occur during their use. When the functioning of the unit is in doubt, the unit should be removed from service until a trained biomedical technician has evaluated the unit and certifies that it is working properly.

Cleaning and Disinfection/Sterilization

The cleaning process has four stages: manual cleaning, disinfection, rinsing, and drying. Cleaning begins at the bedside upon completion of the examination and is an essential step in the procedure. General cleaning can be defined as the removal of gross debris from the outside of the scope and from all working channels. This is accomplished as soon as possible after the procedure. Once protein-based debris is allowed to harden in or on the scope, problems such as scope malfunctioning or even cross-contamination between patients by virtue of adherence of contaminated debris to the endoscope can occur. In the manual cleaning stage, the scope is cleaned by wiping the outside of the scope and brushing all working channels until no visible debris can be identified.

It is very important to leak test the colonoscope before it is immersed in any liquid. Leak testing is done according to the manufacturer's instructions. This step is critical and must be done properly to avoid repairs that are made costlier by exposure of the electrical components of the scope to liquid by immersing a leaking scope. If the scope has passed the leak testing phase, it is then immersed in solution to aid in the cleaning process. A product that will remove protein-based contaminants by enzymatic action is preferable, since flexible endoscopes cannot be placed in a standard ultrasonic machine. Enzymatic solutions will enhance the manual phase of the cleaning process while prolonging the working life of the scope.

Once manual cleaning has been accomplished, the scope is ready for placement in the disinfection solution. Most facilities use an automated processor for the disinfection stage. This is not essential, but it has one distinct benefit: the automation process cannot be interrupted during the disinfection cycle or exposure time. This creates a built-in standard of quality that is reproducible from patient to patient. In an endoscopy unit where the procedure volume is very low, the significant cost of a manual processor can be avoided by purchasing a special soaking pan at a very low cost and using a kitchen timer to regulate the time of exposure to the disinfectant.

The scope is loaded into the automatic processor according to the manufacturer's recommendations to allow for exposure of all surfaces and working channels to the disinfectant. Most new units can accommodate any of the EPA-approved high-level disinfectant solutions currently available. Older units are equipped to handle only glutaraldehyde solutions. A discussion of currently available solutions is provided later in this section. It is important that the automatic processor be set for the correct disinfectant exposure time to achieve high-level disinfection. Most processors will also accommodate biopsy forceps and other immersible accessories, although coiled biopsy forceps should be placed in an ultrasonic cleaner before being exposed to the disinfectant. Some flexible endoscopic accessories can be autoclaved after proper manual cleaning. One should refer to the accessory manufacturer's literature before autoclaving any endoscope accessory.

After exposure to the disinfectant is completed, the scope must be adequately rinsed with water to avoid exposing the patient to any remaining disinfectant. This is accomplished automatically in the automatic processors. All working channels and surfaces are exposed to this rinsing. Sterile water is ideal but not usually practical in the gastroenterology setting. In cases where a soaking pan has been used, another pan with clean water is used to rinse the outside of the scope while an all-channel irrigator rinses the working channels.

The drying stage is accomplished automatically in most processors but may need to be augmented upon removal from the automatic processor. Drying can be accomplished by flushing 70% alcohol through the working channels of the scope followed by air to remove residual alcohol. Care should be taken to avoid vigorous flushing of air through the channels, as damage may result from excessive pressure within the scope. Upon completion of this initial part of the drying stage, the scope should be hung vertically in a well-ventilated closet to prevent damage or contamination. Flexible endoscopes should not be stored coiled in cases or lying flat on a shelf.

Sterilization

Each facility should address the subject of sterilization versus high-level disinfection on an individual basis. In the 1960s, Earl H. Spaulding devised a classification system for levels of disinfection based on the risk of infection inherent in their intended use. Medical equipment and patient care items were classified as critical, semi-critical, and non-critical. Flexible endoscopes fall in the semi-critical category defined as items that "will come in contact with mucous membrane or skin that is not intact." These items require a minimum of high-level disinfection by means of chemical exposure to an approved chemical agent. Sterilization can be achieved using most chemical agents that are used

for high-level disinfection by significantly increasing the exposure time. The chemical agent peracetic acid will provide low-temperature sterilization in a liquid form. Currently in use primarily in automated processors, this chemical provides the added peace of mind of providing a sterilized endoscope to every patient regardless of their history.

It must be remembered that endoscopic procedures are not usually done under medically aseptic surroundings. Equipment and accessories are not handled in a sterile fashion; therefore the only advantage to a sterilized endoscope would be the decreased possibility of cross-contamination between patients. It has been determined that thorough manual cleaning followed by proper exposure to chemical disinfectants for the recommended time will decrease the presence of harmful microorganisms and achieve high-level disinfection. This processing sequence is endorsed by the SGNA, the Association for Professionals in Infection Control and Epidemiology, the American Gastroenterological Association, and the American College of Gastroenterology.

Flexible endoscopes pose a significant challenge when cleaning and disinfecting because of their internal lumens and incompatibility to heat. Disinfectant agents that remain in contact with all internal and external surfaces for the recommended exposure time are considered to achieve high-level disinfection. An automated processor forces disinfectant and then rinse water through all channels during the cycle. Since the cycle is automated, there is a built-in standard of care with regard to exposure time. The only true variables would then be the manual cleaning phase that precedes the automated cycle and the efficacy of the chemical disinfectant being reused.

Chemical Disinfectants

Glutaraldehyde in a 2% solution has been the chemical disinfectant of choice for many years. However, three new disinfectant/sterilants have been introduced in the last few years. These provided exciting new alternatives to glutaraldehyde, whose bothersome fumes require air quality monitoring, special handling, and additional ventilation.

One new disinfectant is a 7.5% hydrogen peroxide and 0.85% phosphoric acid solution marketed under the brand name Sporox (Reckitt & Colman Pharmaceuticals, Richmond, VA). Exposure time for high-level disinfection is 30 minutes, and the agent can be reused for 21 days with a minimum effective concentration of 6% hydrogen peroxide. The major endoscope manufacturers approve this chemical agent as being compatible with their equipment. There is no need to heat the chemical, as the use temperature is 20°C (68°F). Sterilization can be achieved by increasing the exposure time to 6 hours, although this is not usually practical.

Another new disinfectant is a 1% hydrogen peroxide and 0.08% peracetic acid solution marketed under the brand name Cidex PA (Johnson & Johnson, Skillman, NJ). Exposure time for high-level disinfection is 25 minutes, and the agent can be reused for a maximum of 14 days with minimum effective concentration monitored by test strips. Sterilization can be achieved by increasing exposure time to 8 hours at room temperature. Again, this lengthy period of exposure is not entirely practical in a busy gastrointestinal laboratory. This product is also recommended to be used at room temperature.

The last chemical to be discussed here is actually marketed as a liquid sterilant. Steris Laboratories (Phoenix, AZ) has produced a 35% peracetic acid solution that is buffered and diluted to a 0.2% peracetic acid solution in its automated processor. This product is marketed as Steris 20. The automated processor uses a series of filters to achieve the sterile water used for dilution and rinsing after exposure time. This allows the unit to present the user with a sterile endoscope upon completion of the cycle. Exposure time to the chemical agent is 12 minutes. The unit does require water to be heated to 43°C, which is partially accomplished by an internal device that heats the water supply a few degrees. Steris 20 is supplied in a one-time-use container; therefore optimum concentrations are readily available during each cycle.

Evolving technologies and increasing legislation have provided the medical community with safer and more user-friendly choices for disinfectant and sterilant use in a busy healthcare setting.

Recovery Phase

After the successful completion of the colonoscopy, the patient will be transported to the recovery area (postanesthesia care unit) by the RN. On admitting the patient to the postanesthesia care unit, the RN will communicate to the unit's staff the particulars of the procedure: medications given during the procedure, any premedications or antibiotics, the patient's response to the procedure, and the results of a brief assessment done immediately after the procedure. This assessment includes the patient's heart rate and rhythm, respiratory status, abdominal distention, intravenous site, skin temperature and dryness, and ESU grounding pad site.

Most patients can be safely transferred to a recliner upon arrival in the recovery area if they are awake and without significant abdominal distention. The patient may remain lying on his side on the stretcher for a period of time if he is complaining of abdominal distention and not freely passing flatus. It may be necessary to assist the patient into a knee-chest position to facilitate the passage of air from the rectum. Providing for the patient's privacy during this phase is helpful in encouraging the timid patient to expel air that may remain in the colon after the procedure.

Vital signs and level of consciousness should be documented every 15 to 30 minutes during the recovery phase. The patient should stay in the recovery area until he is awake without distress and is able to tolerate oral fluids without nausea. These criteria are often met in 30 to 45 minutes. Care should be exercised to avoid discharging a patient too quickly who has received reversal agents either during the procedure or in recovery. The half-life of the reversal agent is shorter than that of the drug it has been given to reverse. If the patient is discharged too quickly, even if he meets the criteria, resedation can occur in an unmonitored environment.

When the patient is ready for discharge, discharge instructions are reviewed with the responsible adult who will be driving the patient home. The medications used in conscious sedation have an amnesic effect of which the patient is often unaware. It is unwise to allow any patient who has received conscious sedation to drive himself or herself home or even take a taxicab home unaccompanied. There are numerous anecdotes involving patients who did not remember how they got home. It is preferable that someone stay with the patient for a few hours after the procedure, since many postprocedure complications can

arise at a time when the patient may not even remember that discharge instructions were given.
Providing written instructions can reinforce discharge teaching and sometimes procedure findings.

Summary

If the endoscopy team works well together, the patient's discomfort and potential for bad memories
of the procedures can be minimized. All that is
needed is an endoscopy team that is knowledgeable about the procedure and willing to constantly
learn from one another. The team atmosphere can
do much to alleviate some of the anxieties that the
patient may bring to the procedure, and a more relaxed patient often has good memories to bring
back should a return visit be needed. It is the responsibility of each member of the team to keep
up to date with techniques, evolving technologies, and legislation that affect their endoscopic
practice.

Bibliography

American Society for Testing and Materials. Standard
    Practice for Cleaning and Disinfection of Flexible
    Fiberoptic and Video Endoscopes Used in the Exami-
    nation of the Hollow Viscera (ASTM publication
    No. F1518–94). Philadelphia: American Society for
    Testing and Materials, 1994.
Beebe RM, Redd RM, Spathis PL. Endo-Dex: Colon
    Reference Guide. Winston Salem, NC: Wilson Cook
    Medical, 1997.
Federated Ambulatory Surgery Association. Benefits of
    ambulatory surgery centers. Available at: http://www
    .fasa.org/benefits.html. Accessed March 15, 1999.
Federated Ambulatory Surgery Association. The regulation
    of ambulatory surgery centers. Available at: http://www
    .fasa.org/regulation.html. Accessed March 15, 1999.
Rutala WA. Infection control update. Society of Gas-
    troenterology Nurses and Associates 25th Annual
    Course, Denver, CO, May 1998.
Shields N. Changes in disinfectant technology: evaluating
    opportunities. Society of Gastroenterology Nurses and
    Associates 25th Annual Course, Denver, CO, May 1998.
Society of Gastroenterology Nurses and Associates. Gas-
    troenterology Nursing: A Core Curriculum. St. Louis:
    Mosby Year Book, 1993.

2

Anesthesia in Ambulatory Anorectal Surgery

Fatima A. Mawji, M.D., M.B.A.

In the past decade there has been a significant increase in the number of patients undergoing ambulatory surgery. In this era of cost containment, it is estimated that up to 70% of all elective procedures may eventually be performed in ambulatory settings. The development of new and sophisticated technology in medicine and surgery permits safer ambulatory surgery for sicker patients. Advances in anesthesia and drug delivery systems have contributed to the positive outcomes and tremendous growth in ambulatory surgery. The recent introduction of anesthetic agents with ephemeral effects and the development of the laryngeal mask airway have specific places in ambulatory anorectal surgery. Patients undergoing most anorectal procedures should now expect to go home on the same day.

Preoperative Evaluation

It would be ideal for all patients scheduled for surgery to be examined by the anesthesiologist before surgery. This would help to avoid last-minute cancellations and delays. However, it is neither economically effective nor a practical use of resources for all patients to have a preoperative visit. Different organizations have developed innovative methods of interviewing patients before the day of surgery. Telephone interviews are usually adequate for the majority of the patients, but for patients with a more complicated medical history, a personal visit before surgery should be scheduled. The preoperative screening telephone interview and/or onsite visit should be arranged far enough in advance of surgery to allow time for additional laboratory testing or consultations. Members of the nursing staff complete the preoperative questionnaire, which contains pertinent questions on the different organ systems and the social history. The nurses then consult with the anesthesiologists for any particular concerns. In some cases patients request to speak directly with the anesthesiologist. This often decreases the anxiety levels of the patient and family.

During this preoperative visit, the nurses inform the patient about any special dietary modifications that are required. The nurses also instruct the patients on the medications they need to continue or omit on the day of surgery. It is standard practice to continue cardiac medications, antihypertensives, and antidepressants on the day of surgery. Diabetic patients are given specific instructions depending on their medication and dosages. Patients who are taking oral hypoglycemics are instructed to omit the morning dose. Patients who are taking insulin are instructed to bring their insulin with them. A glucometer reading in the preoperative holding area will determine any need for insulin before surgery.

The preoperative telephone interview eliminates the majority of last-minute cancellations. It also helps streamline the admission process and eliminate delays on the morning of surgery. After the interview process, selected patients are asked to come to the facility to undergo a physical examination and ancillary tests. In addition, some patients prefer to visit the facility and become acquainted with the surgery center and the anesthesiologists before the date of surgery.

The process of determining who requires a physical examination and further testing is based on information gleaned from the patient's history and an

TABLE 2.1. (ASA) American Society of
Anesthesiologists physical status classification.

Class	Description
I	Healthy patient
II	Mild disease, no functional limitation
III	Severe disease, functional limitation
IV	Severe disease, constant threat to life
V	Not expected to survive 24 hours, with or without the operation

Source: American Society of Anesthesiologists.

estimation of the patient's physical status. The
American Society of Anesthesiologists (ASA)
physical status classification is the most widely
used (Table 2.1).[1] Virtually all patients with an
ASA physical status classification of I or II are candidates for ambulatory surgery, as are an ever-
increasing number patients classified as ASA III.

The standard in the community regarding laboratory tests for elective anorectal surgery has changed
in recent years. Measurements of the hemoglobin
level and hematocrit and a pregnancy test are recommended for women of childbearing age. Patients
who are taking antihypertensives, heart medications, or diuretics should have their electrolytes
evaluated. Men over age 50 and postmenopausal
women with cardiac risk factors require a screening
electrocardiogram.

Preoperative Medications

Sedation: Diazepam

There has been a considerable change in preoperative sedation techniques for patients undergoing
outpatient surgery. It is important to use medications from which the recovery time is short. Although some anesthesiologists believe that a good
preoperative visit is better than any drug regimen,
our experience suggests that the majority of patients experience a certain amount of anxiety. In
many centers, midazolam (Versed, Hoffmann-
LaRoche Pharmaceuticals, Nutley, NJ), in doses of
1 to 2 mg, is commonly administered IV to allay
anxiety. Midazolam is a short-acting drug that does
not delay awakening. At our facility we use 5 to 10
mg of diazepam (Valium, Roche Pharmaceuticals,
Puerto Rico) by mouth after the patient has signed
consent. It helps the patient to relax, and does not

require intravenous access. In fact, the intravenous
catheter is not inserted until the patient begins to
feel the calming effect of the drug. Another advantage of diazepam is the ability to administer it prior
to the arrival of the surgeon. Unlike intravenous
midazolam, patients taking diazepam are cognizant
enough to converse with the surgeon and are rea-
sonably calm. Diazepam is certainly more cost-
effective, and there is little difference between the
two medications in the recovery phase. With oral
diazepam, precise timing is not as critical to patient
care, and if the surgeon is delayed it does not appear to be as significant an imposition.

Other Medications

Preemptive analgesia has been recommended, and
some have advocated using nonsteroidal anti-
inflammatory medications such as ketorolac. At
our facility we have elected to use propoxyphene
napsylate 100 mg preoperatively unless the patient
is allergic to the drug. Sodium citrate (Bicitra,
Baker Norton Pharmaceuticals, Miami, FL), a non-
particulate antacid, is given to patients who have a
history of hiatal hernia or gastric reflux and to
obese patients, who typically have delayed gastric
emptying time. This antacid neutralizes the acidity
of the gastric juices and decreases morbidity in the
event that the patient aspirates. Another preventive
technique that we use is the aerosolized administration of albuterol breathing treatments in patients
who have a history of chronic heavy smoking,
asthma, or reactive airway disease.

General Anesthesia

Induction: Propofol

Propofol (Diprivan, Zeneca Pharmaceuticals,
Wilmington, DE) has replaced thiopental as the induction agent of choice for general anesthesia in
outpatient surgery for several reasons (Table 2.2).
Propofol (usual dosage, 2.5 mg/kg) produces anesthesia at a rate similar to those of the intravenous
barbiturates.[2] Patients are able to walk sooner after
taking propofol and feel better in the immediate
postoperative period compared with other intravenous anesthetics. Propofol can be used for both
induction and maintenance of anesthesia, and it

TABLE 2.2. General anesthesia.

Advantages	Disadvantages
Rapid onset	Postoperative nausea
Reliability	and vomiting
Patient satisfaction	Aspiration pneumonitis
Rapid emergence with short-	Drug reactions
acting drugs	Sore throat
	Pulmonary edema

TABLE 2.3. Laryngeal mask airway.

Advantages	Disadvantages
Less hemodynamic instability	Aspiration pneumonitis
No need for muscle relaxants	
No sore throat	

which greatly exceeds that of the benzodiazepines and barbiturates.

does not appear to cause cumulative effects or delayed arousal following prolonged infusion. The recovery from propofol is extremely rapid compared with thiopental. Propofol causes greater suppression of airway reflexes and hence facilitates placement of a laryngeal mask airway and better tolerance of the endotracheal tube. Finally, propofol appears to have direct antiemetic effects, and there have been studies revealing a lower incidence of postoperative nausea and vomiting (PONV) when compared to thiopental. These favorable properties are responsible for the extensive use of propofol as a component of balanced anesthesia and for its popularity as an anesthetic in outpatient surgery.

After intravenous administration, distribution occurs with a half-life of 2 to 8 minutes. The drug is rapidly metabolized in the liver by conjugation to glucuronide and sulfate and excreted in the urine. Less than 1% of the drug is excreted unchanged. Total body clearance is greater than hepatic blood flow, suggesting that elimination includes extrahepatic mechanisms in addition to metabolism by liver enzymes. Propofol may potentially cause marked decrease in systemic blood pressure during induction of anesthesia, primarily through decreased peripheral resistance and by its negative inotropic effects on the heart. Apnea and pain at the site of injection are common side effects. The pain experienced during injection can be managed by giving 30 to 40 mg of lidocaine either prior to or in combination with propofol. It is also less painful when propofol is injected into a larger vein. The adult dosage for induction is 2.0 to 3.5 mg/kg, but it is important to remember to reduce the dosage by 25% to 50% in older or debilitated patients. It is also critical to remember that rapid injection may cause hypotension, especially in elderly patients. Muscle movements, hypotonus, and tremors have been reported following its use. A significant disadvantage of prolonged use of propofol is its cost,

Airway Management: Laryngeal Mask Airway

The use of the laryngeal mask airway (LMA) has certainly been a major improvement for outpatient procedures (Table 2.3). The LMA is a short endotracheal tube attached to an ovoid facemask. When properly positioned and inflated, the facemask lies directly over the laryngeal inlet. The benefits of the LMA are numerous. It eliminates the noxious stimulus of laryngoscopy and intubation and the need for muscle relaxants to secure the airway. The patient does not need to be deeply anesthetized toward the end of the surgical procedure because the patient can tolerate the LMA in a much lighter plane of anesthesia. Thus, the possibility of negative pulmonary pressure edema is minimized. The lithotomy position, which is used for most anorectal procedures in our center, is most suitable for placement of an LMA, but for technical reasons, the LMA does not safely secure the airway when the patient is in the prone or jack-knife position. Therefore, because of the impact on airway management and anesthesia it is important to discuss the positioning of the patient with the surgical team before the operation.

Alternate Methods of Airway Management

The traditional neuromuscular blocking agent for short procedures is succinylcholine. The onset of action is rapid within 1 to 2 minutes after an intubating dose of 1.0 to 1.5 mg/kg. The duration of action is approximately 5 minutes after a bolus dose. The neuromuscular blocking action is terminated rapidly by the endogenous enzyme pseudocholinesterase. All of the nondepolarizing muscle relaxants currently in use are longer acting than succinylcholine and may require reversal for short

TABLE 2.4. Pharmacokinetic properties of neuromuscular blocking agents.

Agent	Distribution half-life (min)	Elimination half-life (min)	Clearance (mL/kg/min)	Volume of distribution (L/kg)
Atracurium	2	17–22	5.0–6.0	0.15–0.18
Mivacurium	—*	2–3	53–99	0.15–0.27
Vecuronium	4	65–75	3.6–4.5	0.3–0.4
Rocuronium	1–2	84	4.2	0.25

Data from Rogers, et al.[4] and Wood and Wood.[5]

*Mivacurium is very short acting and the distribution half-life is insignificant.

procedures. The disadvantage of reversal agents (neostigmine and atropine) is the high incidence of PONV. The average duration for anorectal procedures in our center is 30 minutes, and therefore succinylcholine has remained the drug of choice for many anesthesiologists. The low cost of succinylcholine is also advantageous.

The major disadvantage of succinylcholine is postanesthetic muscle pain, particularly in the ambulatory setting. Churchill-Davidson first reported the incidence of myalgia, and noted the higher incidence of "muscle-pains" in patients who walked soon after their procedure (67%) compared with patients who remained in bed (13.9%).[3] This myalgia is most effectively ameliorated with a 3-mg dose of curare before administration of succinylcholine. The other potential side effects of succinylcholine are an increase in the intraocular pressure, malignant hyperthermia, and hyperkalemia.

The nondepolarizing agents favored for intubation and maintenance are atracurium, mivacurium, and vecuronium (Table 2.4).[4,5] For short procedures, mivacurium or atracurium is often used. The major side effect of both of these neuromuscular blocking agents is the release of histamine. Therefore, the author's personal preference is to use a small dose of vecuronium. In the ambulatory surgery center it is critical to avoid life-threatening anaphylactic reactions.

Maintenance: Narcotics and Isoflurane

Traditional maintenance-phase anesthesia consists of a combination of an inhalation agent and a narcotic. Isoflurane is the most widely used inhalation agent. It is critical to turn off the vaporizer early enough in the operation to allow timely extubation. Because of its irritant effect on the airway, desflurane has not replaced isoflurane. Sevoflurane, initially suspect for its nephrotoxicity, fell out of favor until recently, and it is now beginning to gain in popularity for outpatient surgery.

Choice of Narcotics

Fentanyl has stood the test of time and is the most commonly used narcotic in outpatient anesthesia. It is important to administer fentanyl 2 to 5 minutes before the propofol so that the dose of propofol can be minimized and the maximal analgesic effect will be present during surgical and anesthesia stimulation. Fentanyl in doses of 1.0 to 2.0 µg/kg is given at the beginning of the anesthetic to avoid a delay in awakening. Fentanyl can also be used in the immediate recovery period in small incremental doses of 25 to 50 µg intravenously for postoperative analgesia. Muscle rigidity is uncommon at these small doses. Fentanyl is much more cost effective than alfentanil, sufentanil, and remifentanil (Table 2.5).[5–7]

TABLE 2.5. Pharmacokinetic properties of opioids.

Agent	Distribution half-life (min)	Elimination half-life (min)	Clearance (mL/kg/min)	Volume of distribution (L/kg)
Fentanyl	13.4	3.6	11.6	4.2
Sufentanil	17.7	2.7	13.0	1.7
Alfentanil	11.6	1.6	6.4	0.86
Remifentanil	0.94	0.16	41.2	0.39

Data from Wood and Wood,[5] Philip,[6] and Glass et al.[7]

Remifentanil hydrochloride is an ultrashort-acting analgesic with potency similar to fentanyl. It has a high therapeutic index when compared with other narcotics commonly used in anesthesia. The onset of action is within 90 seconds and its effect lasts for 5 to 10 minutes. Its half-life is 8 to 10 minutes. Remifentanil is a phenylpiperidine derivative with opioid agonist effects. The compound is 70% bound to plasma protein and is metabolized by both circulating and tissue-nonspecific esterases. Remifentanil is useful when analgesia is needed for short, painful procedures, such as incision and drainage, dressing changes, etc. It can provide a "cardiac type" anesthetic in patients with compromised myocardial function. Postoperative pain and rapid disappearance of analgesia may be a disadvantage, and local infiltration or other analgesics should be administered before emergence. The initial dose of remifentanil is 0.5 to 1.0 μg/kg per minute when combined with a hypnotic or volatile agent. Anesthesia is maintained with nitrous oxide, isoflurane, or propofol. Quick emergence is a great advantage, although nausea and vomiting are more common than with other analgesics. Remifentanil is also used when intubation is required, such as in prone procedures (e.g., removal of a pilonidal cyst), or when muscle relaxants are not desired. The short half-life permits rapid emergence and return of spontaneous ventilation while avoiding the side effects of muscle relaxants. Remifentanil is certainly one of the more flexible pharmacologic agents available for anorectal surgery.

Alternatives to Narcotic Analgesia

Minimizing patient discomfort in the postoperative period achieves both an early discharge and improved patient satisfaction. Preemptive analgesia has been discussed. Local infiltration is also a good, inexpensive, and effective method of pain control. Subfascial and intramuscular infiltration of local anesthetic is more potent than subcutaneous injection.

Nonsteroidal anti-inflammatory medications, including ibuprofen and ketorolac (Toradol, Syntex International, Palo Alto, CA), are efficacious analgesics. These drugs do not cause drowsiness, nausea, vomiting, or constipation. Therefore, they are especially useful for patients who will be discharged after a few hours. Some caution should be exercised because of side effects that include heartburn and gastric bleeding. Ketorolac should be taken for a maximum of 5 days. These medications have limited potency and are best used as adjuncts in combination with stronger analgesics for very severe pain.

Total Intravenous Anesthesia

Total intravenous anesthesia (TIVA) is an alternative to the traditional combination of a narcotic and a volatile inhalation agent for maintenance anesthesia.[8] With these lipophilic drugs, the dynamic equilibrium between concentration in the plasma and at the effector site is rapid and the intensity of effect becomes proportional to the plasma concentration. This permits a rapid deepening of unconsciousness. One of the recommended protocols for TIVA uses a combination of alfentanil and propofol. A bolus dose of alfentanil 10 μg/kg is followed by an induction or sleep dose of propofol. A continuous infusion of propofol is started at 120 to 200 μg/kg per minute and is adjusted according to the vital signs. The infusion is stopped 5 to 10 minutes before the end of the procedure.

Volatile Induction and Maintenance Anesthesia

Sevoflurane is one of the newest inhalational agents on the market. Although this agent is relatively new to the United States, it has been used extensively in Japan since 1990. Sevoflurane is similar in many ways to isoflurane, the gold standard for inhalational agents in use today, with a few significant differences.

Sevoflurane is a nonflammable fluorinated isopropyl ether. It is less potent than isoflurane with a minimal alveolar concentration (MAC) of 2.0. The greatest benefit of sevoflurane is a rapid onset of action and rapid emergence phase due to its low blood/gas solubility. The tissue solubility, with a fat/blood partition coefficient of 53.4, is also low. This allows rapid elimination and awakening.

Unlike the other gases, the respiratory irritant effects of sevoflurane are minimal, and children, as well as adults, tolerate an inhalation induction with sevoflurane. The cardiovascular and respiratory depressant effects of sevoflurane are similar to those of isoflurane. Sevoflurane causes less hypotension and tachycardia than isoflurane and does not sensitize the heart to catecholamines. The arrhythmogenic threshold for injected epinephrine is between that of enflurane and isoflurane. In one study, with sevoflurane at an MAC of 1.3, the amount of injected epinephrine causing a ventricular arrhythmia was 8.57 μg/kg. The threshold for isoflurane was 9.81 μg/kg, and that of enflurane was 5.17 μg/kg.

Currently, sevoflurane is used as both an induction and a maintenance agent. This is economical, because the high concentration required at the start of the procedure replaces the cost of propofol. In the maintenance phase, less sevoflurane is required because the desired alveolar concentration has already been reached in the induction phase. Additionally, sevoflurane provides ideal conditions for intubation and precludes the need for muscle relaxants. Similarly, it provides good conditions for placement of the LMA.

Another advantage of sevoflurane is in patients who are very frightened of needles. They are induced with inhalation of sevoflurane using the one-breath technique, and the intravenous infusion is deferred until after induction. Patients can be extubated rapidly at the end of surgery and discharged early from the recovery room. Sevoflurane does not provide any analgesia in the immediate postoperative period. It is therefore imperative to use supplemental methods of providing analgesia such as a good perianal block or ketorolac.

Monitored Anesthesia

Monitored anesthesia care is an alternative to general anesthesia (Table 2.6). The goal of this technique is to make the patient comfortable without compromising safety. Some patients do not desire a general anesthetic and wish to be awake but pain free. A combination of midazolam and propofol is used to sedate the patient while the surgeon performs a perianal block with a long-acting local anesthetic, such as bupivacaine. Once the block is in place, the patient is lightly sedated for the rest of the procedure. The critical aspect of the procedure is ensuring that the perianal block is adequate. When there is an ongoing inflammatory process, the local anesthetic may be less effective due to the acidity of the surrounding tissues. As a result, this method is not recommended for incision and drainage of a perirectal abscess. In addition, many surgeons do not like to use this technique for fistulectomies, because of the potential distortion of anatomy that occurs with injection. The local anesthetic is usually injected at the end instead of at the beginning of these procedures.

(*Editor's note:* The addition of hyaluronidase to the local anesthetic promotes rapid diffusion of the agent into the tissues with minimal distortion of the tissues. The muscle relaxation from the local anesthetic and the hemostatic effect of the epinephrine both facilitate the dissection in patients with fistula and/or abscess.)

Propofol may be used for sedation during local or regional anesthesia. After an initial dose of 1 to 2 mg/kg, patients can be kept lightly asleep but easily arousable by a continuous infusion of 3 to 4 mg/kg per hour. Propofol may have an advantage over other sedation techniques because of the ease with which the infusion can be increased, and the anesthetic management can be converted to a general anesthetic from which awakening will be rapid.

Regional Anesthesia

Regional anesthesia is not an ideal choice for ambulatory surgery, because it takes more time to establish the block (Table 2.7). In addition, the quality of the regional block is dependent to a certain extent on the skill of the person performing the block. A major concern with this procedure is the

TABLE 2.6. Monitored anesthesia care.

Advantages	Disadvantages
Hemodynamic stability	Distortion of the anatomy
Rapid recovery	Patient discomfort
Less PONV	
Increased safety	

PONV, postoperative nausea and vomiting.

TABLE 2.7. Regional anesthesia.

Advantages	Disadvantages
No loss of consciousness	Slower onset
Less risk of aspiration	Operator dependence
Less PONV	Spinal headache
Minimal pulmonary complications	

PONV, postoperative nausea and vomiting.

high incidence of spinal headache in young ambulatory patients. Similar problems arise with epidural analgesia because of the occasional occurrence of inadvertent dural puncture. Patient preference is one of the few reasons for performing a regional block, so it is important to fully explain this risk of post–dural puncture headache.

Other Problems

Acquired Immune Deficiency Syndrome

In addition to the infectious complications associated with advanced acquired immune deficiency syndrome (AIDS), there are specific anesthetic complications that are likely to be encountered.[9] Many of these patients are taking zidovudine (AZT) and are at risk for pancytopenia. In addition, both the disease and the drug therapy can cause diarrhea, dysphagia, esophagitis, and electrolyte imbalances that should be corrected before the patient undergoes general anesthesia. Patients with AIDS dementia should not be exposed to commonly used dopaminergic agonists such as droperidol and metoclopramide, which may exacerbate their cognitive dysfunction. The peripheral neuropathy associated with AIDS may be worsened by regional anesthesia. Finally, these patients may have cardiomyopathy or cardiopulmonary dysfunction and should probably undergo surgery in a hospital setting unless their immunologic dysfunction is clinically absent or well controlled.

Postoperative Nausea and Vomiting

Postoperative nausea and vomiting (PONV) is the most common postoperative complication in adults and children. It is the most disliked and most frequently remembered postoperative sequela for patients, family members, and nurses. The prevention of PONV is a high priority for the anesthesiologist.

Prevention should begin with identifying the patients at risk. PONV is more commonly seen in young children and women. Although the incidence of PONV in men is much lower than in women, men with a history of PONV have a very high incidence of recurrence. Postoperative factors that influence PONV include pain, dizziness, motion, early oral intake, and intraoperative or postop-

erative administration of narcotics. Patient factors include obesity, anxiety, a history of motion sickness, a history of PONV, gastroparesis, and a full stomach.

The key to controlling PONV is prevention with the use of antiemetic premedications. The causes of nausea and vomiting are multifactorial, and there does not seem to be any one particular group of drugs that are completely efficacious. Some of the commonly used antiemetic drugs are discussed below.

Promethazine is a phenothiazine that is useful in treating and preventing PONV. The recommended dose range is 25 to 50 mg administered intravenously, intramuscularly, or rectally. The intravenous route can be associated with phlebitis. Sedation is the only side effect that is usually experienced. A promethazine suppository is a good antiemetic and can be used preoperatively for patients with a history of PONV. Promethazine has stood the test of time, has minimal side effects, and is very cost effective.

Droperidol is also used for both the prevention and treatment of PONV. This butyrophenone antagonizes dopamine in the chemoreceptor trigger zone of the brain. Dosages can range from 0.625 to 1.25 mg given intravenously. The extrapyramidal and psychological side effects can be avoided with the lower dose, and droperidol is more cost effective than ondansetron. Droperidol is given at the beginning of the procedure to minimize drowsiness at the end of the procedure.

Metoclopramide prevents PONV by stimulating gastric motility and increasing lower esophageal sphincter tone. A dose of 10 mg given at the end of the procedure appears to be most effective. Rapid administration can result in extrapyramidal effects.

Scopolamine prevents emesis related to motion and is administered via a postauricular patch. This patch can be applied the morning of surgery. Undesirable side effects include dry mouth, dizziness, amblyopia, mydriasis, headache, and sedation.

Ondansetron (Zofran, Glaxo Wellcome Inc., Research Triangle Park, NC) belongs to a new class of antiemetics, the serotonin antagonists. They act by antagonizing serotonin at the 5-hydroxytryptamine type 3 receptor. Ondansetron has no central nervous system side effects and does not stimulate histamine, cholinergic, adrenergic, or dopaminergic receptors. Doses of 4 to 8 mg intravenously are equally effective at decreasing emesis 24 hours after surgery. It is most effective if 4 mg is given about 20 minutes before the end of surgery. It should be noted that 4 mg of ondansetron and 1.25 mg of droperidol are equally effective at prevention of PONV. Because of its high costs, ondansetron is used in patients who have a history of PONV and a successful past result with the drug, in patients who are unresponsive to droperidol, or in patients who experience extreme drowsiness with promethazine.

It is important to hydrate patients at high risk for PONV. It is reported that patients who have been hydrated with 1 L of lactated Ringer's solution do not get postural hypotension and subsequent nausea. (*Editor's note:* The issue of hydration must be carefully balanced in the patient undergoing anorectal surgery due to its relationship with urinary retention. See Chapter 7.) Pain may also contribute to postoperative nausea and vomiting. Pain management is discussed above and is further covered in Chapter 6.

Summary

Anesthesia for ambulatory anorectal surgery is evolving. Newer techniques and medications with fewer side effects are permitting sicker patients to undergo anesthesia safely. Increasingly, anesthetics that are specifically tailored to an individual patient's requirements are becoming the standard of care.

References

1. American Society of Anesthesiologists. New classification of physical status. Anesthesiology 1963;24:111.

2. Kortila K, Ostman P, Faure E, et al. Randomized comparison of recovery after propofol-nitrous oxide versus thiopentone-isoflurane-nitrous oxide anesthesia in patients undergoing ambulatory surgery. Acta Anaesthesiol Scand 1990;34:400–403.

3. Churchill-Davidson HC. Succinylcholine and muscle pains. BMJ 1954;74(1):74–75.

4. Rogers MC et al. (eds). Principles and Practice of Anesthesiology. St Louis: Mosby, 1993, pp 1053–1086, 1151–1154, 1518–1540.

5. Wood M, Wood A. Drugs and Anesthesia. Baltimore: Williams & Wilkins, 1990, pp 129–78, 179–224, 225–270, 271–318.

6. Philip BK. Opioids in outpatient anesthesia. Anesthesiology Reviews 1991;18(S1):4–8.

7. Glass PSA, Hardman D, Kamiyarna Y, et al. Preliminary pharmacokinetics and pharmacodynamics of an ultra-short-acting opioid: remifentanil (G178084B). Anesth Analg 1993;77:1031–1040.

8. Healy TEJ (ed). Total Intravenous Anesthesia (Monographs in Anesthesiology). New York, Elsevier Science, 1991, pp 1–11.

9. Berkowitz ID. Evaluation of the patient with acquired immunodeficiency syndrome and other serious infections. In Rogers MC et al (eds). Principles and Practice of Anesthesiology. St Louis: Mosby, 1993, pp 410–427.

10. Barash PG, Cullen BF, Stoelting RK (eds). Clinical Anesthesia, 2nd ed. Philadelphia: JB Lippincott, 1992, pp 1401–1402.

11. Katzung BG. Basic and Clinical Pharmacology. Stamford, CT, Appleton & Lange, 1998, pp 421–422.

Acknowledgments

The author is grateful for the assistance of Pat Alford, M.S., C.R.N.A.; Gay Abangan, C.R.N.A.; Marilyn Bartlett, C.R.N.A.; Lisa Palattzi, S.R.N.A.; and Karen Scheske, R.N. in gathering the information presented in this chapter.

3

Selection, Preoperative Assessment, and Education of the Patient for Ambulatory Surgery

Michael J. Snyder, M.D.

The preoperative evaluation of the ambulatory anorectal surgery patient determines his or her relative risk for the proposed procedure. Since its beginnings at the University of California, Los Angeles, in 1962,[1] ambulatory surgery has evolved to include increasingly complex and invasive procedures. In addition, advances in the medical therapy of a variety of disorders have allowed patients with multiple medical problems to undergo surgical procedures safely. Improvements in preoperative evaluation and postoperative management have been the cornerstone permitting many patients with complex medical problems to have surgery in the outpatient setting. Although fewer patients are excluded from undergoing ambulatory surgery, it is imperative that high-risk patients are carefully screened with a thorough and appropriate evaluation.

General Considerations

Patient selection for ambulatory anorectal surgery is based on the physical status of the individual. The physical status classification system established by the American Society of Anesthesiologists (ASA) consists of five categories (see Table 2.1).[2] Patients with a physical status class of I or II are ideal candidates for ambulatory surgery, and those with a physical status of III may also undergo surgery if the medical condition in question is stable and will not be significantly exacerbated by the proposed procedure or anesthetic technique. Although there is no age limit to having ambulatory surgery, the functional capabilities and projected short-term disability in elderly patients must be carefully considered. The type of surgical procedure and the anticipated duration of the operation are important considerations. Patients who may experience significant blood loss or require invasive cardiac monitoring should probably not have surgery in the outpatient setting. Procedures with high complication rates that may require laparotomy should also be avoided. Other considerations in choosing between the ambulatory and inpatient setting include the anticipated need for injectable analgesics, antibiotics, or intravenous fluids postoperatively.

Patients who are actively abusing alcohol or other recreational drugs have a higher rate of anesthetic complications. Cocaine and amphetamines increase the risk of spastic myocardial ischemia during induction. Alcohol tolerance changes the expected dose and response to anesthetic agents, especially the benzodiazepines. These patients may have outpatient surgery if there has been no recent abuse; otherwise they are optimally treated as inpatients.

Inpatient observation may also be necessary if the patient is unable to arrange for transportation or carry out preoperative instructions, especially regarding bowel preparation. A responsible adult must be present during the first 24 hours to help care for the patient after the procedure. For the elderly or disabled patient, social services can help arrange visiting nurses and other critical assistance. Given sufficient time and preparation, few logistical problems cannot be solved, except possibly for the elderly and for patients with psychosocial pathology.

Cardiovascular Disease

Many patients undergoing ambulatory anorectal surgery have known and silent cardiovascular disease. Hypertension is one of the most common disorders in the general population. Newly diagnosed or poorly controlled hypertension should be adequately treated before any elective surgery because of the higher incidence of chronic dehydration in these patients. This can lead to hypotension and subsequent ischemia upon induction of general anesthesia.[3] Patients receiving long-term diuretic therapy should be evaluated for electrolyte abnormalities, especially hypokalemia. If hypertensive patients on diuretic therapy require a bowel preparation, a polyethylene glycol regimen is preferred to minimize intestinal electrolyte depletion. Lastly, hypertension is an independent risk factor for significant coronary artery disease and may be an indication for further cardiac evaluation.

The prevalence of coronary artery disease continues to increase as our population ages. Annually, 20,000 deaths occur from perioperative myocardial infarctions in the United States. Although some patients with coronary artery disease are asymptomatic, the perioperative risk of myocardial infarction in asymptomatic patients is only 0.15%.[4] Asymptomatic patients under age 50 without risk factors for coronary artery disease do not require further cardiac evaluation for anorectal surgery. Asymptomatic patients over age 50, men over age 40 with cardiac risk factors, and postmenopausal women with cardiac risk factors should have a baseline electrocardiogram. A careful history and physical examination and the judicious use of ancillary tests are necessary to remove high-risk patients from the ambulatory surgery arena. Symptomatic patients or asymptomatic patients with abnormal electrocardiograms should be evaluated by an internist or cardiologist before elective surgery. Such medical evaluation helps avoid emergency consultations in the intraoperative or perioperative period for possible myocardial ischemia. Further evaluation of high-risk patients should be guided by the patient's cardiologist. Patients who have undergone angioplasty or coronary artery bypass grafting are candidates for ambulatory surgery if they have a good functional result. Patients who may require invasive intraoperative cardiac monitoring or postoperative telemetry for arrhythmias should undergo their operations in an inpatient setting.

Valvular heart disease, overall, has declined markedly with the advent of penicillin therapy for rheumatic fever; however, aortic stenosis is becoming more prevalent. Aortic stenosis is the most important valvular abnormality to detect preoperatively, as it is associated with a 13% incidence of perioperative mortality.[5] Patients with artificial valves are usually taking warfarin for anticoagulation. Close consultation with the patient's cardiologist on the timing of stopping and resuming warfarin is critical. Patients with prosthetic cardiac valves are also at high risk for bacterial endocarditis following gastrointestinal procedures. Other patients have valvular abnormalities such as mitral valve prolapse with regurgitation and bicuspid aortic valves that create turbulence. These abnormalities place them at moderate risk for bacterial endocarditis in the face of transient bacteremia. Antibiotic prophylaxis is recommended for high-risk patients and is optional for moderate-risk patients undergoing anorectal surgery.[6] The current recommendations for antibiotic prophylaxis with anorectal procedures are noted in Table 3.1.

TABLE 3.1. Prophylactic regimen for patients with valvular heart disease undergoing anorectal procedures.

Situation	Agents	Regimen
High risk	Ampicillin + gentamicin	Ampicillin 2.0 g IM or IV, plus gentamicin 1.5 mg/kg, 30 min before procedure, amoxicillin 1 g PO 6 hr after procedure
Moderate risk	Amoxicillin	Amoxicillin 2.0 g PO 1 hr before procedure
High risk, penicillin allergic	Vancomycin + gentamicin	Vancomycin 1.0 g IV, plus gentamicin 1.5 mg/kg, 30 min before procedure
Moderate risk, penicillin allergic	Vancomycin	Vancomycin 1.0 g IV, 30 min before procedure

Adapted from Dejani AS, et al.[6]

IM, intramuscularly; IV, intravenously; PO, by mouth.

Pulmonary Disease

Asthma and chronic obstructive pulmonary disease (COPD) are becoming increasingly prevalent in our society. General anesthesia has the potential to exacerbate these conditions. If the patient with pulmonary disease is well controlled medically and has good exercise tolerance, then he or she can safely undergo ambulatory anorectal surgery. Patients regularly using aerosolized bronchodilators should be instructed to take their medications the morning of surgery. In addition, intraoperative and perioperative nebulizer therapy should be available.

Patients with poor exercise tolerance, a history of intubation, or current steroid use may benefit from further evaluation by an internist or pulmonologist to maximize their pulmonary reserve. If the patient is believed to require intravenous medications or possible ventilator weaning in the perioperative period, then the operation should not be performed in the ambulatory setting.

Preoperative chest radiography for anorectal surgery rarely changes the perioperative management or outcome. In 1979, a landmark study was completed on preoperative chest radiography by the Royal College of Radiologists.[7] This study concluded that for asymptomatic patients undergoing nonthoracic surgery, the preoperative chest radiograph did not influence the choice of anesthesia or the decision to perform surgery. In addition, the chest radiograph was of little value as a baseline study and did not predict postoperative respiratory complications. For patients with underlying pulmonary disease such as COPD, however, the chest radiograph may be useful to rule out coexisting pneumonia. In patients with suspected coronary artery disease, the chest radiograph may also be of benefit in the diagnosis of cardiomegaly.

Renal Disease

Patients receiving dialysis for chronic renal failure will often have significant comorbidities such as hypertension, diabetes mellitus, and advanced atherosclerosis. The incidence of coronary artery disease is high in dialysis patients. However, if other medical factors are stable, merely being on dialysis does not disqualify the patient from ambulatory surgery. The operation should be performed soon after dialysis to ensure a normokalemic and nonacidotic state, as this will minimize anesthetic complications. Patients on dialysis have two abnormalities that lead to problems with blood clotting. The first of these is the residual heparin remaining following dialysis. The second is a platelet abnormality. The number of platelets is usually normal, but the platelet function is deficient. For procedures with a significant risk of postprocedure bleeding, platelets for possible transfusion and deamino-D-arginine vasopressin (DDAVP) should be available.

Other Disorders

Other high-risk patients include those with obesity, liver disease, diabetes mellitus, and acquired immune deficiency syndrome (AIDS). Obese patients have a high incidence of cardiopulmonary disease. A good assessment of the airway is imperative if ventilation by mask is considered. Because of the lipid-soluble nature of many anesthetic agents, care must be taken in choosing the ideal agents for short anorectal surgical procedures in obese patients.

Diabetes mellitus is a disorder of glucose metabolism associated with premature accelerated atherosclerosis involving the brain, heart, kidneys, and nervous systems. A thorough preoperative workup is crucial to prevent perioperative complications. An electrocardiogram is recommended except in very young diabetic patients because of the high incidence of silent ischemia.[8] The timing of insulin administration and oral hypoglycemic medication before surgery is discussed below under Patient Education. Patients with poorly controlled or brittle diabetes should not be considered for ambulatory anorectal surgery.

The patient with advanced liver disease has potential deficiencies in nutrition, coagulation, and drug metabolism. Portal hypertension is the hallmark of the disease, and the anorectum may contain large varices. Although newer anesthetic agents are significantly less hepatotoxic than older agents such as halothane, the decreased hepatic blood flow that occurs with general anesthesia for even short procedures can precipitate postoperative liver failure. The risk of significant postoperative complications in patients with advanced liver disease is high, and inpatient surgery should be strongly considered.

TABLE 3.2. Centers for Disease Control classification system for HIV infection.

Group	Description
I	Acute infection
II	Asymptomatic infection
III	Persistent generalized lymphadenopathy
IV	AIDS-related disease

Source: Centers for Disease Control.[9]

The human immunodeficiency virus (HIV) is a retrovirus that infects and consumes the helper-inducer (T4) lymphocytes. After a variable latency period, HIV produces declining immunologic function that culminates as AIDS. In 1986, the Centers for Disease Control (CDC) presented a classification system for HIV disease (Table 3.2).[9] Although this system was revised in 1993 to include stratification based on T4 cell counts (Table 3.3),[10] the important surgical aspect of both of these classification systems is that early-stage patients have an adequately functioning immune system. With advancements in treatment, the survival of HIV-seropositive patients has been prolonged, primarily due to drugs that maintain them for longer periods at an earlier stage of disease.

Several studies have demonstrated that asymptomatic HIV-seropositive patients can be expected to have adequate wound healing with few complications after anorectal surgery.[11,12] Many surgeons, however, have discovered that patients with an advanced stage of HIV infection have poor results with any type of operative therapy. The high incidence of morbidity and significant mortality in patients with advanced HIV disease reflects their altered immune status.[13,14] Some authors have advocated using T4 cell counts to help determine which asymptomatic or minimally symptomatic patients will exhibit normal wound healing. The critical level for the T4 cell count may be above 200 lymphocytes per milliliter. Recently, the ability to take accurate measurements of the viral load

TABLE 3.3. Revised CDC classification system for HIV infection and expanded AIDS surveillance case definition for adolescents and adults.

CD4 cell count	Clinical categories		
	(A)	(B)	(C)
1. 500/μL or greater	A1	B1	C1
2. 200–400/μL	A2	B2	C2
3. less than 200/μL	A3	B3	C3
	Asymptomatic HIV infection • Acute retroviral syndrome • Persistent generalized lymphadenopathy • Acute (primary) HIV infection	Symptomatic not (A) or (C) • Bacillary angiomatosis • Candidiasis, oral or vaginal • Cervical dysplasia • Hairy leukoplakia, oral • Herpes zoster infection • Idiopathic thrombocytopenia purpura • Listerosis • Pelvic inflammatory disease • Peripheral neuropathy	AIDS, opportunistic infections • Candidiasis, pulmonary, esophageal • Cervical cancer • Coccidiomycosis • Cryptococcosis, extrapulmonary • Cryptosporidiosis • Cytomegalovirus, chronic or esophageal • Histoplasmosis • Isosporiasis • Kaposi's sarcoma • Lymphoma • Mycobacteria, avium • Mycobacteria, kansaii • Mycobacteria, tuberculosis • Pneumocystis carinii • Pneumonia, recurrent • Progressive, mulfifocal leukoencephalopathy • Salmonellosis

Source: Centers for Disease Control.[10]

has supplanted T4 counts as the most sensitive indicator of disease activity in the asymptomatic patient.

The ambulatory setting is suitable for early-stage (CDC groups I and II) HIV-seropositive patients. Good surgical technique, including the judicious handling of sharps, will ensure that the operation is safe for both the patient and the surgeon. Because of their attenuated immune function, late-stage patients (CDC groups III and IV) should be observed as inpatients for possible septic complications.

Bowel Preparation

Since the 1950s, preoperative mechanical bowel preparation has been widely used for patients undergoing major colon and rectal surgery.[15] In addition, the efficacy of prophylactic antibiotics in rectal surgery has been well documented.[16] For major anorectal surgery such as sphincter repair, rectovaginal fistula repair, operations for rectal prolapse, and full-thickness transanal excision of rectal tumors, a combination of mechanical cleansing and prophylactic antibiotics is crucial to provide a clean operative site and minimize infectious complications.

Several techniques can provide a satisfactory mechanical preparation of the colon and rectum. A lavage solution of polyethylene glycol and electrolytes or a cathartic containing sodium phosphate are the two most widely used regimens. Both methods are effective and safe for most patients. A significant percentage of patients have difficulty ingesting the entire (4-L) polyethylene glycol mixture.[17] In addition, more gastrointestinal cramping and bloating occur with the polyethylene glycol preparation.[17] The sodium phosphate solution is contraindicated in patients with congestive heart failure, chronic renal insufficiency, ascites, or congenital megacolon. Cardiac arrhythmias can occur after taking the sodium phosphate solution in patients who are hypokalemic and are receiving digitalis and diuretics.[18] The author's preferred regimen for bowel preparation for major anorectal surgery is shown in Table 3.4.

Prophylactic antibiotics are administered to patients undergoing major anorectal surgery. Oral and systemic antibiotics appear to have equal efficacy in intestinal surgery.[14] A combination of the two offers a theoretical if unproven advantage. Neomycin and metronidazole are the most frequently administered oral antibiotics, and their dosage is noted in Table 3.4. Erythromycin can be substituted for the metronidazole, but it may be associated with severe nausea and emesis in a significant percentage of patients. Systemic antibiotics are begun just before surgery and are continued for 24 hours postoperatively. The ideal agent is long acting and provides both anaerobic and aerobic coverage. Currently, a second-generation cephalosporin is the most commonly used agent. For penicillin-allergic patients, a combination of intravenous ciprofloxacin and metronidazole is often employed.

The recent introduction of antibiotics such as trovafloxacin (Trovan, Pfizer Pharmaceuticals, New York, NY) provide high blood levels of antibiotic, cover both aerobes and anaerobes, and can be taken once daily. Such agents may allow more complex procedures to be performed in the ambulatory setting.

Patients undergoing minor anorectal surgery who are at high risk for wound complications because of immunosuppression or prior radiation therapy should also have a full mechanical bowel preparation with prophylactic antibiotics. For other patients

---

TABLE 3.4. Mechanical and antibiotic bowel preparation.

1. The patient consumes a clear liquid diet on the day before the procedure.
2. The patient stops drinking at 2:00 P.M. and takes nothing by mouth until 3:30 P.M.
3. The patient takes one Reglan 10-mg tablet by mouth at 3:30 P.M.
4. The patient begins polyethylene glycol preparation at 4:00 P.M. The patient drinks one 8-ounce glass every 15–20 minutes until the 4 L are consumed or the effluent is clear.
5. After consuming the polyethylene glycol, the patient takes four bisacodyl tablets.
6. The patient may resume clear liquids until midnight.
7. The patient takes nothing by mouth after midnight.
8. The patient takes neomycin 1.0 g by mouth at 1:00, 2:00, and 11:00 P.M. on the day before surgery for a morning case.
9. The patient takes metronidazole 1.0 g by mouth at 1:00, 2:00, and 11:00 P.M. on the day before surgery for a morning case.
10. The patient receives cefotetan 2.0 g intravenously after being called to the operating room.

undergoing minor anorectal surgery, adequate cleansing of the anus and rectum can usually be accomplished with phosphate or saline enemas. Antibiotics are not routinely necessary in these patients.

Deep Venous Thrombosis Prophylaxis

Deep venous thrombosis (DVT) and subsequent pulmonary embolism are largely preventable complications. The risk factors for the development of DVT are listed in Table 3.5. Patients undergoing major anorectal surgery lasting longer than 2 hours should receive DVT prophylaxis.

Many effective prophylaxis regimens exist. The most widely used consist of either intermittent sequential compression devices or low–molecular weight heparin. A combination of both is recommended in patients with multiple risk factors. Either treatment reduces the incidence of DVT by up to 60%.[19]

Intermittent sequential compression devices should be applied before the induction of anesthesia and removed when the patient is walking. Patient compliance is occasionally a problem with these devices that are also not easily used in the ambulatory surgery environment. Low–molecular weight heparin is injected subcutaneously 1 to 2 hours before surgery and is repeated daily until discharge. The incidence of complications may be less than with standard mini-dose heparin.

Preoperative Testing

Many authors have concluded that routine preoperative testing of asymptomatic patients is a costly and ineffective method of detecting disorders that

TABLE 3.5. Risk factors for deep venous thrombosis (DVT).

Previous DVT or pulmonary embolism
Age greater than 40 years
Obesity
Malignancy
Pelvic surgery
Estrogen therapy
Length of surgery > 2 hours
Hypercoagulable states

will have an impact on patient care during anesthesia and surgery. Laboratory and ancillary tests, such as chest radiographs and electrocardiograms, are useful to define and maximize a patient's condition before surgery, but they have important inherent deficiencies. Abnormalities identified during preoperative testing are often incompletely evaluated or ignored, a situation that could lead to potential medicolegal consequences. Testing may be falsely positive, resulting in costly delays and cancellation of surgery, as well as unnecessary, potentially invasive evaluations. Finally, nonselective tests may not uncover significant pathology and may result in a false sense of security. A good history and physical examination remain the best screening tools, for which no amount of testing can be substituted. Finally, in this age of cost containment, the additional expense of unnecessary testing can no longer be condoned.

No consensus exists as to the most appropriate preoperative testing regimen. Testing should be based on the results of the history and physical examination, the age of the patient, the proposed operative procedure, the prevalence of the abnormality, and the relevance of the abnormality in changing the anesthetic or surgical management (Figure 3.1).

Laboratory

The incidence of unsuspected anemia in patients undergoing anorectal surgery is less than 5%. High-risk groups include menstruating women, patients with a history of bleeding, and men over age 60 years. Hemoglobin screening of these groups of patients should be performed. Rarely, however, is a complete blood count (CBC) indicated. Several authors have found that the incidence of preoperative neutropenia and thrombocytopenia is less than 0.1%.[20] A CBC should be ordered for patients who have recently undergone chemotherapy, those with known bone marrow abnormalities, and chronic alcoholics.

Although coagulation tests are useful in patients at higher risk for bleeding complications, they have no value in screening asymptomatic patients undergoing outpatient surgery.[21] Again, the history and physical examination will usually identify patients in need of further evaluation for coagulation abnormalities. These tests are indicated in patients with a

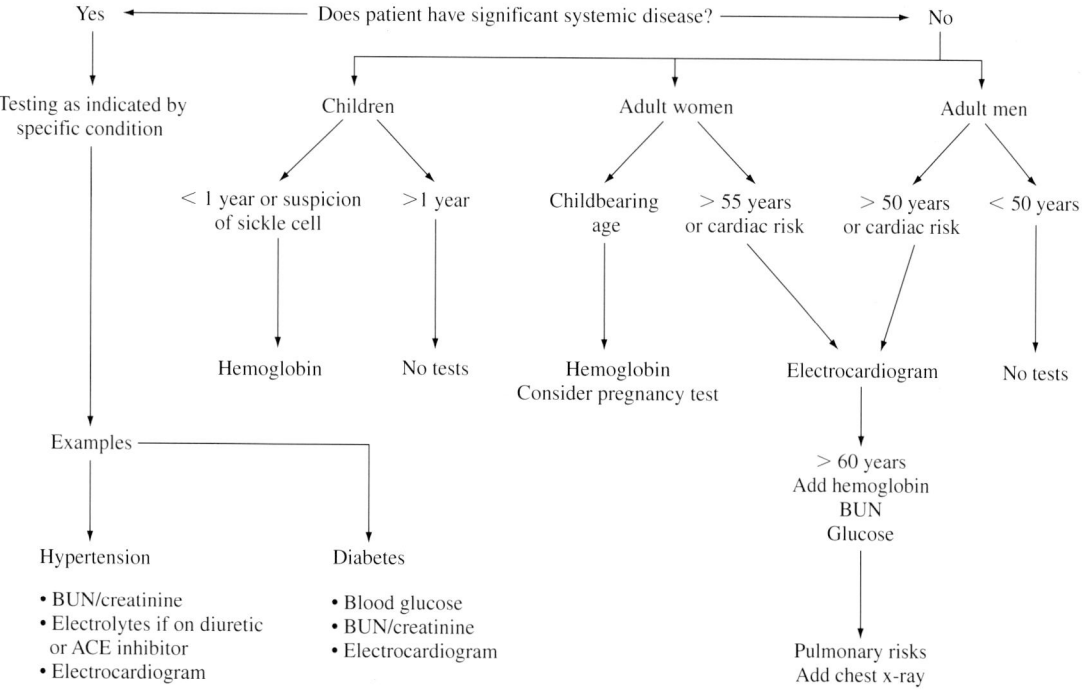

FIGURE 3.1. Preoperative testing algorithm. Adapted from Twersky RS. The Ambulatory Anesthesia Handbook. St. Louis: CV Mosby, 1995, Appendix III.

history of a bleeding disorder, liver disease, or use of anticoagulants.

Biochemical panels are unnecessary, costly and often lead to further testing in the asymptomatic patient. On a 20-test panel more than 50% of the normal population will have a reported abnormality. This is because the confidence limits for normal values are set at 95%, meaning that 5% of the normal population will have abnormal values. This not only leads to additional testing, but also presents a possible liability problem for a seemingly ignored test. Measurement of electrolyte levels should be ordered based on the findings of the history and physical examination. The electrolyte levels of greatest concern to the anesthesiologist and surgeon are those of potassium and magnesium because of the cardiac affects of these electrolyte. Indications for potassium screening include chronic diuretic therapy, a history of renal insufficiency, a history of new-onset hypertension, digoxin therapy, and a history of cardiac arrhythmias. Magnesium should be analyzed in patients with a history of hypokalemia and cardiac arrhythmias.

Abnormalities are frequently found on routine urinalysis and are often ignored.[22] A urinalysis is indicated in the anorectal surgery patient undergoing complex fistula-in-ano surgery and when inflammatory bowel disease is suspected. Elderly patients should be screened for asymptomatic bacteriuria because of its high prevalence. All women of childbearing potential should be asked about the possibility of pregnancy, and if any question exists, she should have a urine pregnancy test.

The indications for electrocardiography and chest radiography are discussed in the sections on the preoperative evaluation of cardiovascular and respiratory disease, respectively.

Prior Testing

There have been few studies evaluating the length of time a laboratory or ancillary test can be used before a subsequent study is indicated. Macpherson has suggested that normal laboratory values do not warrant repeating the tests within 1 year.[23] However, patients with prior abnormal laboratory values have a significant likelihood of having changes on subsequent screening that would affect the anesthetic management. Chest radiographs should only be redone if a change in the respiratory status has occurred in the interim. Repeating preoperative electrocardiograms in asymptomatic, low-risk patients younger than age 50 years is unnecessary.[24] However, in patients at higher risk, an electrocardiogram within 2 to 3 months is prudent to detect any interim change.

Patient Education

Education of the anorectal surgery patient undergoing ambulatory surgery is crucial for a successful outcome. A well-informed patient recovers faster and develops fewer complications. Issues of pain control and anxiety are improved by better understanding of the expected results. Complications, when they occur, are more easily managed in the properly educated patient.

The education begins with a detailed discussion of the implications of the medical diagnosis, the options for treatment, and the recommended surgical operation. This part of the preoperative teaching should be done by the operating surgeon to ensure that all questions are appropriately and completely answered. This is followed by very specific instructions on diet, bowel preparation, and the need for social support. For most ambulatory procedures, unless they are to be performed without sedation, a responsible adult must be available to drive the patient home and preferably to stay with the patient for 24 hours. Most anorectal procedures require no dietary instructions other than to take nothing by mouth after midnight the evening before surgery. However, for any patient requiring mechanical bowel preparation, careful oral and written instructions must be provided.

Most cardiac and antihypertensive medications should be taken the morning of surgery with a sip of water. Aspirin, however, should be discontinued at least 1 week before surgery. Diabetic patients should not take their oral hypoglycemic agent or full dose of insulin on the morning of surgery. Decisions regarding warfarin dosing and the interval of stopping and restarting are best made after careful consultation with the patient's internist or cardiologist. With the recent development of improved heparin preparations, fewer patients will need to undergo the classic "heparin window" for elective procedures. These instructions, both written and oral, are discussed in the physician's office and then reinforced by the nursing and anesthesiology personnel in the ambulatory surgery unit.

The next phase of education usually occurs in the ambulatory surgery unit. The patient and family meet with the surgeon, anesthesiologist, and nursing staff. The anesthetic technique is discussed, as well as an explanation of the projected length of the operation and the duration of postoperative stay in the unit. Many of the postoperative instructions can also be given to the patient and family at this time before the patient is under the influence of amnestic medications.

The postoperative instructions include details regarding activity in the immediate postoperative period, dietary restriction, the expected duration of the local perianal nerve block, and how to take sitz baths. Ambulation is strongly encouraged for most patients to minimize DVT and other musculoskeletal complaints. Driving, operating heavy machinery, or making major life decisions are strongly discouraged until the anesthetic agents have cleared.

An explanation of the possible complications of the procedure is reiterated. For expected minor complications, instructions about how to manage these at home will suffice. For more serious problems, information needs to be provided in a written format, including telephone numbers for contacting the surgeon and the surgical unit. Follow-up, to include timing of suture removal and wound care, should be clearly stated.

Methods of patient education are evolving as the surgical profession embraces the information age. Regardless, verbal discussion between the surgeon and the patient remains the cornerstone of education. Enough time in a busy office must be set aside to answer all the myriad questions and concerns. Not all the information is retained by the patient during the first discussion. For this reason, it is advantageous to restate much of the information in the ambulatory surgical unit. Verbal information should also be reinforced by written instructions that can be used as a reference by patients and family. Such instructions should be written in lay terms and frequently updated to reflect both the standard of care and individual surgeon preferences. It is essential that the verbal and written material be consistent. Recently, computer programs and videotapes containing preoperative instructions have become available and will undoubtedly become more important adjuncts in the future.

Conclusion

Thorough preoperative evaluation and education of the ambulatory surgery patient are crucial to a successful outcome. As technology in caring for sicker patients improves, we will be challenged to provide outpatient management for these increasingly complex patients. Our ability to meet this challenge relies on combining objective physiologic measurements and sound surgical judgment to determine the right operation for the right patient in the right setting.

References

1. Davis JE. History of major ambulatory surgery. In Davis JE (ed). Major Ambulatory Surgery. Baltimore: Williams & Wilkins, 1986, pp 3–31.
2. American Society of Anesthesiologists. New classification of physical status. Anesthesiology. 1963;24:111.
3. Goldman L, Caldera D. Risk of general anesthesia and elective operations in hypertensive patients. Anesthesiology 1979;50:285–292.
4. Freeman WK, Gibbons RJ, Shub C. Preoperative assessment of cardiac patients undergoing noncardiac surgical procedures. Mayo Clin Proc 1989;64:1105–1117.
5. Golman L, Caldera DL, Southwick FS, et al. Cardiac risk factors and complications in non-cardiac surgery. Medicine 1978;57:357–370.
6. Dajani AS, Taubert KA, Wilson W, et al. Prevention of bacterial endocarditis. Recommendations by the American Heart Association. JAMA 1997;277:1794–1800.
7. National Study by the Royal College of Radiologists. Preoperative chest radiography. Lancet 1979;2:83–86.
8. Milaskiewicz R, Hall B. Diabetes and anesthesia: the past decade. Br J Anaesth 1992;68:198–206.
9. Centers for Disease Control: Classification system for human T-lymphocyte virus type III/-lymphadenopathy-associated virus infections. MMWR Morb Mortal Wkly Rep 1986;35:334–339.
10. Centers for Disease Control: 1993 Revised classification system for HIV infection and extended surveillance case definitions for AIDS among adolescents and adults. MMWR Morb Mortal Wkly Rep 1992;41:1–19.
11. Carr ND, Mercey D, Slack WW. Non-condylomatous perianal disease in homosexual men. Br J Surg 1989;76:1064–1066.
12. Beck DE, Jaso RG, Zajac RA. Surgical management of anal condylomata in the HIV-positive patient. Dis Colon Rectum 1990;33:12–15.
13. Wexner SD, Smithy WB, Milsom JW, Dailey TH. The surgical management of anorectal disease in AIDS and pre-AIDS patients. Dis Colon Rectum 1986;29:719–723.
14. Buchmann P, Seefeld V. Rubber band ligation for piles can be disastrous in HIV-positive patients. Int J Colorectal Dis 1989;4:57–58.
15. Bartlett JG, Condon RE, Gorbach SL, et al. Veterans Administration cooperative study on bowel preparation for elective colorectal operation: impact of oral antibiotic regimen on colonic flora, wound irrigation cultures and bacteriology of septic complications. Ann Surg 1978;188:259–254.
16. Conte JE Jr, Jacob LS, Polk HC Jr. Antibiotic Prophylaxis in Surgery. A Comprehensive Review. Philadelphia: JB Lippincott, 1984.
17. Oliveira L, Wexner SD, Daniel N, et al. Mechanical bowel preparation for elective colorectal surgery: a prospective randomized, surgeon-blinded trial comparing sodium phosphate and polyethylene glycol-based oral lavage solutions. Dis Colon Rectum 1997;40:585–591.
18. Gupta SC, Gopalswamy N, Sarkar A, et al. Cardiac arrhythmias and electrocardiographic changes during upper and lower gastrointestinal endoscopy. Mil Med 1990;155:9–11.
19. NIH Consensus Development Conference. Prevention of venous thrombosis and pulmonary embolism. JAMA 1986;256:744–749.
20. Turnbull JM, Buck C. The value of preoperative screening investigations in otherwise healthy individuals. Arch Intern Med 1987;147:1101–1105.
21. Suchman AL, Mushlin, AI. How well does the activated partial thromboplastin time predict postoperative hemorrhage? JAMA 1986;256:750–753.
22. Heiman GA, Frohlich J, Bernstein M. Physician's response to abnormal results of routine urinalysis. Can Med Assoc J 1975;2:486–489.
23. Macpherson DS, Snow R, Lofgren RP. Preoperative screening: value of previous tests. Ann Intern Med 1990;113:969–973.
24. Rabkin SW, Horne JM. Preoperative electrocardiography: its cost-effectiveness in detecting abnormalities when a previous tracing exists. Can Med Assoc J 1979;121:301–305.

4

Positioning the Patient for Anorectal Surgical Procedures

Part A: The Prone Jack-Knife Position: The Gold Standard

Richard E. Karulf, M.D., F.A.C.S.
and
Stanley M. Goldberg, M.D., F.A.C.S.

Surgeons pride themselves on their ability to adapt to unforeseen circumstances. New situations are stimulating and prompt the surgeon to stop and to focus on basic principles. However, common procedures, which lack the luster of new and challenging cases, may become routinized because of the tyranny of a busy practice. The choice of the position of a patient during anorectal surgery is an example of a detail that may become a matter of habit rather than a conscious decision. This subchapter focuses on the prone jack-knife position, the rightful gold standard for anorectal surgery. It describes the appropriate use of this position during anorectal surgery and factors that would prompt the surgeon to use an alternative position.

Position

The prone jack-knife position, also known as the Buie position, was first popularized in the United States by Dr. Louis A. Buie, a prominent colon and rectal surgeon at the Mayo Clinic, who was also one of the founding members of the American Board of Colon and Rectal Surgery. It has been used successfully since that time by generations of colon and rectal surgeons for anorectal surgery. The correct prone jack-knife position requires that the patient be prone with the crests of the ilia just below the break in the operating table (Figure 4.1). Although many surgeons break (or flex) the table, it is not necessary for the majority of anorectal procedures. Pads should be placed under the insteps of the feet, the knees, and the pelvis as well as the head and chest. A patient's ability to sense and express discomfort is diminished or abolished during conscious sedation and general anesthesia. Monitoring the patient and avoiding pressure to vulnerable body parts, such as the genitalia, breasts, peripheral nerves, and face, is essential.

Patient Factors

Patient factors are those that are associated with the unique emotional needs and physical limitations of individuals as they face anorectal surgery. The fears and concerns of a patient related to his or her

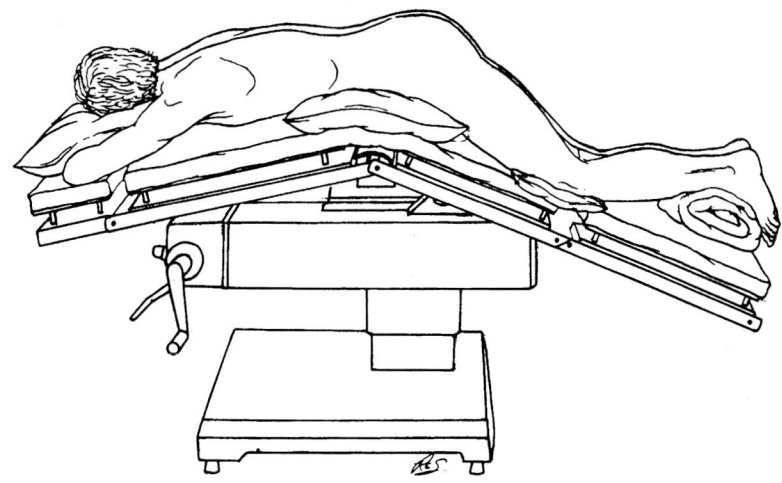

FIGURE 4.1. The prone jack-knife position.

position during surgery deserve mention. Embarrassment is a common reaction to the prone jack-knife position, especially in an office setting. Although proper draping allows most patients to overcome these feelings, for other patients the vulnerability and lack of modesty resulting from the prone jack-knife position is an important deterrent to its use. Dealing compassionately with patients and naming their fears, whether it is simple modesty or memories of an assault, will usually allow them to overcome their objections to this position for anorectal surgery. Comfort is also a prime concern of patients. Prolonged time in the prone jack-knife position, although uncomfortable in an office setting, is well tolerated in the operating theater when the patient is properly positioned.

Individual physical limitations of patients occasionally prevent the use of the prone jack-knife position. Physical factors that would prevent a patient from lying prone on the operating table, such as obesity, pregnancy, and tense ascites, may require the use of a different position. Orthopedic considerations, such as hip and knee joint problems, long leg casts, and kyphosis may be contraindications to this position. In these relatively rare circumstances, consideration should be given to the lateral position as described by Sims (also called the lateral recumbent position) (Figure 4.2). Cardiac and pulmonary considerations are discussed elsewhere in this chapter.

Perhaps the single most important patient factor is one described by Nivatvongs.[1] The shape of the buttocks (or depth of the gluteal cleft) was found to be an important factor in determining the patient position and type of anesthesia for anorectal surgery. Although Nivatvongs preferred the prone jack-knife position for all three patient types, he believed this position to be essential for "type B" patients with high buttock mounds (Figure 4.3).

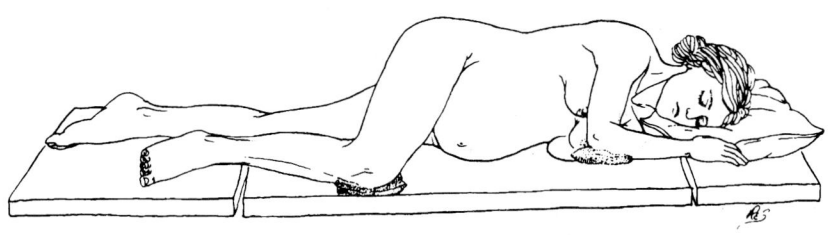

FIGURE 4.2. Sims' position (the lateral recumbent position).

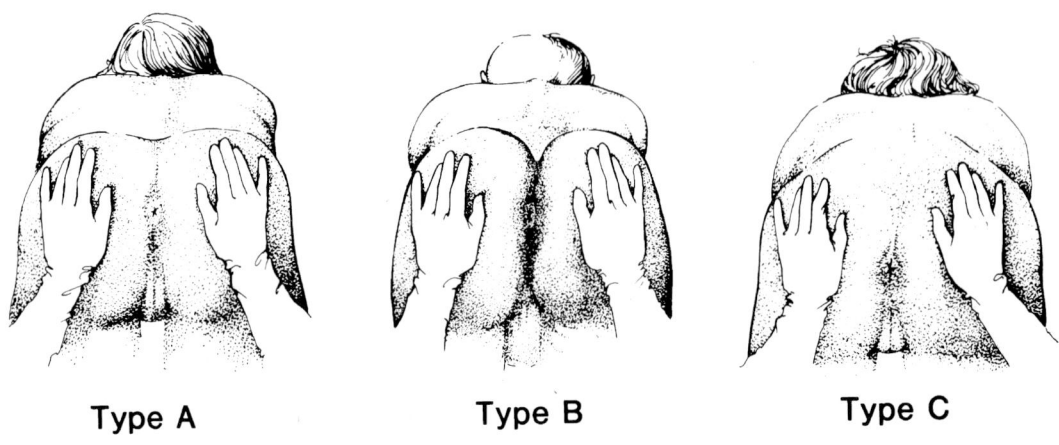

Type A   Type B   Type C

FIGURE 4.3. The different shapes of the buttocks. Reproduced with permission from Nivatvongs.[1]

Surgeon Factors

The primary reason that many surgeons prefer the prone jack-knife position is the excellent visibility provided during anorectal procedures. The exposure provided for office procedures, such as excision of thrombosed external hemorrhoids or drainage of abscesses is not equaled by other positions. In the operating room, whether the surgeon is dissecting the rectum off of the prostate or vagina in an abdominoperineal resection or preserving the internal sphincter during a mucosectomy for ulcerative colitis, visibility and lighting are key factors. Since the gluteal cleft is in a horizontal rather than a vertical orientation in the prone jack-knife position, illumination can be provided with overhead lights rather than headlamps. Similarly, more than one person can visualize the operating field without crowding or being in an awkward body position. New equipment for anorectal procedures, such as the Lone Star Retractor™ (Lone Star Medical Products, Houston, TX), can further improve the excellent exposure created by taping the buttocks apart without damaging the anal sphincter.

Many authors have made the observation that less blood loss occurs in procedures in the prone jack-knife than in other positions. Despite the frequency of this observation, blood loss has rarely been compared in series of similar cases with different operating positions. One author noted that measured blood loss during mucosectomy for ileoanal anastomosis in the lithotomy position was 2.5 times greater than when the procedure was performed in the prone jack-knife position.[2]

Perhaps the best testimonial to the prone jack-knife position is the wide variety of procedures that are performed in this position. Procedures that are the mainstay of colon and rectal surgery, such as hemorrhoidectomy, fistula procedures, pilonidal surgery, and transanal excision of tumors, are commonly performed in the Buie position. Many less common procedures are also performed in this position, including endorectal repair of rectocele[3] and rectourethral fistula, sphincteroplasty[4] and levatoroplasty, conventional and laparoscopic-assisted perineal rectosigmoidectomy,[5] and portions of abdominoperineal resection of the rectum and the ileal pouch–anal anastomosis.[6] One author noted that even thought the operative time was 2.4 hours shorter for a restorative proctocolectomy using a two-team approach in the lithotomy-Trendelenburg position, their institution preferred the prone jack-knife position because of the improved access to the anal canal and the ability to perform meticulous mucosectomy.[7]

Although it is not the focus of this book, it is noteworthy that there are many gynecologic procedures that may be suitable for the prone jack-knife position. Specifically, cystocele repairs and procedures to treat rectocele or vaginal prolapse could be done comfortably in this position but are traditionally done in the lithotomy position.

Anesthesia Factors

One of the most common concerns about the prone jack-knife position is the safety of the airway during anesthesia. Patients are occasionally placed in lithotomy position rather than the preferred prone jack-knife position because of the concern for the airway.[8] While patient safety is a prime concern, there are no reports of the loss of control of airway during repositioning. Although this lack of evidence does not exclude individual episodes, it does indicate that the heightened awareness has probably minimized the risk to the patient to an acceptable level.

Perhaps because of the concern for the patient's airway, there have been a number of reports of alternatives to general anesthesia for anorectal surgery. The usual options include pure local anesthesia, local anesthesia with conscious sedation, epidural anesthesia, and various forms of spinal anesthesia. One type of spinal anesthesia that seems to be ideal for many limited anorectal procedures is hypobaric spinal anesthesia with bupivacaine[9] or lidocaine.[10] Reports indicate that with hypobaric spinal anesthesia there is a dense block of the sensory nerves with minimal changes in heart rate and blood pressure.

Physiologic Factors

Careful positioning of patients when they are under anesthesia is crucial. Most surgeons focus on avoiding damage to peripheral nerves from prolonged pressure when positioning patients. However, an even more significant risk to overall patient well-being can result from the unintended consequences of anesthesia that may affect patient physiology. They include compression of arteries, impairment of venous return, limitation of ventilation, and blood pooling. Many authors have examined the prone jack-knife position to assess the potential physiological impact.

There are mixed reports about the cardiac effects of the prone jack-knife position. If the patient is improperly positioned, transmitted pressure on the vena cava may cause blood pooling in the lower extremities and result in decreased venous return.[11] In one study, when patients were turned from the supine to the prone position there was a temporary decrease in cardiac index; however, when the patients were placed in the prone jack-knife position the cardiac index returned to the level seen in the supine position. There was no change in heart rate, mean arterial pressure, and systemic vascular resistance with change from the supine position to the prone jack-knife position, but there was a decrease in the left ventricular stroke work index and a significant increase in the pulmonary capillary wedge pressure.[2] Overall, the effects of the prone jack-knife position were comparable to other surgical positions and were believed to be manageable by experienced anesthesiologists.

The effect of posture on pulmonary physiology in general and the specific effect of the prone jack-knife position on vital capacity has been examined. When patients in the sitting position are considered to be at baseline, there is a 9% decrease in vital capacity in the supine position, a 12.5% decrease in the jack-knife position, and an 18% decrease in the lithotomy position. The reduction in vital capacity is due to obstruction of the movement of the diaphragm and to a lesser extent to the restriction of the anteroposterior movement of the ribs.[11] This modest decrease is tolerated by most patients but merits careful monitoring during conscious sedation and general anesthesia.

Possible Complications

Avoidance of complications is one of the goals of every procedure. There are many positions that appear to be similar to the prone jack-knife position. Each of the alternative positions comes with its unique set of advantages and disadvantages.

The prone position is reported to be associated with a number of complications. Visceral hypoperfusion and rhabdomyolysis have been reported in prolonged procedures.[12] Macroglossia has been reported, especially when the prone position is combined with the Trendelenburg position.[13] Optic neuoropathy[14] and retinal artery occlusion have been reported when there is improper positioning and pressure on the globe.

The knee-chest position is an exaggerated version of the prone jack-knife position in which there is greater flexing of the hips and more weight in the knees during surgery (Figure 4.4). This position has the same risks as the prone jack-knife position in addition to an increased risk of impaired lower-extremity blood flow.[15] This position, although listed as an option by many authors, is in practice of

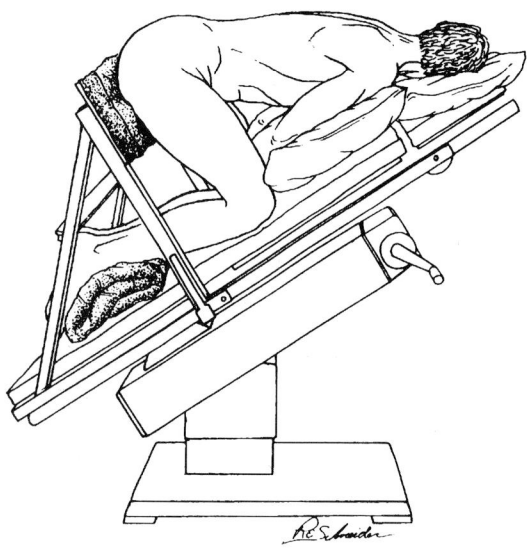

FIGURE 4.4. The knee-chest position.

historic interest only and is not used by modern colon and rectal surgeons.

Summary

The prone jack-knife position is the gold standard for anorectal surgical procedures. It provides the best exposure to the surgeon for the majority of patients. An assistant can both see and comfortably reach the surgical field during complex anorectal procedures. Blood loss may be reduced. Anesthetic options are not limited in this position, and the hypobaric spinal anesthesia is especially effective. The physiological impact is manageable and the risk of complications is low when the patient is properly positioned. Given the weight of all these factors, the reasonable surgeon realizes that the prone jack-knife position is the only way to go for anorectal surgical procedures.

References

1. Nivatvongs S, Fang DT, Kennedy HL. The shape of the buttocks: a useful guide for selection of anesthesia and patient position in anorectal surgery. Dis Colon Rectum 1983;26:85–86.

2. Hatada T, Kusunoki M, Sakiyama T, et al. Hemodynamics in the prone jackknife position during surgery. Am J Surg 1991;162:55–58.

3. Khubchandani IT, Clancy JP, Rosen Let al. Endorectal repair of rectocele revisited. Br J Surg 1997;84:89–91.

4. Block IR, Rodriguez S, Olivares AL. The Warren operation for anal incontinence caused by disruption of the anterior segment of the anal sphincter, perineal body and rectovaginal septum: report of five cases. Dis Colon Rectum 1975;18: 28–34.

5. Reissman P, Weiss E, Teoh T, et al. Laparoscopic-assisted perineal rectosigmoidectomy for rectal prolapse. Surgical Laparoscopy & Endoscopy 1995;5:217–218.

6. Pang AS, Chung MR, Lee KK, Schraut WH. An analysis of 50 cases of restorative proctocolectomy. Ann Acad Med Singapore 1994;23:76–82.

7. Horai T, Kusunoki M, Shoji Y, et al. Clinicopathological study of anorectal mucosa in total colectomy with mucosal proctectomy and ileal anastomosis. Eur J Surg 1994;160:233–8.

8. Smith LE. Ambulatory surgery for anorectal diseases: an update. South Med J 1986;79:163–136.

9. Maroof M, Khan RM, Siddique M, Tariq M. Hypobaric spinal anesthesia with bupivacaine (0.1%) gives selective sensory block for ano-rectal surgery. Can J Anaesth 1995;42:691–694.

10. Bodily MN, Carpenter RL, Owens BD. Lidocaine 0.5% spinal anaesthesia: a hypobaric solution of short-stay perirectal surgery. Can J Anaesth 1992;39:770–773.

11. Courington FW, Little DM. The role of posture on anesthesia. Clinical Anesthesia 1968;3:24–54.

12. Ziser A, Friedhoff RJ, Rose SH. Prone position: visceral hypoperfusion and rhabdomyolysis. Anesth Analg 1996;82:412–415.

13. Pivalizza EG, Katz J, Singh S, et al. Massive macroglossia after posterior fossa surgery in the prone position. J Neurosurg Anesthesiol 1998;10: 34–36.

14. Dilger JA, Tezlaff JE, Bell GR, et al. Ischaemic optic neuropathy after spinal fusion. Can J Anaesth 1998;45:63–66.

15. Laakso E, Ahovuo J, Rosenberg PH. Blood flow in the lower limbs in the knee-chest position: ultrasonographic study in unanaesthetised volunteers. Anaesthesia 1996;51:1113–1116.

Part B: The Dorsal Lithotomy Position: Preferred by Surgeon and Anesthesiologist

H. Randolph Bailey, M.D., F.A.C.S.

Proper positioning of the patient for anorectal surgical procedures is essential to the success of the operation. Three positions are commonly used. The lithotomy position has been widely used in countries influenced by the British tradition.[1] The prone jack-knife position has been popular in the United States, largely because of the influence of Fansler and his followers.[2,3] The left lateral position, described by Sims, has been largely used at the Ferguson Clinic and by its trainees.[4] A fourth position, the left anterolateral, has been described by Nivatvongs, to avoid the pain over the pubis and the backache that may accompany the jack-knife position.[5] We will not discuss this position.

A surgeon's choice of position is largely influenced by his or her experiences during the years of surgical training. I may be unique in that my training encompassed procedures on patients in all three of the positions. My medical school and early surgical training was in Dallas, Texas, where the prone position was the standard. My general surgical years were spent in Houston, Texas, where most surgeons used the lithotomy position. Finally, my fellowship in colon and rectal surgery was in Grand Rapids, Michigan, at the Ferguson Clinic, where I was exposed to the lateral position. My ultimate decision to use the lithotomy position for the majority of anorectal surgical procedures was the result of my experience with all three options and careful weighing of the advantages and disadvantages of each.

Anesthetic Considerations

From the standpoint of the safety and ease of administration of the anesthetic for the surgical procedure, the lithotomy position is clearly the winner.

Access to the airway as well as overall simplicity of the administration of the anesthetic are clearly greater with a patient lying on his back rather than on his face or side. In the lithotomy position, the patient's airway can be managed with a mask, endotracheal intubation, or laryngeal mask airway. If the endotracheal tube is omitted, the patient does not need to be paralyzed and may awaken more quickly at the end of the procedure. Managing the airway in the lateral position requires skill and experience that few anesthesiologists possess. The anesthesia department at the Ferguson Hospital was particularly skilled in this technique and experienced few complications. Other institutions, however, do not have such expertise, and most anesthesiologists are uncomfortable managing the airway in the lateral position. It is clearly not possible to deal with the airway of the anesthetized patient in the prone position without an endotracheal tube. Putting the patient to sleep on the stretcher, intubating the patient, and then turning the patient onto the operating table in the prone position require more time, personnel, and risk than do the other positions. Although the prone position does work well for the majority of patients managed by conscious sedation and local anesthesia, if the patient responds excessively to the sedation and hypoventilates, regaining control of the airway suddenly becomes an emergency.

Of course, another anesthetic option for perineal surgery is regional block with spinal, caudal, or epidural technique. The use of hypobaric spinal anesthesia has been reported for patients in the prone position, but we have no experience with the technique.[6,7] In our institution, the time required for administration of regional anesthesia is greater than that for general anesthesia or conscious sedation.

These techniques also carry some risk of postoperative headache and require longer periods of observation in the postanesthesia care unit as the block wears off. Finally, because of the sympathectomy that frequently accompanies regional block, most anesthesiologists are reluctant to limit intravenous fluids in patients who have regional anesthesia. Clearly, the rate of postoperative urinary retention is related to the amount of intravenous fluids the patient receives, and patients receiving regional anesthesia do have a higher incidence of urinary retention.

Technique of Lithotomy Position

Before discussing the other advantages of the lithotomy position, I will describe in detail how the patient may be optimally positioned. I continue to be surprised to hear the criticisms of the lithotomy position such as difficulty of exposure and inability of the assistants to view the procedure. I recently saw a video of a British surgeon performing an anorectal procedure in the lithotomy position. The legs of the patient were over the surgeon's shoulders, and the assistants were reaching over the legs to provide retraction. I would agree that the above-mentioned criticisms are applicable to the position used in the video. Although the position described above has been used successfully by gynecologists for decades, most of their work is done deep inside the vagina and not on the surface of the anal canal. Thus, their angle of view needs to be substantially different from that of the anorectal surgeon.

Instead of using the Lloyd-Davies stirrups (or the Allen stirrups) as used by the British and by gynecologists, we use the candy-cane stirrups. These stirrups avoid pressure on the patient's calf and allow the hips to rotate externally (Figure 4.5). The patient's buttocks are pulled down well below the edge of the table so that they protrude a few inches. The stirrups are positioned so the patient's heels are parallel to the end of the table. The stirrups are raised high enough to allow about 90° of flexion of the knees. (Figure 4.5) It is obviously necessary to prevent pressure between the patient's legs and the stirrups but it is generally not necessary to pad the stirrups. In the lithotomy position it is also unnecessary to go through the checklist of the myriad pressure points that must be padded and checked

each time a patient is turned prone. The stirrups are rotated outward and raised to avoid pressure points. In male patients, the scrotum is suspended out of the operative field by the use of a wet surgical towel.

The angle of the anus and distal rectum to the perineum is quite different than that of the vagina. Gynecologists usually sit high on a stool to get the proper perspective. For anorectal procedures, we suggest that the surgeon sit on a low stool, approximately 18 inches above the floor, with an instrument tray on his or her lap. Some degree of Trendelenburg position is needed for proper visualization of the anal canal. The angle can be steepened to view the anterior anus and decreased to view the posterior anus or rectum. The head-down position also pulls the legs away from the stirrups and helps avoid pressure injury. The angle of the anus also causes blood to pool in the rectum rather than on the surgeon's tray. External bleeding can be handled nicely with a straight-tipped suction device. The head-down position may increase the risk of aspiration in patients with reflux, but some risk of aspiration also exists in the prone position as it is usually practiced.

Lighting is achieved by bringing the overhead lights down and shining them over the surgeon's shoulders. Our preference is also to use a headlight, but we use the headlight for practically all of our operations, regardless of position.

Advantages for the Surgeon

The exaggerated lithotomy position actually makes more room around the entire circumference of the anus than either of the other positions for the handle of the retractors. There is ample room between the legs for the surgeon and one or two assistants, all with a direct view of the operative field. The sitting position is also, in my opinion, less fatiguing and easier on the surgeon's back. It is not necessary to lean over the field to get the midline view, as is required with the patient in the prone position. Although it is usually necessary to tape the buttocks apart to facilitate exposure in the prone position, this maneuver is rarely required in the lithotomy position. As the thighs are pulled upward and outward, the buttocks separate quite readily. Avoiding the use of tape on the buttocks may also obviate the

FIGURE 4.5. The exaggerated lithotomy position with the surgeon seated comfortably on a low stool. The inset shows the perineal view obtained in this position without taping the buttocks.

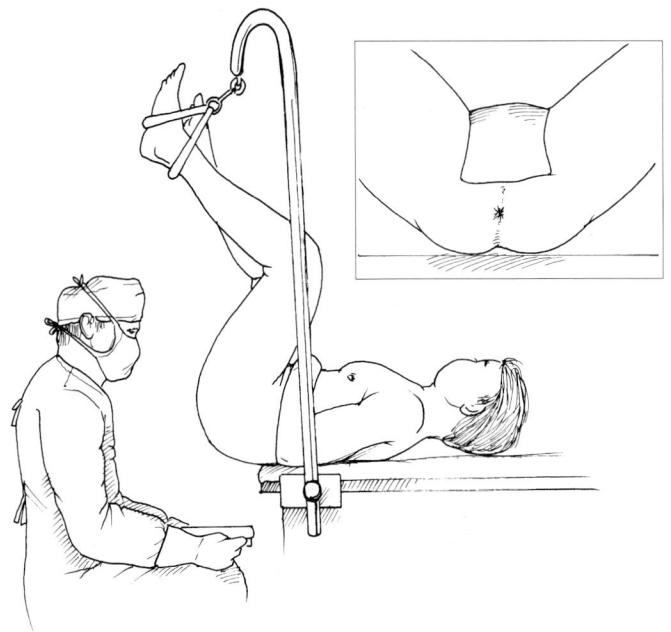

need for shaving the buttocks, a potential source of itching and irritation for several weeks after anorectal surgery.

Personnel and Cost Advantages

From a personnel standpoint, the lithotomy position is also advantageous. The lateral position requires a person to retract the buttock and another to assist with the instruments. The prone position also requires retraction and assistance with the instruments. With the patient in the lithotomy position and the surgeon sitting, a lap tray allows access to the instruments while the scrub person can function as an assistant.

Unless the patient operated on in the prone position is managed by conscious sedation and local anesthesia instead of general anesthesia, the time required to position the patient before starting the procedure as well as turning the patient back onto the stretcher following the procedure adds to the operating room costs and the total cost of medical care. If the anesthesiologist feels that chest rolls are necessary for proper ventilation of the prone, anesthetized patient (as do our anesthesia staff), positioning becomes even more cumbersome and time consuming.

With operating-room time costs in the range of $20 per minute, shorter anesthetic induction and turnover times will save both hospital cost and the surgeon's time. This saved time may allow the surgeon to perform more procedures per day, get to the clinic earlier, or experience free time with his or her family.

Patient Considerations

While it is obvious that the patient's legs should not be forced into position in the stirrups, it is rare to find a patient whose legs and hips do not allow proper positioning. The risk of injury in the lithotomy position, if one uses common sense and care, is quite low. In the past 25 years, the author has performed more than 5000 operations in the lithotomy position without a single neurologic or orthopedic injury of which we are aware.

Patients who have had lower-extremity amputations require special consideration. Certainly, in these patients the prone position can be used, but the lithotomy position is also a possibility. A below-knee stump can usually be held by the stirrup without difficulty. The patient can also wear his prosthesis to the operating room, where the foot of the prosthesis is placed in the stirrup. Above-knee stumps can be managed by suspending the thigh from the stirrup with strips of tape.

With regard to the shape of the perineum and its suitability for various operative positions, Nivatvongs et al. have described three types of buttocks[8] (Figure 4.3). Of the three types of buttock shapes described, Nivatvongs believes that two ("type A" and "type C") are suitable for lithotomy position, whereas the third is not. In our experience, patients with what Nivatvongs describes as "type B" buttocks can be better visualized in the lithotomy position than in prone positions.

The prone position has been particularly touted for operations involving the anterior anus or distal rectum, such as rectovaginal fistula or sphincter repairs. I prefer the lithotomy position for the performance of these procedures as well. It is my feeling that access to the vaginal portion of the fistula is much easier in the lithotomy position than in the prone position, as is mobilization of the anterior rectum from the sphincters. For anterior endorectal advancement flaps, deepening the Trendelenburg position allows good visualization of the anterior anal and rectal mucosa. We would, however, concede that the prone position is preferable for operations involving the sacrococcygeal areas, such as pilonidal disease or retrorectal tumors.

Potential Disadvantages

For procedures performed with conscious sedation and local anesthesia, the patient may experience more leg discomfort in the lithotomy position than in the prone position. This discomfort is noted primarily in procedures that take more than 30 minutes to complete, such as hemorrhoidectomy. Since the number of operative hemorrhoidectomies performed in our practice is quite low, leg discomfort is only a minor disadvantage.

In each position there is an area of the anal canal that is more awkward than others to approach surgically. In the lithotomy position, the right anterior hemorrhoidal column is more difficult to suture than are the other columns. I am somewhat ambidextrous and solve the problem by suturing this wound with my left hand. Other solutions include standing and suturing with the right hand or taking each stitch in two bites.

In our clinic we do use the modified jack-knife position on the tilt table for office examinations and treatments. This change of orientation can result in possible confusion with regard to location of lesions when the patient is later examined in the lithotomy position.

Complications of the Lithotomy Position

The literature contains a significant number of reports of complications following operations in the lithotomy position. These include compartment syndrome,[9–15] peroneal nerve palsy,[16,17] femoral nerve palsy,[18,19] sciatic nerve injury,[20,21] and rhabdomyolysis.[22–24] Of these, compartment syndrome is by far the most commonly reported. This complication seems to be associated with prolonged operations with the legs in the Lloyd-Davies stirrups with some pressure on the calf muscle. There is reduction in both mean arterial pressure and oxygen saturation in the calf muscle with the legs elevated in the Lloyd-Davies stirrups.[25] The mechanism of injury is probably ischemia[26] followed by reperfusion and subsequent edema. We hasten to add that the compartment syndrome has not been reported after anorectal operations of short duration in the lithotomy position.

Peroneal nerve injury can be a result of mild and unrecognized compartment syndrome or direct pressure on the nerve as it passes around the head of the fibula. Awareness of the need to avoid pressure in this area will essentially eliminate the problem. Femoral nerve injury seems to be associated with forceful abduction of the thighs, a problem that does not occur with the candy-cane stirrups. With the candy-cane stirrups, the hips externally rotate to prevent forceful abduction.

Sciatic nerve injury has also been reported after operations in the lithotomy position. At least one report has shown the incidence of sciatic stretch to be no higher after use of the lithotomy position than after the use of other operating positions.[27] The lithotomy position is similar to some of the back-stretching exercises recommended for those with lumbosacral strain. Needless to say, we have not seen either compartment syndrome or rhabdomyolysis.

Conclusions

Although more surgeons in the United States use the prone position than the lithotomy position in performing anorectal operations, I feel that this difference might disappear if proper use of the lithotomy position were taught to surgical trainees. The anesthetic advantages are clearly in favor of the lithotomy position, as are the economic benefits as described. A surgeon who uses the lithotomy position will finish his or her operating schedule earlier, experience less fatigue, and place his or her patients at less risk of anesthetic complications. Try it; you will like it!

References

1. Milligan ET, Morgan CN, Jones LE, Officer R. Surgical anatomy of the anal canal, and the operative treatment of haemorrhoids. Lancet 1937;2:1119–1124.
2. Atkinson KG, Baird RM. Modified Buie amputation for extensive hemorrhoidal disease. Am J Surg 1978;135:862–864.
3. Fansler WA, Anderson JK. A plastic operation for certain types of hemorrhoids. JAMA 1933;101:1064–1066.
4. Ferguson JA, Mazier WP, Ganchrow MI, Friend WG. The closed technique of hemorrhoidectomy. Surgery 1971;70:480–484.
5. Nivatvongs S. Alternative positioning of patients for homorrhoidectomy. Dis Colon Rectum 1980;23:308–309.
6. Maroof M, Khan RM, Siddique M, Tariq M. Hypobaric spinal anesthesia with bupivacaine (0.1%) gives selective sensory block for ano-rectal surgery. Can J Anaesth 1995;42:691–694.
7. Bodily MN, Carpenter RL, Owens BD. Lidocaine 0.5% spinal anaesthesia: a hypobaric solution of short-stay perirectal surgery. Can J Anaesth 1992;39:770–773.
8. Nivatvongs S, Fang DT, Kennedy HL. The shape of the buttocks. A useful guide for selection of anesthesia and patient position in anorectal surgery. Dis Colon Rectum 1983;26:85–86.
9. Scott JR, Daneker G, Lumsden AB. Prevention of compartment syndrome associated with dorsal lithotomy position. Am Surg 1997;63:801–806.
10. Tuckey J. Bilateral compartment syndrome complicating prolonged lithotomy position [see comments]. Br J Anaesth 1996;77:546–549.
11. Goldsmith AL, McCallum MI. Compartment syndrome as a complication of the prolonged use of the Lloyd-Davies position. [Review] [26 refs]. Anaesthesia 1996;51:1048–1052.
12. Reddy PK, Kaye KW. Deep posterior compartmental syndrome: a serious complication of the lithotomy position. J Urol 1984;132:144–145.
13. Moses TA, Kreder KJ, Thrasher JB. Compartment syndrome: an unusual complication of the lithotomy position. [Review] [8 refs]. Urology 1994;43:746–747.
14. Neagle CE, Schaffer JL, Heppenstall RB. Compartment syndrome complicating prolonged use of the lithotomy position. [Review] [18 refs]. Surgery 1991;110:566–569.
15. Khalil IM. Bilateral compartmental syndrome after prolonged surgery in the lithotomy position. J Vasc Surg 1987;5:879–881.
16. Leff RG, Shapiro SR. Lower extremity complications of the lithotomy position: prevention and management. J Urol 1979;122:138–139.
17. Herrera-Ornelas L, Tolls RM, Petrelli NJ, et al. Common peroneal nerve palsy associated with pelvic surgery for cancer. An analysis of 11 cases. Dis Colon Rectum 1986;29:392–397.
18. Tondare AS, Nadkarni AV, Sathe CH, Dave VB. Femoral neuropathy: a complication of lithotomy position under spinal anaesthesia. Report of three cases. Canadian Anaesthetists Society Journal 1983;30:84–86.
19. Roblee MA. Femoral neuropathy from the lithotomy position: case report and new leg holder for prevention. Am J Obstet Gynecol 1967;97:871–872.
20. Batres F, Barclay DL. Sciatic nerve injury during gynecologic procedures using the lithotomy position. Obstet Gynecol 1983;62:92s–94s.
21. Flanagan WF, Webster GD, Brown MW, Massey EW. Lumbosacral plexus stretch injury following the use of the modified lithotomy position. J Urol 1985;134:567–568.
22. Biswas S, Gnanasekaran I, Ivatury RR, et al. Exaggerated lithotomy position-related rhabdomyolysis. [Review] [23 refs]. Am Surg 1997;63:361–364.
23. Bildsten SA, Dmochowski RR, Spindel MR, Auman JR. The risk of rhabdomyolysis and acute renal failure with the patient in the exaggerated lithotomy position. J Urol 1994;152:1970–1972.
24. Muret J, Farhat F, Jayr C. [Rhabdomyolysis after prolonged surgical procedure in the lithotomy posture]. [French]. Ann Fr Anesth Reanim 1994;13:262–265.
25. Svendsen LB, Flink P, Wojdemann M, et al. Muscle oxygen saturation during surgery in the lithotomy position. Clin Physiol 1997;17:433–438.
26. Canterbury TD, Wheeler WE, Scott-Conner CE. Effects of the lithotomy position on arterial blood flow in the lower extremities. W V Med J 1992;88:100–101.
27. Clarke AM, Stillwell S, Paterson ME, Getty CJ. Role of the surgical position in the development of postoperative low back pain. J Spinal Disord 1993;6:238–241.

Part C: The Left Lateral Decubitus (Sims') Position: The Middle Position

Martin A. Luchtefeld, M.D., F.A.C.S.

The left lateral decubitus position has been the position of choice for most anorectal procedures at the Ferguson Clinic since at least 1971.[1] Sims' position, a modification of the lateral position, dates back to 1857 when a prominent New York City gynecologist, J. Marion Sims, began to use the position for operations on the perineum, rectum, vagina, and bladder.[2]

Positioning the Patient

For the left lateral decubitus position the patient is completely lateral with the left side down (Figure 4.6). The buttocks are brought to the edge or even a bit slightly over the edge of the table to allow for optimum visualization. Both arms are extended and the hips and knees are both flexed with the patient being in essentially a knee-chest position. The back is flexed slightly. The patient needs to be positioned relatively near the foot end of the operating table or else the final position of the buttocks will be too far away from the foot of the bed for the assistant at that position to provide any help with exposure, suction, or passing of instruments. If the lower portions of the legs are allowed to lie parallel with the opposite side of the table, this will allow for a relatively large flat surface to place instruments. A safety strap is always needed to ensure that the patient does not roll off the table. In addi-

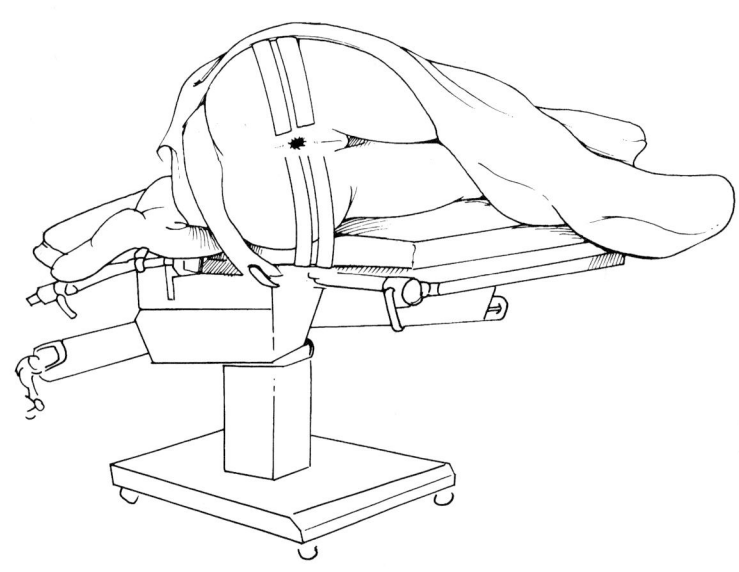

FIGURE 4.6. The lateral position for anorectal surgery as utilized at the Ferguson Clinic. Redrawn from Mazier WP.[3]

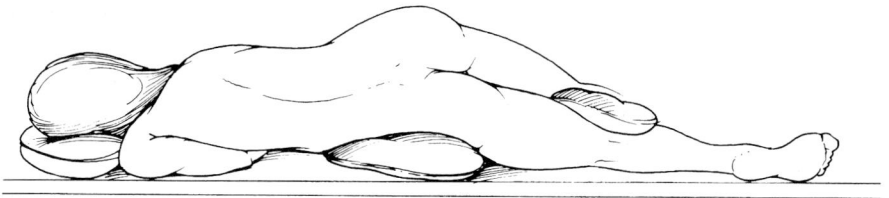

FIGURE 4.7. Sims' position as described by J. Marion Sims in 1857.[2]

tion, the upper buttock can be pulled up with tape to keep it from falling into the field of vision. An additional piece of tape over the lower portion of the legs is also sometimes used to help maintain proper positioning to optimize visualization of the operative field. The table needs to be positioned with the head down and rotated slightly away from the surgeon. Once the head is brought down, the foot of the table should also be cranked down so that there is a slight break in the table at the level of the buttocks. This will keep the surface for the instruments in a level plane. If it is anticipated that the anesthesia will last for very long, an axillary roll should be placed as well to minimize the stretch on the suprascapular nerve and compression of the neurovascular bundle on the left side.

Sims' position (Figure 4.7) is a slight variation on this alignment. With this position, the patient is in more of a left anterolateral position. The left leg and thigh are maintained in an extended position with the right thigh and leg flexed on a pillow.

Physiology

There are some slight changes in the respiratory physiology of a patient in the left lateral decubitus position compared with the supine position. When the patient is in the left lateral decubitus position, the dependent lung has a moderate decrease in functional residual capacity and, as a result, is predisposed to atelectasis. The nondependent lung may actually have an increased functional residual capacity.[4]

Hydrostatic gradients can occur between the two hemothoraces in the low-pressure pulmonary circuit. Most of the downside lung lies below the level of the atrium whereas most of the upside lung lies above it, leading to relative vascular congestion of the downside lung and relative hypoperfusion of the upside lung. The result of the relative compres-

sion of the dependent side and decompression of the nondependent side can lead to excessive ventilation of the underperfused upside lung and hypoventilation of the congested downside lung. In a patient with significant pulmonary disease, this can lead to the potential for clinically significant ventilation-perfusion mismatch.[5]

If the legs were maintained at the same level of the body, there would be essentially no pressure gradient along the great vessels from head to foot. If, however, the legs are allowed to flex and remain below the level of the heart, there can be a tendency for blood to pool in the lower extremities. Thus, it is important to keep the patient in a slight Trendelenburg position to allow for adequate venous return. In addition, the cervical spine of the patient should be carefully maintained in alignment with the thoracolumbar spine so that there will be no pressure gradient between the head and the mediastinum. Improper support of the head with significant angulation in the lower neck can bring about obstruction of flow in the jugular vein.[5]

Advantages and Disadvantages

The left lateral decubitus position offers a number of advantages but it is not the optimum position for all circumstances. All patients seen in the Ferguson Clinic are examined in the left lateral decubitus position. This is an excellent position not only for an anorectal examination but for sigmoidoscopy as well. When operating on these same patients, the alignment of any identified pathologic lesion is exactly the same as was seen in the office. When the surgery is for hemorrhoids this position offers excellent visualization of the right anterior and left lateral quadrants; however, the right posterior quadrant can be relatively difficult to see. For any kind of operation in the anterior midline, such as a post-obstetrical sphincter repair, the visualization is excellent. However, for relatively complex procedures that need to be done in the posterior midline, such as an advancement flap for a high fistula or local excision for rectal cancer, the left lateral decubitus position can be quite awkward because of a poor field of vision in the direct posterior midline.

If the patient is properly positioned toward the foot of the operating table, the assistant at the foot of the bed should have an excellent view of the operative field as well as ready access to assist with the operation. One disadvantage of Sims' position is that for the surgeon to have optimal visualization and exposure, a second assistant is needed on the side of the patient opposite the surgeon to pull up the upper buttock. This can be obviated to a certain degree by taping the buttock up or, alternatively, by using towel clips to hold the Hill-Ferguson retractors in place, as described by Chen et al.[6] The second assistant, who retracts the upper buttock, has a very limited view of the operative field.

Airway management in the left lateral decubitus position is straightforward. Because the airway is relatively accessible, the anesthesiologists are comfortable with giving heavy intravenous sedation while the local block is being applied. General anesthesia by mask or endotracheal tube is also possible. Intubation can also be performed in the left lateral decubitus position without difficulty. The blades of the laryngoscope are designed to push the tongue and soft tissues to the left of the pharynx with the laryngoscope blade and light source on the right side away from the soft tissue. In the left lateral decubitus position, gravity naturally takes the soft tissue to the left side and facilitates placement of the laryngoscope. This makes intubation relatively straightforward if the sedation becomes so deep as to require assisted ventilation.

Conclusions

The lateral position (Sims' position) provides excellent exposure for the majority of anorectal operations. Once the technique is learned by the operating room staff, the positioning of the patient can be accomplished rapidly. The physiologic stresses on the patient in the lateral position may be less than with any of the other commonly used positions for this type of surgery. Although anesthesia personnel often approach the lateral position with trepidation, with brief experience they become confident that they can adequately ventilate the patient and maintain control of the airway.

References

1. Ferguson JA, Mazier WP, Ganchrow MI, Friend WG. The closed technique of hemorrhoidectomy. Surgery 1971;70:480–484.
2. Sims JM. Silver Suture in Surgery: The Anniversary Discourse Before the New York Academy of Medicine, November 18, 1857, New York, Samuel Ellis and William Wood, 1858.
3. Mazier WP. Hemorrhoids. In Mazier WP, Levien DH, Luchtefeld MA, Senagore AJ (eds). Surgery of the Colon, Rectum, and Anus. Philadelphia: WB Saunders, 1995, p 234.
4. Benumof JL. Respiratory physiology and respiratory function during anesthesia. In Miller RD (ed). Anesthesia, 3rd edition. New York: Churchill Livingstone, 1990, pp 505–549
5. Martin JT, Warner, MA. Patient positioning. In Barash PG, Cullen BF, Stoelting RK (eds). Clinical Anesthesia, 3rd edition. Philadelphia: Lippincott-Raven, 1997, pp 606–610.
6. Chen HH, Chen JS, Changchien CR, et al. Hemorrhoidectomy with self-retaining retraction. Dis Colon Rectum 1996;39:1058–1059.

5

Postoperative Management

M. Parker Roberts, M.D., F.A.C.S.

A patient scheduled for an anorectal surgical operation may be facing the experience of surgery for the first time in his or her life. The surgeon, on the other hand, deals with such situations on a daily basis and is quite familiar with what the patient may experience after surgery. Thus, it is important that the surgeon share this practical knowledge with patients when preparing them for the surgical experience and allaying fears, many of which may be based on misinformation. Unlike other aspects of medicine, there are few mass media resources that publicize anorectal diseases or serve as references. During the initial preoperative visit there is rarely sufficient time to allow explanation of every detail of the postoperative course. In addition, the patient is unlikely to retain all of the significant information that is provided. As a result, it is critical that the verbal information be reinforced with clearly written instructions or even a videotaped presentation. It is important to periodically review these instructions for completeness and keep them updated.

The postoperative instructions for ambulatory anorectal surgery should contain information regarding what the patient may expect in the immediate postoperative period and how to deal with possible complications. Topics addressed should include management of pain, wound care, means of providing a soft stool and regular bowel evacuation, level of physical activity, and diet. Potential complications of anorectal surgery—such as bleeding, urinary retention, pain unrelieved by the prescribed medication, fever, and constipation—should be discussed. A concise explanation of each complication in lay terms, along with an appropriate algorithm, is helpful. The underlying principle

guiding these postoperative instructions is to anticipate and answer many of the common questions and problems that may arise. What follows are some specific concepts that can be incorporated into a set of postoperative instructions.

The Immediate Postoperative Period

Dressings

Many surgeons use dressings or even packing in the anal canal after operations such as hemorrhoidectomy and fistulotomy. Routine use of packing is not recommended, as it is seldom necessary for hemostasis and may precipitate urinary retention. Packing is ideally employed only in a large open wound after incision and drainage of a perirectal abscess or pilonidal cyst and should be removed within 24 hours. Almost every anorectal operation results in some bloody drainage. A small dressing, such as one or two 4×4 inch gauze sponges, placed or taped between the buttocks will absorb such discharge and avoid soiling of the patient's clothing. This dressing is used as long as there is any drainage from the wound. A female sanitary pad or panty liner may also work well as a perineal dressing. Understandably, many male patients are embarrassed and reluctant to wear such pads. If the patient requires wound packing, clear instructions should be provided detailing the method and time of removal of the packing, and describing the possible complications after removal; for example, pain and bleeding.

Urinary Retention

Some patients have difficulty urinating after an anorectal operation. Although this condition is transient, it may be aggravated by rapid bladder expansion during and after the operation. To avoid urinary retention, intraoperative fluids should be minimized, and patients are instructed to limit oral fluid intake until successful voiding occurs. Many patients are informed by friends or family to "drink lots of water so urine will come out." This misinformation should be specifically discouraged in the postoperative instructions. Sitting in a warm sitz bath will help relax the pelvic muscles and bladder outlet, thus allowing urination.[1] If still unable to void, the patient is instructed to call the surgeon. Arrangements can be made for insertion of a Foley catheter in the office or emergency room. The catheter is left in place for 24 to 48 hours to allow the bladder to regain tone and the patient's pain level to subside. The patient is either instructed on how to remove the catheter at home at the appropriate time or else is scheduled for an office visit for its removal. A recurrent voiding problem may respond to re-catheterization, but at this point a visit to a urologist is reasonable.

Pain Control and Readmission

An ice pack applied to the operative site may be an effective adjunct to pain medication during the first 12 to 24 hours after surgery. It is initially placed while the patient is in the recovery room and is continued at home. The type and strength of pain medications are tailored to the patient and the operation. Hemorrhoidectomy is the anorectal operation that typically generates the most postoperative pain. Postoperative pain, however, is often based on the patient's personal perception and is unique in every case. Most patients should have a potent pain medication, usually a narcotic, available for the first few postoperative days. Occasionally, standard oral analgesics are inadequate for control of pain. Increasing the dose of analgesic or adding an anxiolytic/muscle relaxant such as diazepam is usually effective. In addition, sitz baths, as described below, are helpful in controlling pain. Readmission for pain control is an option that may be discussed preoperatively with the patient. A plan for this eventuality should be in place before

the patient calls. It is important to know the readmission rate for each particular operation so the patient may be adequately prepared preoperatively.

Expected Postoperative Care

Sitz Baths

Sitting in either a bathtub or a small pan containing warm water placed on the toilet confers excellent pain relief for most patients. As discussed, it is also useful in relieving urinary retention.[1] Sitz baths are started as early as the evening of surgery and may be taken as often as the patient desires. Plain, comfortably warm water is suggested, without soaps, disinfectants, or salts. Mild lavage with a hand-held shower head, squirt bottle, or bidet can additionally help keep complex anal wounds clean.

First Bowel Movement

The amount of time before the first postoperative bowel movement is not important. If a bowel preparation is used or if the patient has been on bowel rest preoperatively, it may be several days before the first bowel evacuation occurs. The patient needs to be reminded and encouraged to have a bowel movement whenever the urge occurs. Delaying a bowel movement until later in the postoperative period is tempting, as patients believe there will be less pain. Unfortunately, such a delay can lead to the development of a fecal impaction. The surgeon should advise the patient that many anorectal operations cause tenesmus. Differentiating between the real urge for a bowel movement and the lower-intensity, but more constant, urge of tenesmus is important and can be learned.

The use of bulk-forming laxatives such as psyllium or methylcellulose is optimally begun in the preoperative or immediate postoperative period. Such agents produce a soft, bulky stool that is ideal for many patients. If the patient uses other laxatives fairly frequently, discontinuing them in the early postoperative period is not recommended. In the case of laxative-dependent patients, the agents are either stopped far in advance of surgery or after the anal wound is completely healed.

Diet

There is probably more variation among surgeons concerning dietary instructions than any other aspect of postoperative anorectal care. Patients may be advised to eat a regular diet as soon as the effects of anesthesia have dissipated. Alternatively, they may be restricted to a low-residue or no-residue diet for a week or two, as this will potentially delay the onset of bowel movements and secondary pain. Other physicians encourage "confining" the bowels by adding constipating medications like codeine. The important concept underlying nutritional management is not when food intake should start, but when bowel action should resume. Bowel movements in the immediate postoperative period do not cause deleterious effects on the results following most anorectal operations. An early bowel movement may be painful, but the first bowel movement is painful whenever it occurs. Many patients may desire to limit their oral intake in the postoperative period to diminish the possibility of having a bowel movement. Although delay of bowel function may not cause damage, patients should clearly understand not to ignore the urge to have a bowel movement whenever it occurs. (*Editor's note:* It is our preference to resume a regular diet promptly following anorectal operations. It is our feeling that stool passage through the anal canal is beneficial in preventing postoperative anal stenosis. It also seems best for patients to get the first bowel movement "behind them" to alleviate the fear and apprehension that often precede the first bowel movement.)

The consumption of caffeine either in coffee or other beverages should not be discontinued in the postoperative period. Besides the severe headaches and possible mood changes that often accompany caffeine withdrawal, many patients use caffeine as a gastrointestinal stimulant.

Exceptions to these dietary suggestions apply to patients who have undergone operations in which exposure of the anorectum to stool in the early postoperative period may be undesirable. These operations include transanal excision of low rectal tumors, perineal repair of rectal prolapse, anal sphincter repair, and anoplasty. In these situations it may be best to avoid early bulky bowel movements. A clear liquid diet for a week postoperatively and enema programs are helpful. Our suggested program is a daily tap water enema to allow a soft evacuation. The patient, a family member, or another caregiver is instructed how to administer the enema preoperatively. This routine is continued for up to a month postoperatively to allow the tissues to heal before exposing them to a "normal" bulky bowel movement.

Activity

Activity need not be severely restricted after anorectal surgery. The resumption of normal activity often accelerates healing and return of bowel function. The patient's own discomfort is usually an adequate limitation to most postoperative activities. Obviously, sexual activity should be limited after operations that involve reconstruction near the vagina, such as anal sphincter or rectovaginal fistula repair. In addition, sports activities likely to directly traumatize the perineum such as bicycle, horseback, or motorcycle riding should be avoided for several weeks after anorectal surgical procedures.

Employment Restrictions

The recommended period away form work varies widely depending on the patient, the nature of the job, and the extent of surgery. Most patients want a reasonable estimate of any employment restrictions and time off from work so they can make arrangements with their employer. The estimate is based on the experience of the individual surgeon. For nonstrenuous employment, the expected time off from work ranges from 1 day for colonoscopy, 2 to 3 days for fissure and minor fistula repairs, and from 1 to 3 weeks for hemorrhoidectomy, complex fistulae, sphincteroplasty, and perineal repairs of prolapse. The patient, however, is often the best judge of when to return to full employment.

Postoperative Complications

Bleeding

A small amount of bleeding can occur after any anorectal operation, and it is very important to mention this during the preoperative counseling.

The patient is instructed not to take aspirin or aspirin-containing preparations for 2 weeks after most operations (including colonoscopic polypectomy). Although 6 days was the average time period reported in one study,[2] delayed hemorrhage can occur up to 3 weeks after anorectal surgery. It is often difficult to determine the amount and severity of bleeding based on the patient's observations as reported over the telephone. Arrangements should be made to see the patient immediately if the bleeding is profuse or ongoing or if the patient is significantly concerned. The bleeding patient is optimally evaluated in the office or the emergency room. Vital signs and a baseline hemoglobin level are obtained. Any symptoms of volume depletion or vasovagal syncope are taken seriously, as such patients are often best admitted for observation and serial hemoglobin levels. Typically, it is very difficult to perform a satisfactory anal examination in the early postoperative period because of the pain and anxiety associated with the examination. Intravenous administration of midazolam and/or narcotics and infiltration of the anal canal with local anesthetic agents may allow adequate examination and management of the bleeding site in the emergency department. The examination is started using a proctoscope. Suction should be available to allow evacuation of clots and blood from the rectum. Once a bleeding site is identified, it may be controlled either through the proctoscope if suction and cautery are available, or through the anoscope if the location is favorable. Anal canal packing can be placed at the bedside, but this technique has a high incidence of recurrent bleeding reported in one study.[2] The bleeding site may be suture ligated under direct vision through an anoscope. A Brinkerhoff retractor (a conical anoscope with a removable panel along one side) may allow easy access to a bleeding site for suture placement. A trip to the operating room may be necessary if the bleeding cannot be controlled with the measures described above or if the examination is difficult because of an uncooperative patient.

Fecal Impaction

Fecal impaction may produce significant morbidity after anorectal surgery. Limiting potent narcotic analgesics to the first 2 to 3 days postoperatively may be helpful in reducing the incidence of fecal impaction. Early ambulation of the patient and the judicious use of stool softeners, as well as the avoidance of dehydration, are helpful preventive measures. The patient with an impaction reports a recurring sharp cramping pain in the rectum or lower abdomen. There may or may not be an urge to have a bowel movement. The cramps usually occur at about 8- to 10-minute intervals, and there may be no pain in between the cramps. Patients with an impaction may have small, loose stools or pass mucoid, diarrheal stools. The patient will frequently report that he or she is unable to hold an enema, or if an enema is given it usually passes virtually unaltered almost immediately. A digital examination is usually diagnostic of fecal impaction but is often difficult to perform in a patient 1 week after anorectal surgery. Topical or injected local anesthetic is frequently necessary to allow for diagnosis and treatment. If the patient can tolerate examination, the impaction can be fragmented with the finger. Alternatively, a catheter or nasogastric tube can be passed proximal to the impaction and a high enema administered to promote evacuation. If these measures fail or if the patient is uncooperative, a trip to the operating room may on rare occasions be necessary for disimpaction.

Conclusion

The postoperative period can be a difficult time for the patient undergoing ambulatory anorectal surgery. It is the responsibility of the surgeon, office personnel, and staff at the ambulatory surgical center to provide comprehensive care for the patient and answer any questions or concerns. By taking a proactive approach and fully informing and educating the patient before surgery, postoperative complications may be minimized or more easily managed and the patient will achieve greater satisfaction with the operative procedure.

References

1. Shafik A. Role of warm water bath in inducing micturition in postoperative urinary retention after anorectal surgery. Urol Int 1993;50(4):213–217.
2. Rosen L, Sipe P, Stasik JJ, et al. Outcome of delayed hemorrhage following surgical hemorrhoidectomy. Dis Colon Rectum 1993;36(8):743–746.

6

Management of Pain After Anorectal Surgery

Part A: Postoperative Pain Management

Ernest Max, M.D., F.A.C.S.

No matter how skillfully conducted or successful the result, almost all surgical procedures produce tissue trauma and pain.[1] Postoperative pain and its management become factors in the patient's recovery and the ultimate success of the procedure. Compared with patients whose postoperative pain is inadequately or haphazardly managed, patients with an effective postoperative pain management plan experience earlier ambulation and mobility, a more rapid recovery, and a decreased need for analgesics. In addition, a decreased incidence of lingering chronic pain, a reduced incidence of postoperative complications, and lower overall cost can be realized.[2,3] Finally, these patients are much more likely to adhere to prescribed regimens and be satisfied with the operative procedure and their surgeon.[4-7]

Eliminating all postoperative pain is neither realistic nor advisable. Postoperative pain is an inextricable part of the healing process. Overly aggressive use of opioids may be associated with complications in excess of those associated with the pain itself, including respiratory depression and decreased bowel motility. In addition, excessively vigorous blunting of the pain pathway may obscure and delay the diagnosis of infectious complications, for which increased pain is a reliable indicator.

Nevertheless, studies continue to demonstrate that it is considerably more likely that after surgery a patient will be undermedicated rather than overmedicated. Many patients return home from an operation with little or no understanding of the amount and kind of pain to expect postoperatively or of the options available to address the pain.[8,9] This lack of an appropriate pain management plan adversely affects recovery.

Of the anorectal procedures addressed in this volume, hemorrhoidectomy is the procedure most often associated with significant postoperative pain. Accordingly, this subchapter focuses on pain management after hemorrhoidectomy. However, the principles of pharmacologic and nonpharmacologic pain control described below are equally relevant for other outpatient anorectal surgical procedures.

Preoperative Preparation

The single most important aspect of managing postoperative pain is a frank preoperative discussion with the patient about what to expect. Whenever pain management is discussed in detail with the patient preoperatively by the surgical team, the patient rates his or her postoperative pain significantly lower, uses less analgesics, and feels more satisfied with the surgical experience compared with patients who did not receive such preparation.[4-7]

This "psychological preparation" should include detailed descriptions of normal postoperative pain, how long to expect the pain, and what methods, pharmacologic and nonpharmacologic, are available to manage the pain. Patients vary significantly in their response to pain and in their willingness to discuss pain. It should be made clear that the surgical team is available to work with each patient individually to develop the best pain management plan for that patient. Consequently, it is important that the members of the surgical team have a specific and coordinated plan to treat postoperative pain (Figure 6.1), and that they regularly reassess their approach based on new developments in the field of pain management.

Preoperatively is the optimal time to discover any sensitivities to pain medications and any concerns by the patient regarding addiction to narcotics. Before surgery is also the best time to review postoperative care and the management of pain with both the patient and the family member or friend who will be assisting the patient. The patient can be instructed in the use of relaxation methods that can be useful in reducing pain. A clear set of written instructions including whom to call concerning postoperative pain management should be given to every patient.

Postoperative Management of Pain

Postoperative pharmacologic pain management begins during surgery and in the immediate postoperative period. After any outpatient anorectal procedure, it is preferable that the patient feel little or no pain for the first few postoperative hours. Such pre-

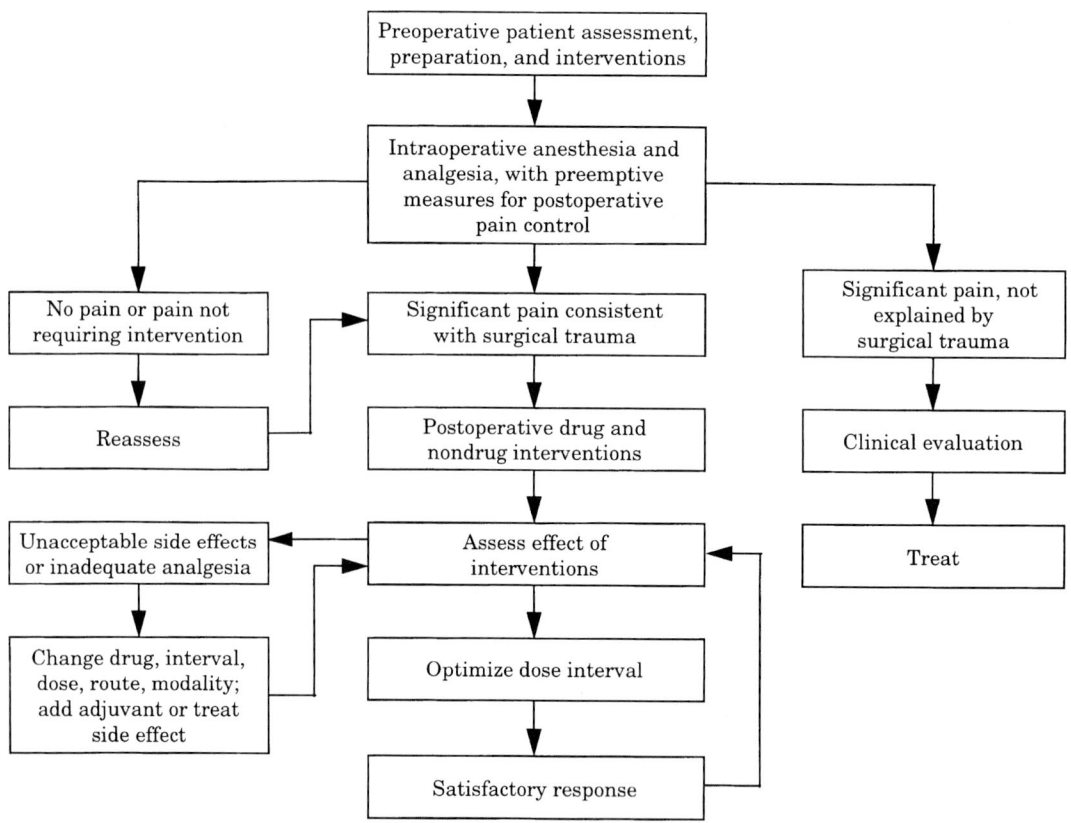

FIGURE 6.1. Flow chart for effective pain management. Reprinted from Acute Pain Management Guideline Panel. Acute Pain Management in Adults: Operative Procedures: Quick Reference Guide for Clinicians. AHCPR Pub. No. 92–0019. Rockville, MD: Agency for Health Care Policy and Research, Public Health Service, U.S. Department of Health and Human Services, February 1993.

emptive pain control has been shown to reduce subsequent postoperative pain significantly, probably by interrupting the initial pain pathway as well as by allowing the patient sufficient time to be, in effect, "in control of the pain." For a closed, Ferguson-type hemorrhoidectomy, we utilize general anesthesia or conscious sedation and infiltrate the anal canal and anal sphincter with bupivacaine hydrochloride (0.25% with epinephrine 1:200,000). Approximately 50 mL of the local anesthetic is used. In the postanesthesia care unit, the patient receives ketorolac (Toradol, Syntex International, Inc., Palo Alto, CA) 30 mg given intravenously or intramuscularly. Ketorolac, a potent nonsteroidal anti-inflammatory drug (NSAID), has been found to be similar in analgesic effect to narcotics and is used for the control of moderately severe, acute pain. Ketorolac is associated with fewer complications than commonly prescribed narcotics.[10] This regimen allows the patient to wake up with no pain, be driven home by a friend or family member, and be comfortable before any pain begins. In general, such a regimen will prevent pain for 4 to 6 hours after surgery.

(*Editor's note:* Although I have practiced with Dr. Max for almost 25 years, he and I do some things slightly differently. I routinely add 300 U of hyaluronidase to the bupivacaine solution to allow more rapid diffusion of the anesthetic into the tissues. This reduces the edema of the tissues and also results in more rapid onset of the action of the anesthetic. Postoperatively, I use an ice bag applied to the anal area for the first 8 to 12 hours after surgery. The ice slows absorption of the local anesthetic and prolongs its duration of action. It also probably reduces postoperative swelling.)

Although we have found the combination of bupivacaine and ketorolac to be effective for perioperative pain control, slightly different approaches are used at other centers. Differing strategies include general anesthesia and local infiltration with ketorolac (60 mg) into the perirectal tissues, followed by parenteral or oral ketorolac,[10,11] pudendal nerve blocks, and epidural bupivacaine injection. A patient-controlled subcutaneous morphine pump begun in recovery[12] has also been used to control perioperative pain. However, an increase in complications, especially urinary retention, is associated with morphine therapy following anorectal procedures.[10]

Once the patient is home, a combination of ketorolac 10 mg taken every 6 hours and propoxyphene napsylate (Darvocet N–100, Eli Lilly & Co., Indianapolis, IN) one or two tablets taken every 4 hours, beginning shortly after arrival home, is effective in controlling pain. Ketorolac should not be taken for more than 5 days because of the increased risk of side effects when taken for a longer period. For most patients, we authorize a single prescription for 20 tablets of ketorolac and renew the prescription for propoxyphene as necessary. For patients who undergo an open anorectal procedure in which bleeding is a concern, we generally prescribe propoxyphene tablets alone, because ketorolac inhibits platelet function.

Spasm of the external and internal anal sphincter muscles is often a key element in the development of pain after anorectal procedures. We recommend a warm sitz bath every 3 to 4 hours during the first few days postoperatively and as desired thereafter. Sitz baths may help relax the anal and urinary sphincters, encourage bowel and bladder emptying, and relieve muscle spasms that exacerbate pain. Although adequate pain medication, combined with relaxation strategies and warm sitz baths, is generally sufficient to relieve muscle spasm, some patients may require additional measures. Diazepam, at a dose of 5 mg three or four times daily, is frequently effective in relieving muscle spasm. Diazepam and other muscle relaxants may, however, exacerbate urinary retention as a result of relaxation of the detrusor muscle of the bladder. They should therefore be used cautiously until the patient is voiding satisfactorily.

In addition to minimizing sphincter spasm, it is important to avoid constipation by restoring and maintaining good bowel function. Constipation exacerbates postoperative pain and may lead to fecal impaction. For most patients, a high-fiber diet, sufficient oral fluid intake, and regular warm-water sitz baths are sufficient. Most hemorrhoidectomy patients experience their first bowel movement approximately 2.5 days after surgery.

A variety of nonpharmacologic strategies such as slow rhythmic breathing, relaxation exercises, distraction by personally preferred music, guided imagery, and biofeedback therapies have been used in the management of postoperative pain. The use of transcutaneous electrical nerve stimulation has also been reported. Several publications have demonstrated the efficacy of these techniques in reducing self-reported postoperative pain and the need for analgesics.[4,13–15]

Other Considerations

Increasing pain or a significant change in the nature of postoperative pain may signal the development of complications that require treatment. Patients should be instructed to report any significant alteration in the quality or magnitude of their pain or the presence of fever. The most common complications that result in increased postoperative pain are fecal impaction and infection. Bleeding is not generally accompanied by increased pain unless a hematoma develops.

Analgesic agents are not without risk. Patients with known sensitivities, elderly persons, and patients with coexisting medical conditions should be managed cautiously. All patients should be asked specifically about any sensitivities to medications and be advised of potential side effects as well as symptoms of allergic reaction for any medication prescribed. Elderly patients are particularly at risk for both undertreatment and overtreatment of pain.[4,16] The elderly experience altered distribution and clearance of many medications. They are also at increased risk for adverse effects from opioids as well as gastric, liver, and renal toxicity from nonopioid analgesic drugs, including NSAIDs and acetaminophen. Side effect from opioids include sedation, respiratory depression, constipation, urinary retention, cognitive impairment, and exacerbation of Parkinson's disease. In addition, special care in choosing a pain management protocol is critical in patients with respiratory, renal, or liver disease, as such coexisting conditions increase the risk of adverse effects from analgesics. Although addiction to opioids following their short-term use for acute pain is uncommon, patients who express concern about this issue or who have a history of substance abuse are ideally managed with a plan that avoids narcotics.

The cost of appropriate outpatient pain management, including analgesics and other adjuncts we have mentioned, is generally reasonable and affordable. This is especially true since the ambulatory surgery environment may significantly reduce the overall cost of treatment. The more expensive pain management therapies, such as patient-controlled morphine infusion or transcutaneous electrical nerve stimulation, have been used after ambulatory anorectal surgery, but because simpler, less costly, and generally more effective treatments are available, the use of these therapies is warranted only in unusual circumstances.

References

1. Hargreaves KM, Dionne RA. Evaluating endogenous mediators of pain and analgesia in clinical studies. In Max M, Portnoy R, Laska E (eds). Advances in Pain Research and Therapy: The Design of Analgesic Clinical Trials. New York: Raven Press, 1991, pp 579–598.
2. Moskowitz L. Psychological management of post-surgical pain and patient adherence. Hand Clinics 1996;12:129–137.
3. Jain S, Datta S. Postoperative pain management. Chest Surg Clin N Am 1997;7:773–799.
4. Acute Pain Management Guideline Panel. Acute Pain Management: Operative of Medical Procedures and Trauma. Rockville, MD: Agency for Health Care Policy and Research, U.S. Department of Health and Human Services, 1992.
5. Fortin F, Kirouac S. A randomized controlled trial of preoperative patient education. Int J Nurs Stud 1976;13:11–24.
6. Jamison RN, Ross MJ, Hoopman P, et al. Assessment of postoperative pain management: patient satisfaction and perceived helpfulness. Clin J Pain 1997;13:229–236.
7. Carpenter RL. Optimizing postoperative pain management. Am Fam Physician 1997;56:835–844, 847–850.
8. Moote CA. Postoperative pain management—back to basics. Can J Anaesth 1995;42:453–457.
9. Rose DK, Cohen MM, Yee DA. Changing the practice of pain management. Anesth Analg 1997;84:764–772.
10. O'Donovan S, Ferrara A, Larach S, et al. Intraoperative use of Toradol facilitates outpatient hemorrhoidectomy. Dis Colon Rectum 1994;37:793–799.
11. Milito G, Cortese F, Brancaleone C, Casciani CU. Effect of ketorolac in the management of posthemorrhoidectomy pain. Available at: http://www.csgen.it/medicina/articoli/961full/p004.htm. Accessed March 9, 1999.
12. Goldstein ET, Williamson PR, Larach SW. Subcutaneous morphine pump for postoperative hemorrhoidectomy pain management. Dis Colon Rectum 1993;36:439–446.
13. Wells N. The effect of relaxation on postoperative muscle tension and pain. Nurs Res 1982;31:236–238.
14. Flaherty GG, Fitzpatrick JJ. Relaxation technique to increase comfort level of postoperative patients: A preliminary study. Nurs Res 1978;27:352–355.
15. Good M. Effects of relaxation and music on postoperative pain: A review. J Adv Nurs 1996;24:905–914.
16. Egbert AM. Postoperative pain management in the frail elderly. Clin Geriatr Med 1996;12:583–599.

Part B: Innovative Approaches to Pain Management

Sergio W. Larach, M.D., F.A.C.S.
and
Joseph Gallagher, M.D.

Many anorectal procedures are currently being performed on an outpatient basis. One million people present to physicians each year with symptomatic hemorrhoids, and approximately 10% of them will require surgery.[1] A radical three-quadrant hemorrhoidectomy is considered major anorectal surgery and maintains this status in spite of innovative surgical and anesthesia techniques. For patients undergoing surgical hemorrhoidectomy, the most feared element is the postoperative pain.[2,3] Because there is a disproportionate amount of pain compared to the size of the operative wounds, pain control after hemorrhoidectomy continues to be an elusive problem to resolve.

As individual patients respond quite variably to posthemorrhoidectomy pain, it is difficult to predict patient response or standardize medication doses. During the first 24 hours after surgery, drug consumption can vary by a factor of 20 among similar patients.[4] Different techniques have been used in attempting to reduce complications, such as urinary retention and fecal impaction, that can be triggered by uncontrolled pain. We discuss a variety of ideas that have been proposed and studied in attempts at reducing pain and its consequences following surgical hemorrhoidectomy. The ultimate goals of pain management after hemorrhoidectomy are to minimize pain, minimize complications, achieve a high degree of patient satisfaction, shorten or eliminate hospital stay, and reduce cost.

Sphincterotomy

The association between elevated resting pressure of the anal canal and the etiology of hemorrhoids is not clear. After surgery, the anal wound may provoke reflex spasm of both the involuntary internal sphincter and the voluntary external sphincter. Sustained spasm of the anal sphincter may start a vicious cycle with increased anal pain as well as painful bowel action and resultant fissure formation.[3,5,6] Sphincterotomy may help with postoperative pain by decreasing spasm of the sphincter. Pain relief may, however, be at the expense of incontinence. Watts et al.,[7] in a trial evaluating different hemorrhoidectomy techniques, noted that one predictor of decreased postoperative pain was the addition of anal stretch to the procedure. Unfortunately, these authors did not report the incidence of incontinence when anal stretch was added to hemorrhoidectomy. Asfar et al.[8] showed the superiority of open sphincterotomy to anal stretch. In their study, anal stretch was associated with long-term impaired sphincter control in 24% of patients. The open sphincterotomy group, however, had only a 6.4% incidence of fecal soiling for an average of 4.5 weeks and no long-term incontinence.[8] Reversible "sphincterotomy" by topical application of glycerol trinitrate may be beneficial for posthemorrhoidectomy pain control. Glycerol trinitrate 0.2% causes a reduction in anal canal pressures of 20% to 30%[9] and is comparable to the 26% to 58% reduction reported after a surgical sphincterotomy.[10–13] Trimebutine (Proctolog), a smooth-muscle relaxant[14] that may be administered as a suppository, lowers the mean resting anal pressure by up to 35%. In a randomized trial of 160 patients to evaluate the effects of trimebutine on postoperative pain after a hemorrhoidectomy, there was no difference in postoperative pain compared with controls.[15] Due to the lack of clear benefit, the use of any type of sphincterotomy as an adjunct to pain control has not gained widespread acceptance.

Open Versus Closed Technique

There is still controversy over the relationship between open and closed hemorrhoidectomy technique and postoperative pain. Since Ferguson[16] reported his closed technique of hemorrhoidectomy in 1959, it has gained wide acceptance in North America. This modification of hemorrhoidal technique, moving from open-wound hemorrhoidectomy (Milligan-Morgan) to closed wound, (Ferguson) has been reported to decrease postoperative pain.[16,17] Parks[18] described a submucosal technique and reported limited postoperative pain. Parks' successful results with pain reduction could not, however, be duplicated in later studies.[7,19] Seow-Choen et al.[20] reported a prospective randomized trial comparing conventional scissor excision/ligation versus diathermy excision without ligation. The study revealed that overall subjective pain control was equivalent, but the diathermy patients used less oral pain medication. His conclusion implied that the effect of coagulation on the pain receptor caused a reduction in postoperative pain. Patel and O'Connor[21] compared suture ligation technique to the Milligan-Morgan hemorrhoidectomy and found a significantly decreased linear analog pain scale ($P < 0.05$) in the ligation group.

Use of Lasers in Hemorrhoidectomy

The use of lasers in anal surgery has also sparked considerable debate. Senagore et al.,[22] in a prospective randomized study, compared treatment of advanced hemorrhoidal disease with cold scalpel versus contact neodymium:YAG laser. They concluded that there was no significant difference in postoperative pain.[22] Leff,[23] in an outpatient trial, compared carbon dioxide laser hemorrhoidectomy to standard closed technique and also found no significant difference between the two groups. The laser is an advancement in technology frequently requested by patients; however, it adds additional cost to any surgical procedure and has not been shown to be of benefit in pain control in hemorrhoidectomy.

Role of Defecation

It has become standard practice to give patients laxatives in an attempt to reduce the postoperative pain associated with bowel movements. London et al.[24] showed that patients who took lactulose for 4 days before their hemorrhoidectomy defecated earlier and had more frequent bowel action during the first week after surgery. The pain during the initial 24 hours following surgery was no different between the two groups, but thereafter the patients who received the lactulose had less pain. The advantage in pain control was presumed to be secondary to less constipation.[24]

A significant amount of postoperative pain is directly associated with defecation. Fecal impaction occurs in up to 5% of posthemorrhoidectomy patients and is a significant source of morbidity. To facilitate defecation, the stool should be kept bulky and soft. The use of fiber supplements, including plain bran, psyllium, methylcellulose, and calcium polycarbophil has become the standard of care.[25] Stool softeners such as docusate calcium and mild stimulant laxatives (senna concentrate) are also frequently used in the postoperative period. Wheat fiber produces a more satisfactory bowel movement postoperatively than do traditional laxatives, such as magnesium sulfate or mineral oil. The use of fiber has been shown by Johnson et al. to decrease the incidence of fecal leakage and reduce defecation pain after hemorrhoidectomy.[26] All of our patients undergo a standard protocol including both bulk fiber and a mild stool softener postoperatively.

Wound Care

A clean wound reduces irritation of the surgical site and the incidence of infection. Soaking the anus and perianal tissue in warm water (sitz bath) two to three times a day for 5- to 10-minute intervals may relieve muscle spasm and reduce pain. However, prolonged periods of soaking may lead to maceration of the perianal skin.[27]

Metronidazole appears to decrease postoperative pain by helping to reduce infection in the anal wounds. Carapeti et al.,[28] in a double-blinded randomized trial, evaluated the efficacy of metronidazole taken for 1 week following anorectal surgery. Their brief study included only a small number of patients and suggested that postoperative pain is reduced toward the end of the first week, specifically on days 5 through 7. All patients were also given diclofenac (an NSAID) suppository at the end of the procedure and also 0.2% glyceryl-trinitrate anal ointment applied three times daily for 2 weeks.[28] Nausea, a potential side effect of metronidazole, may have an impact on patient compliance and satisfaction. Other antibiotics may offer benefits similar to metronidazole without producing nausea.

Analgesics

Traditionally, the treatment for pain after hemorrhoidectomy was by the use of parenteral meperidine, morphine sulfate, or an epidural catheter during the first 24 to 48 hours postoperatively. The patient would then be given oral analgesics such as oxycodone or propoxyphene. This postoperative pain management method required hospitalization, and therefore new strategies needed to be developed.

Local Anesthetic

Bupivacaine, an amide local anesthetic, is a potent agent that provides prolonged anesthesia. For anal surgery, the 0.25% solution with adrenaline 1:200,000 is commonly used. Chester et al.[29] compared 40 patients who underwent Milligan-Morgan hemorrhoidectomy and received bupivacaine 1.5 mg/kg with 1:200,000 adrenaline or just the 1:200,000 adrenaline at the time of surgery. All patients received lactulose daily, and opiates on demand. The study found that the local anesthetic increased only the time before the first demand of additional analgesia and concluded that the benefits of locally injected bupivacaine are marginal.[29] The delay in the onset of pain, however, may allow the patient to void more easily postoperatively. Smith and Simon[30] proposed viscous lidocaine, delivered through a catheter positioned with the tip just above dentate line, as a posthemorrhoidectomy analgesic.[30]

Narcotics

Opiates act through opioid receptors and have significant side effects, such as constipation and respiratory depression, as well as significant potential for abuse. Narcotics are usually given intermittently, with the resultant peaks and troughs in analgesic efficacy.[31]

Nonsteroidal Anti-inflammatory Medications

Ketorolac tromethamine (Toradol, Syntex International, Palo Alto, CA) is an NSAID that blocks the formation of prostaglandins by inhibiting the cyclooxygenase pathway of production. Doses of 30 to 60 mg injected intramuscularly, followed by 10 mg orally every 6 hours, are recommended. Side effects of chronic use include inhibition of platelet aggregation and prolongation of bleeding time, abnormalities of liver function, fluid retention, edema, and impaired renal function. The most serious complications of the use of ketorolac include gastrointestinal ulceration, bleeding, and perforation, Because of these potential side effects, it is recommended that ketorolac be administered for no more than 5 days after surgery.

Ketorolac can be administered by direct injection into the exposed sphincter at the time of surgery. In 100 patients so treated, Reichmann[32] found 83% improvement in pain relief and only 2% incidence of urinary retention. Reichmann's work has been duplicated in our institution by O'Donovan et al.[33] Three groups of patients were studied for a period of 5 days. The three arms of the study included patients receiving oral narcotics only, those using a subcutaneous morphine pump, and those treated with ketorolac alone. In our series, the ketorolac group achieved pain control equivalent to the narcotic groups, had a higher satisfaction rating, and had no increase in complications. Urinary retention did not occur in the ketorolac group, possibly as a result of blunting of the pain reflex response mediated by prostaglandins. The ketorolac regimen allows safe same-day discharge after hemorrhoidectomy. Another advantage noted in the ketorolac patients when compared to both narcotics groups was less constipation, as measured by the time to first bowel movement.[33]

Patient-Controlled Analgesia

Patient-controlled analgesia (PCA) was first introduced in 1972 and has become widely accepted.[34] PCA permits immediate access to narcotics via an intravenous access with doses tailored to the patient's perception of pain. PCA is effective and safe and has excellent patient acceptance. A change in the access route from intravenous to subcutaneous confers no advantage for patients undergoing elective abdominal or extremity surgery.[35] Goldstein et al.[36] at our institution reviewed the use of the subcutaneous PCA pump for posthemorrhoidectomy pain management in the outpatient setting. A butterfly needle was placed in the subcutaneous tissue and connected to an ambulatory infusion pump (CADD-PCA Model 5800, Pharmacia Deltec, Inc., Saint Paul, MN) with a programmed dosage administration. The pump has a lockout feature to prevent overdosing with both continuous and bolus modes. Use of the pump requires daily visits by a home health nursing service. The study demonstrated effective pain control, no correlation between pain level and morphine dose, and high patient acceptance. The incidence of urinary retention was high compared with other studies by our same group. Other side effects of the morphine were present in a small number of patients.[36]

Transdermal Fentanyl

Transdermal fentanyl provides an alternative form of pain management that has been effectively used in the treatment of chronic pain. The transdermal delivery system for fentanyl uses a stacked array of five layers that allows for rate-controlled delivery and maintains serum drug concentrations for a prolonged period (mean half-life of 17 hours). Using a randomized double-blind study, Kilbride et al.[37] evaluated the use of transdermal fentanyl to assist with pain control following a hemorrhoidectomy. The placebo group required more narcotics after surgery and had higher recorded pain scores.[37] The concerns for using transdermal fentanyl are the possibility of variable absorption and the long half-life, which could lead to serious complications.

Suggested Strategy

Our current strategy for performing a hemorrhoidectomy is as follows. During surgery the patient is under monitored anesthesia care or conscious sedation, usually using propofol, with local infiltration of the perianal region using bupivacaine with adrenaline for a complete anal block. We utilize a closed hemorrhoidectomy technique with intraoperative intramuscular injection of ketorolac. Postoperative management consists of oral ketorolac limited to 5 days and narcotic analgesics as needed. All patients receive a perioperative laxa-

tive, bulking agents, and sitz baths. Patients are seen in the clinic 7 days after their procedure. Based on our preoperative assessment of the patient, certain patients are selected for the use of the subcutaneous morphine pump with home health support.

Successful management of patients who have undergone surgical hemorrhoidectomy on an outpatient basis relies on multiple different pain management strategies. The perception of pain varies depending on individual patient tolerance, operative technique, presence of infection, and other factors. Outpatient management relies on the patient's abilities to follow instructions, to help recognize problems, and to communicate these problems to the surgical team.

References

1. Johanson JF, Sonnenberg A. The prevalence of hemorrhoids and chronic constipation, an epidemiologic study. Gastroenterology 1990;98:380–386.
2. Goligher JC. Surgery of Anus, Rectum and Colon. 5th ed. London: Bailliere Tindall, 1984, p 98.
3. Parks AG. The surgical treatment of hemorrhoids. Br J Surg 1956;43:337–351.
4. Lehmann KA, Gordes B, Hoeckle W. Postoperative on-demand analgesia with morphine [in German]. Anaesthetist 1985;34(10):494–501.
5. Eisenhammer S. Proper principles and practices in the surgical management of hemorrhoids. Dis Colon Rectum 1969;12:288–305.
6. Allgower M. Conservative management of hemorrhoids. Part III. Partial internal sphincterotomy. Clinical Gastroenterology 75;4:608–618.
7. Watts JM, Bennett RC, Duthie HL, Goligher JC. Pain after hemorrhoidectomy. Surg Gynecol Obstet 1965;121:1037–1042.
8. Asfar SK, Juma TH, Ala-Edeen T. Hemorrhoidectomy and sphincterotomy—a prospective study comparing the effectiveness of anal stretch and sphincterotomy in reducing pain after hemorrhoidectomy. Dis Colon Rectum 1988;31:181–185.
9. Loder PB, Kamm MA, Nicholls RJ, Phillips RKS. 'Reversible chemical sphincterotomy' by local application of glyceryl trinitrate. Br J Surg 1994;81: 1386–1389.
10. Arabi Y, Alexander-Williams J, Keighley MRB. Anal pressures in hemorrhoids and anal fissure. Am J Surg 1977;134:608–610.
11. McNamara MJ, Percy JP, Fielding IR. A manometric study of anal fissure treated by subcutaneous lateral internal sphincterotomy. Ann Surg 1990;211: 235–238.

12. Arabi Y, Gatehouse D, Alexander-Williams J, et al. Rubber band ligation or lateral subcutaneous sphincterotomy for treatment of hemorrhoids. Br J Surg 1977;64:737–740.

13. Schouten WR, Blankensteijn JD. Ultra slow wave pressure variations in the anal canal before and after lateral internal sphincterotomy. Int J Colorectal Dis 1992;7:115–118.

14. Nagasaki M, Homori S, Ohashi H. Effect of trimebutine on voltage activated calcium current in rabbit ileal smooth muscle cells. Br J Pharmacol 1993;110:399–403.

15. Ho YH, Seow-Choen F, Low JY, et al. Randomized controlled trial of trimebutine (anal sphincter relaxant) for pain after hemorrhoidectomy. Br J Surg 1997;84:377–379.

16. Ferguson JA, Heaton JR. Closed hemorrhoidectomy. Dis Colon Rectum 1959;2:176–179.

17. Vernava AM, Dean P. Preoperative and postoperative management. In Beck DE, Wexner SD (eds). Fundamentals of Anorectal Surgery. New York: McGraw-Hill, 1992, pp 50–55.

18. Parks A. The surgical treatment of hemorrhoids. Br J Surg 1956;43:337–351.

19. Roe AM, Bartolo DC, Velacott KD, et al. Submucosal versus ligation haemorrhoidectomy: a comparison of anal sensation, anal sphincter manometry and postoperative pain and function. Br J Surg 1987;74:948–951.

20. Seow-Choen F, Ho Y-H, Ang H-G, Goh H-S. Prospective, randomized trial comparing pain and clinical function after conventional scissors excision/ligation vs. diathermy excision without ligation for symptomatic prolapsed hemorrhoids. Dis Colon Rectum 1992;35:1165–1169.

21. Patel N, O'Connor T. Suture hemorrhoidectomy: a day-only alternative. Aust N Z J Surg 1996;66(12): 830–831.

22. Senagore A, Mazier WP, Luchtefeld MA, et al. Treatment of advanced hemorrhoidal disease: a prospective, randomized comparison of cold scalpel vs. contact Nd:YAG laser. Dis Colon Rectum 1993;36:1042–1049.

23. Leff EI. Hemorrhoidectomy—laser vs. nonlaser: outpatient surgical experience. Dis Colon Rectum 1992;35:743–746.

24. London NJM, Bramley PD, Windle R. Effect of four days of preoperative lactulose on post hemorrhoidectomy pain: results of placebo controlled trial. BMJ 1987;295:363–364.

25. Beck DE, Cataldo TE, Larach SW. Non-operative treatment of hemorrhoidectomy disease. In Hicks TC (ed). Complications of Colon & Rectal Surgery. Baltimore: Williams & Wilkins, 1996, pp 173–180.

26. Johnson CD, Budd J, Ward AJ. Laxative after hemorrhoidectomy. Dis Colon Rectum 1987;30(10): 780–781.

27. Mazier WP, Wolkomir AF. Hemorrhoids. Seminars in Colon and Rectal Surgery 1990;1(4):197–206.

28. Carapeti EA, Kamm MA, McDonald PJ, et al. Double-blind randomized controlled trial of effect of metronidazole on pain after day-case hemorrhoidectomy. Lancet 1988;351:169–172.

29. Chester JF, Stanford BJ, Gazet JC. Analgesic benefit of locally injected bupivacaine after hemorrhoidectomy. Dis Colon Rectum 1990;33:487–489.

30. Smith SL, Simon R. Viscous lidocaine as a post-hemorrhoidectomy analgesic. Dis Colon Rectum 1979;22:40–41.

31. Dodson ME. A review of methods for relief of postoperative pain. Ann R Coll Surg Engl 1982;64: 324–327.

32. Reichmann IM. Use of Toradol in anorectal surgery. Dis Colon Rectum 1993;36:295–296.

33. O'Donovan S, Ferrara A, Larach SW, et al. Intraoperative use of Toradol facilitates outpatient hemorrhoidectomy. Dis Colon Rectum 1994;37: 793–799.

34. Keeri-Szanto M, Heaman S. Postoperative demand analgesia. Surg Gynecol Obstet 1972;134:647–651.

35. Urquhart ML, Klapp K, White P. Patient-controlled analgesia: a comparison of intravenous versus subcutaneous Hydromorphone. Anesthesiology 1988;69: 428–432.

36. Goldstein ET, Williamson PR, Larach SW. Subcutaneous morphine pump for postoperative hemorrhoidectomy pain management. Dis Colon Rectum 1993;36:439–446.

37. Kilbride M, Morse M, Senagore A. Transdermal Fentanyl improves management of postoperative hemorrhoidectomy pain. Dis Colon Rectum 1994;37: 1070–1072.

7

Prevention of Urinary Retention After Anorectal Surgery

Stuart D. Hoff, M.D., F.A.C.S.

Postoperative urinary retention after anorectal surgery is a feared but largely preventable complication. It can occur with any anorectal operation but is most commonly associated with hemorrhoidectomy. By understanding the factors involved with bladder emptying, the surgeon is able to alter operative and perioperative management to greatly reduce the incidence of urinary retention. Reduction or elimination of urinary retention may then allow the vast majority of anorectal surgeries to be performed in the outpatient setting and result in lower cost and greater patient comfort.

Structure and Function of the Bladder and Urethra

Anatomy

The major components of the bladder are the body and the base. The body lies above the ureteral orifices and is the main collecting and storage area. The bladder base consists of the posterior trigone (which extends between the ureteral orifices and the internal urethral meatus), the deep detrusor, and the inferior aspect of the anterior bladder wall. The bladder base, along with the proximal urethra and the external urethral sphincter, forms the bladder outlet. This area is histologically and biochemically distinct from the body of the bladder.[1]

The body of the bladder wall is made up of interlacing fibers of the detrusor muscle. This meshwork of smooth muscle, upon contraction, allows for a reduction of the bladder in all dimensions and, thereby, complete evacuation. The spherical geometry of the bladder permits a relatively slow increase in wall tension as urine volume increases.[1]

The bladder wall is richly innervated by an excitatory, parasympathetic nerve supply. Contributions from levels S2 through S4, conveyed by the pudendal nerve and the pelvic plexus, provide both sensory and motor fibers to the bladder. Stretch receptors in the wall of the bladder send afferent impulses to spinal reflex centers and to cortical areas that modulate voluntary control of micturition.[1,2]

Although sympathetic nerves are found along the blood supply to the bladder, they do not appear to play a significant role in the innervation of the smooth muscle of the bladder itself.[3] The detrusor muscle, however, is indirectly inhibited by sympathetic stimulation. This probably takes place in the interconnecting nerves of the pelvic plexus, where sympathetic nerves can modulate parasympathetic outflow to the detrusor muscle via feedback loops.[1,2]

As previously noted, the smooth muscle of the bladder outlet is histologically and histochemically distinct from the detrusor. In the bladder base, the deep muscle layer is continuous with the detrusor, but rather than having an interconnecting meshwork arrangement as is seen in the bladder body, it exhibits a predominantly circular orientation. A layer of longitudinal muscle bundles is found more superficially in the area of the trigone. Although no obvious sphincter exists in the bladder base, these muscular arrangements form a functional basis for its role as a sphincter.[1] The muscles in this area receive sparse parasympathetic input, but they receive a rich supply of sympathetic, α-adrenergic nervous input.[3]

Whether the detrusor or trigonal muscles extend into the urethra is still a matter of debate. In men, the thin, smooth muscle layer of the membranous urethra is continuous with the prostatic urethra. Near the prostatic apex, an outer layer of circularly oriented striated muscle forms a horseshoe configuration around the urethra, sparing its posterior surface. This is the external urethral sphincter, or rhabdosphincter, which is innervated by the pudendal nerve, containing motor axons from S2 through S4. The external urethral sphincter is, in turn, surrounded by the periurethral striated muscle of the pelvic floor.[1]

Women differ in the arrangement of muscle bundles in this area. In women, the external urethral sphincter does exist, but in an attenuated form. As in men, it is deficient posteriorly. In addition, two other muscle bundles, the compressor urethrae and the urethrovaginal sphincter, are present, as is the periurethral muscle of the pelvic floor.[1]

In addition to smooth muscle, skeletal muscle along the urethra and in the pelvic floor plays a role in micturition and urinary continence. The pudendal nerve innervates these muscles, which are composed of a heterogeneous mixture of slow- and fast-twitch muscle cells. They exert their greatest pressure in the membranous urethra in men and in the mid-urethra in women. Two effects on contraction of these muscle are apparent: the urethra is supported, lengthened, and compressed, and the detrusor motor nucleus is inhibited. Conversely, contraction of this muscle group is inhibited when the detrusor motor nucleus fires, and the relationship between these muscles and the detrusor is apparent.[1] In fact, stimulation of the pudendal nerve or anal muscles has been used in the past to treat uninhibited detrusor activity.[4]

Micturition

The micturition cycle involves an involuntary sacral reflex with central voluntary and involuntary modulation. As urine empties into the bladder, intravesicular pressure slowly rises until approximately 200 to 250 mL of urine is present. This is generally the volume at which the initial desire to void is noted. Above this volume, pressure begins to increase rapidly as more urine is collected. Stretch receptors in the bladder wall then send impulses to the sacral cord and the detrusor motor nucleus, which in turn results in a reflex contraction of the detrusor. This further increases bladder pressure and augments this reflex. After a brief period of sustained contraction, the detrusor relaxes and the bladder pressure falls. As more urine empties into the bladder, this cycle is repeated. Additionally, reflex mechanisms stimulate contraction of the external urethral sphincter, and when the bladder is filled near its capacity, firing in the pudendal nerve increases along with the tone of periurethral muscles and pelvic floor muscles to maintain continence.[1]

Once the bladder pressure is high enough to force open the bladder outlet, another reflex, passing through the pons (spino-bulbospinal reflex) occurs to inhibit hypogastric and pudendal nerve firing. Relaxation of the smooth muscle of the bladder outlet and skeletal muscle of the pelvic floor occurs, and micturition results. Sustained contraction of the detrusor continues until the bladder is fully emptied. In the intact individual, the timing of micturition is influenced by higher brain centers. Cortical and brainstem centers exert an inhibitory influence on the spino-bulbospinal micturition reflex and facilitate contraction of the periurethral and pelvic muscles to allow micturition to occur at an acceptable time.[1]

Incidence of Urinary Retention After Anorectal Surgery

The incidence of urinary retention after anorectal surgery varies greatly,[5–15] and it is very difficult to determine the true frequency of occurrence. In some larger series of patients the incidence of urinary retention requiring catheterization has been as high as 52%,[7] whereas in other series the incidence has been very low.[5,11–13] The 52% incidence reported by Prasad and Abcarian[7] was noted in a medical audit of hemorrhoidectomy patients at Cook County Hospital. This audit prompted a prospective study of the incidence of urinary retention following anorectal surgery for benign disease. In the prospective study, the authors found an incidence of only 1.17% overall and 10.5% in hemorrhoidectomy patients.[7]

There may be several factors that cause this wide variation in reported frequency of urinary retention.

Many series, particularly those reporting a low incidence of retention, use techniques aimed at decreasing the incidence of urinary retention.[5,11-13] As will be presented later, perioperative management plays a large role in the development, or the avoidance, of postoperative urinary retention. Another factor in the equation is the percentage of hemorrhoidectomy or other extensive operations of the anorectal area contained in each series. A higher incidence of urinary retention has been noted after hemorrhoidectomy than after operations associated with less postoperative discomfort, such as abscess drainage, fistula surgery, or internal anal sphincterotomy.[5,7,12] Unfortunately, most studies do not separate patients according to procedure, or report only posthemorrhoidectomy urinary retention.

The threshold at which the patient and physician feel that urinary retention is present may also influence its reported incidence. Misinterpretation of symptoms may lead to a high reported incidence of urinary retention. Many patients will have pelvic muscle spasm immediately after anorectal surgery and will report a sensation of bladder fullness even when little urine is present upon catheterization.[15]

It is also possible that patients in some series actually had a moderate, usually voidable, amount of urine in the bladder and were temporarily unable to empty the bladder due to factors that will be discussed. Many of these patients may have been able to void later and would not have required catheterization if enough time had been allowed to pass. This is illustrated in a 1957 report by Salvati and Kleckner,[16] who decreased the incidence of catheterization after anorectal surgery from 48.5% to 20.2% simply by delaying catheterization. Patients were catheterized only when the bladder was palpable, and not when the patient initially complained of bladder fullness. Few series follow the example of Petros and Bradley,[15] who did not consider a patient to have urinary retention unless at least 400 mL of urine was present in the bladder at the time of catheterization.

In summary, the incidence of urinary retention after anorectal surgery has varied greatly in reported series over the years. Older series tend to report a higher incidence of urinary retention than do more recent series. This is probably the result of better understanding of the problem today, and of the means of avoiding it. It is unfortunate that many

surgeons are hesitant to perform anorectal surgery on an outpatient basis because of concerns about the incidence of urinary retention reported in these older series.

Etiology of Postoperative Urinary Retention

There is probably no single cause of urinary retention after anorectal surgery, just as there is no single factor causing the diseases for which these patients have surgery. There are a host of factors that can "tip the scales" to cause urinary retention in any patient after anorectal surgery. By understanding these factors, measures can be taken to avoid or reduce this complication.

Neural Factors Affecting the Bladder Outlet

Neural factors obviously play an important role in the development of urinary retention, as the bladder and other structures of micturition are simply muscular tissues under nervous control. The musculature of the bladder outlet is rich in stimulatory sympathetic, α-adrenergic receptors that act to close the bladder outlet to the flow of urine.[1-3] A role for these receptors in postoperative urinary retention is almost certain. Stress and postoperative pain generate generalized adrenergic stimulation, causing α-adrenergic stimulation of the muscles of the bladder outlet. More direct adrenergic stimulation of these muscles may result from reflex stimulation of the α_{1A} receptors in the bladder outlet mediated by the pudendal nerve in response to anal pain or anorectal distention. There is evidence pointing to stimulation of the smooth muscle of the bladder outlet and proximal urethra as a major cause of retention. In a urodynamic study by Barone and Cummings of patients with acute urinary retention after anorectal surgery, findings were consistent with bladder outlet obstruction rather than detrusor dysfunction as the cause of retention.[17]

It has been known for many years that pharmacologic blockade of postsynaptic α-adrenergic receptors can lead to a decrease in the incidence of urinary retention in men with prostatism.[18] Phenoxybenzamine, a nonselective α-adrenergic antagonist, was one of the first drugs used to treat urinary retention associated with prostatism, but its many adverse effects, including postural hypotension and tachycardia, have limited its use.[19] Additionally, Goldman et al.[20] showed phenoxybenzamine to be effective in treating postherniorrhaphy urinary retention in a prospective, randomized study. None of 58 patients receiving the drug developed retention, compared with 59% retention in the control group.[20]

Research on bladder outlet physiology has led to the development of agents designed to selectively block α_1-adrenergic receptors, such as terazosin (Hytrin, Abbott Laboratories, North Chicago, IL) and doxazosin (Cardura, Roerig Division, Pfizer Pharmaceuticals, New York, NY). Although these agents have been effective in improving urine flow in men with prostatism, side effects similar to those of phenoxybenzamine limit their usefulness in some patients. More recent evidence suggests that the α_1 receptor subtype α_{1A} is the important functional receptor in the smooth muscle of the bladder outlet. This has led to the development of tamsulosin (Flomax, Yamanouchi U.S.A., Inc., White Plains, NY) , which is a specific antagonist of this receptor and has fewer side effects than earlier agents.[19]

However, although the α-adrenergic blocker phenoxybenzamine has been successfully used in prevention of urinary retention in postherniolasty patients,[20] results of studies using α-adrenergic blocking agents to prevent urinary retention in patients undergoing anorectal surgery have been mixed. In the study by Eftaiha et al., the use of oral phenoxybenzamine did not significantly influence the incidence of postoperative urinary retention (20% incidence with phenoxybenzamine versus 22.8% incidence in the control group).[21] Leventhol and Pfau reported success with this medication, although no numerical data were available in their report.[22]

Neural Factors Affecting the Detrusor Muscle

Inhibition of detrusor muscle function is another possible mechanism of urinary retention after anorectal surgery. In an elaborate series of experiments, Pompeius[23] demonstrated an abnormal detrusor function in response to anal pain and dis-

tention. This was believed to be the result of a reflex mechanism involving the pudendal nerve, sacral spinal cord, and pelvic parasympathetic nerves.[23] Additionally, stimulation of pelvic sympathetic nerves is known to have an inhibitory effect on the parasympathetic motor supply to the detrusor.[1]

Although parasympathomimetic agents, particularly bethanechol, have been shown to stimulate detrusor function, studies of clinical usefulness have had mixed results.[24] Reports by Bowers et al.[25] and Eftaiha et al.[21] failed to demonstrate significant improvement in postoperative urinary retention when using this agent after anorectal surgery. However, a prospective, blinded, randomized study by Gottesman et al.[26] on 132 patients with acute posthemorrhoidectomy urinary retention demonstrated a significant reduction in the need for catheterization with the use of bethanechol. In their algorithm, 69% (26 of 38) of the patients receiving bethanechol voided within 30 minutes of the injection, whereas none of the placebo group voided. "Mild reactions, including flushing, excess salivation, and sweating" which lasted 30 minutes or less occurred in 17% of their patients.[26]

Perioperative Fluid Intake

Fluid intake plays a critical role in the development of urinary retention. It is self-evident that the less fluid (oral or intravenous) a patient receives, the less urine the patient will produce, and the longer the period of time after surgery before the bladder will become distended. If urine production can be kept to a minimum until factors causing detrusor or bladder outlet dysfunction subside, urinary retention may be avoided.

The restriction of fluids after anorectal surgery was first championed by Hopping,[27] and many studies have confirmed this therapy.[5,7,12,13,15,25,27–30] Bailey and Ferguson[12] reported a reduction of postoperative urinary retention from 15% to 4% by restricting both intravenous and oral fluids perioperatively. Hoff et al.[5] reported an incidence of urinary retention of 0.53% in their series of 190 consecutive outpatient hemorrhoidectomies using similar fluid restriction.

Perioperative fluid restriction can reduce the production of urine to 20 to 25 mL/h. The desire to void typically occurs at bladder volumes of 250 to

300 mL, with normal bladder capacity being 400 to 500 mL. Therefore, many hours can pass before the patient needs to void the bladder. Additionally, the lack of bladder distention will prevent stretching of the detrusor and the resultant muscle dysfunction.[1]

Pharmacologic Agents

Many pharmacologic agents that are typically used in the perioperative period may contribute to the development of acute postoperative urinary retention. Anticholinergics can block the muscarinic receptors of the detrusor and directly lead to detrusor dysfunction. Atropine is commonly used for anesthetic management in the perioperative period, and urinary retention with this agent is well described. Doyle and Briscoe[31] found that atropine abolished detrusor contractions in some, but not all, patients. Therefore, the effect on urinary retention may vary within a patient population. Scopolamine and many antihistamines are other commonly used medications that may be associated with urinary retention.

Opiate drugs, commonly used for postoperative pain relief, have been shown to decrease detrusor function and to increase urethral sphincter tone.[31] Epidural morphine is a potent analgesic, but it is associated with a high incidence of urinary retention.[32–35] Although the effect of oral narcotic dosing on bladder function is not clear, the possibility that it may contribute to urinary retention must be inferred. As might be expected, the use of the opioid antagonist naloxone is effective in increasing detrusor tone and decreasing urethral sphincter tone. This produces urinary urgency even in patients who have not received exogenous opioids.[36,37]

Several series have implicated spinal anesthesia as a factor in postoperative urinary retention in a large percentage of patients.[15,16] Prasad and Abcarian, however, found no correlation between spinal anesthesia and urinary retention.[7] Spinal anesthesia probably blunts reflex pathways to the structures involved with micturition. Shorter-acting agents, such as lidocaine, are less frequently associated with retention than are longer-acting agents, such as bupivacaine, but even with short-acting agents, the retention rate is substantial.[15]

(*Editor's note:* Spinal anesthesia often produces some degree of sympathetic blockade. A large volume of intravenous fluid may then be administered by the anesthesiologist in an attempt to prevent or treat the hypotension so frequently associated with the sympathectomy. This fluid then leads to early bladder fullness.)

Other Factors

Several other factors in the postoperative period may lead to the development of urinary retention. It often appears that an anxious patient is more prone to develop this complication. Anxiety may be an important element, perhaps by increasing sympathetic discharge or influencing higher cortical centers that modulate micturition. However, the study by Gottesman et al.[26] failed to show any benefit of using diazepam in patients with postoperative urinary retention, although diazepam was given only after retention developed.

Discharging the patient soon after surgery to a less anxiety-producing home environment may also be important.[5] In the comfortable and familiar surroundings of home, the patient has prompt access to oral analgesics and ready access to the sitz bath. In addition, not having a nurse frequently asking about voiding and mentioning catheterization plays a large role in the low rate of urinary retention in our patients.

Pain can contribute in a number of ways to urinary retention. The pudendal nerve not only conveys pain from the anal area, but it also is involved in innervation of the urethral musculature. Pain may thus indirectly stimulate the muscles that produce bladder outlet obstruction. Additionally, pain leads to anxiety, with its attendant sympathetic discharge, and to the use of narcotics for analgesia, both of which are probably important pieces of the puzzle.[5] The role of endogenous endorphin release in postoperative urinary retention is unknown, but it may be a contributing factor, as bladder activity can be induced by naloxone blockade of opioid receptors.[34]

Rectal distention is a known cause of retention. The incidence of urinary retention is high in patients with a fecal impaction. Therefore, the use of rectal packing after surgery should be avoided whenever possible. In the vast majority of anorectal surgery cases, packing of the anal canal or rectum is unnecessary.[16]

Prevention of Urinary Retention

With proper perioperative care, the patient undergoing anorectal surgery faces a minimal risk of postoperative urinary retention. This may be of benefit to the surgeon, who saves a great deal of personal time and worry over his or her patients. The patient obviously benefits, as most are anxious about the possibility of catheterization. The health care system, as a whole, also benefits, as fewer resources are used when a procedure can be performed on an outpatient basis and no postoperative emergency room visit is needed.

Perioperative Fluid Restriction

It is critically important that the patient void before surgery and enter the operating room with a nearly empty bladder. As noted above, many studies have shown that the restriction of fluids in the perioperative period has a significant effect on the incidence of urinary retention. It is sometimes difficult to persuade our anesthesiology colleagues to restrict fluids, as most habitually give the patients liberal intravenous fluids based on the perception that the patient is volume depleted. Obviously, if the patient is hemodynamically unstable, then volume repletion is important. However, this is usually not the case.

A goal of infusing less than 250 mL of intravenous fluids can be achieved in a high percentage of cases. The intravenous fluid infusion should be ordered to start at a minimal rate (20 mL/h) in the preoperative area. In the operating room, fluid boluses may be needed for administration of drugs. If it is difficult for the anesthesiologist to remember to slow infusion rates down after giving the induction medications, then the use of a smaller-volume bag of intravenous fluids, or wasting 500 to 750 mL of a 1000-mL bag in the preoperative area can serve as a reminder to limit fluids. Additionally, the use of a "mini-drip" infusion set can serve as a reminder to minimize fluids.

In the recovery room, the intravenous infusion is decreased to 20 mL/h, and the fluids are stopped as soon as the patient is awake. Very importantly, oral intake of fluids should also be restricted in the postoperative setting until the patient voids satisfactorily for the first time. The time to initial voiding may be 12 to 16 hours after surgery. Once the patient has voided, fluids may be taken *ad libitum*.[5,12]

Pain Management

Another important aspect of postoperative care is the management of pain. Pain increases anxiety and directly interferes with micturition. In the operating room, the perianal area should be liberally infiltrated with a long-acting local anesthetic, such as bupivacaine. This allows the patient to arouse from the anesthetic with less pain, and if the patient is discharged within a few hours after surgery, he or she will have a more comfortable ride home. Once the effect of this local anesthetic dissipates, the patient will be in a comfortable home environment and presumably less anxious.

The patient should be given an oral dose of pain medication, typically propoxyphene napsylate with acetaminophen, just before discharge. This agent can be continued at home and supplemented with ibuprofen. An ice bag is generally applied to the operative site in the recovery room and is continued for 4 to 8 hours postoperatively. The purpose of the ice is to lessen swelling and slow absorption of the local anesthetic. Following this period of time, the patient may begin sitz baths in plain, warm water. The baths are often effective in relieving the muscle spasm associated with surgery. The patient is told that urinating in the bathtub is perfectly acceptable, as the warmth will often relax the urinary sphincter and stimulate the urge to void. A shower is an acceptable alternative. Sitz baths should be continued at least three times a day for 7 days following surgery. Many patients will spend much more time in the sitz bath than suggested because of the comfort it provides.[5]

The intraoperative use of ketorolac (Toradol, Syntex International, Palo Alto, CA) deserves special mention. Ketorolac is a nonsteroidal anti-inflammatory drug that is available in both oral and injectable forms. It can be injected into the anal musculature at the time of surgery, and it acts by blocking prostaglandin production at the site of the pain. At the end of the procedure, 30 to 60 mg of ketorolac is injected into the anal muscles, and studies have shown it to provide effective postoperative pain control. Low rates of urinary retention are associated with ketorolac.[38,39] (*Editor's note:* We have used ketorolac both intramuscularly, as described above, and by the intravenous route and find no difference in pain relief with either technique. Because of the simplicity of administration, we now use the intravenous route.)

Perioperative Nursing Care

Nursing personnel should make every effort to produce an environment that is as comfortable and supportive as possible. Anxiety plays an important role in postoperative urinary retention, and a quiet, calm environment is helpful in its prevention. The nurses in the outpatient surgery department should be educated on the mechanisms of postoperative urinary retention and should attempt to minimize its occurrence as a result of this understanding.

Nurses should be instructed not to continually inquire about the patient's need to void. This will often create anxiety in the patient, and the answer to the question "What will happen if I can't urinate?" ("catheterization") will only serve to further increase the anxiety. If the patient inquires, reassurance should be given that urination will occur and that patience will be needed. Additionally, since many patients will not void for many hours postoperatively if fluids have been properly restricted, the requirement for voiding should be removed from the discharge criteria.

Operative Technique

Good operative technique is important to minimize pain postoperatively. As mentioned above, ketorolac and a long-acting local anesthetic may be injected into the anal muscles intraoperatively for improvement in postoperative pain.

Good surgical technique with a minimal amount of tissue destruction is also important. The use of the electrocautery, particularly in the "coagulation" mode, should be minimized, as this may lead to a great deal of tissue necrosis and subsequent pain and spasm. Tissues should be handled gently to minimize trauma. The use of packing in the rectum or anal canal is rarely necessary and may lead to increased discomfort and a significant risk of urinary retention.

Patient Education

The patient who knows what to expect after surgery is less anxious about the events unfolding before him or her. A detailed oral explanation as well as written material should be given to the patient well in advance of surgery. This information should be reiterated to the patient and family after surgery. The possibility of some difficulty in voiding postoperatively should be briefly mentioned, but not dwelled upon. (For example, the physician could tell the patient, "You may find it difficult to urinate for the first time after surgery, but if you follow these instructions it should not be a problem.")

After surgery the patient and family are informed that fluids may be ingested initially only to take pain medication or keep the mouth moist. After the patient voids, fluids may be taken liberally. The patient and family should be reassured that the patient may not void for some hours and that sitting in a bath of warm water will often allow the patient to void. They should also be instructed that pain and spasm in the operative site and pelvic muscles will give the patient the sensation that the bladder is full, and that the warm baths will often relieve this sensation.

Above all, the patient needs to be reassured that all is well, and that by going home he or she will be more comfortable than at the hospital. Pain medications and sitz baths are more readily available at home, the surroundings are more familiar, and the bed and furniture are more comfortable. The food at home is usually not only better than that at the hospital, but it is also more to the liking of the patient. Reassurance that the surgeon is always available if needed will usually relieve the patient's fear of not being able to contact a health care professional. The program we have outlined will make the outpatient surgery as pleasant as possible and will significantly decrease the risk of urinary retention.[5]

Summary

The fear of postoperative urinary retention after anorectal surgery is to a great degree unfounded. By following a set of simple surgical guidelines, the great majority of anorectal operations can be performed on an ambulatory basis with little fear of this complication. This will result in a more pleasant surgical experience for the patient, will save time and concern for the surgeon, and will save health care dollars for society as a whole.

References

1. Steers W. Physiology of the urinary bladder. In Walsh P, Retik A, Staney T, Vaughan E (eds). Campbell's Urology. Philadelphia: WB Saunders, 1996, pp 142–176.
2. Gosling J. The structure of the bladder and urethra in relation to function. Urol Clin North Am 1979; 6:31–36.
3. Gosling J, Dixon J, Lendon R. the autonomic innervation of the human male and female bladder neck and proximal urethra. J Urol 1977;118:302–305.
4. Merrill D, Conway C, De Wolfe W. Urinary incontinence—treatment with electrical stimulation of the pelvic floor. Urology 1975;5:67–71.
5. Hoff S, Bailey R, Butts D, et al. Ambulatory surgical hemorrhoidectomy—a solution to postoperative urinary retention? Dis Colon Rectum 1994;37: 1242–1244.
6. McConnell J, Khubchandani I. Long-term follow-up of closed hemorrhoidectomy. Dis Colon Rectum 1983;26:797–799.
7. Prasad M, Abcarian H. Urinary retention following operation for benign anorectal diseases. Dis Colon Rectum 1978;21:490–492.
8. Bleday R, Pena J, Rothenberger D, et al. Symptomatic hemorrhoids: current incidence and complications of operative treatment. Dis Colon Rectum 1992;35:477–481.
9. Leff E. Hemorrhoidectomy—laser vs. nonlaser: outpatient surgical experience. Dis Colon Rectum 1991;35:743–746.
10. Wang J, Chang-Chien C, Chen J, et al. The role of lasers in hemorrhoidectomy. Dis Colon Rectum 1991;34:78–82.
11. Campbell E. Prevention of urinary retention after anorectal operations. Dis Colon Rectum 1972;15: 69–70.
12. Bailey HR, Ferguson J. Prevention of urinary retention by fluid restriction following anorectal operations. Dis Colon Rectum 1976;19:250–252.
13. Scoma J. Catheterization in anorectal surgery. Arch Surg 1975;110:1506.
14. Crystal R, Hopping R. Early postoperative complications of anorectal surgery. Dis Colon Rectum 1974;17:336–341.
15. Petros J, Bradley T. Factors influencing postoperative urinary retention in patients undergoing surgery for benign anorectal disease. Am J Surg 1990;159:374–376.
16. Salvati E, Kleckner M. Urinary retention in anorectal and colonic surgery. Am J Surg 1957;94:114–117.
17. Barone J, Cummings K. Etiology of acute urinary retention following benign anorectal surgery. Am Surg 1994;60:210–211.
18. Caine M, Perlberg S, Shapiro A. Phenoxybenzamine for benign prostatic obstruction: review of 200 cases. Urology 1981;17:542–546.
19. Lieber M. Pharmacologic therapy for prostatism. Mayo Clin Proc 1998;73:590–596.
20. Goldman G, Leviav A, Mazor A, et al. Alpha-adrenergic blocker for post hernioplasty urinary retention. Arch Surg 1988;123:35–36.
21. Eftaiha M, Amshel A, Shonberg I. Comparison of two agents in prevention of urinary retention after benign anorectal surgery. Dis Colon Rectum 1980;23: 470–472.
22. Leventhol A, Pfau A. Pharmacologic management of postoperative urinary distention of the bladder. Surg Gynecol Obstet 1976;146:347–348.
23. Pompeius R. Detrusor inhibition induced from anal region in man. Acta Chir Scand Suppl 1966;351:1–54.
24. Finkbeiner A. Is bethanechol chloride clinically effective in promoting bladder emptying? A literature review. J Urol 1985;134:443–449.
25. Bowers F, Hartmann R, Khanduja K, et al. Urecholine prophylaxis for urinary retention in anorectal surgery. Dis Colon Rectum 1980;23:470–472.
26. Gottesman L, Milsom J, Mazier W. The use of anxiolytic and parasympathomimetic agents in the treatment of postoperative urinary retention following anorectal surgery. Dis Colon Rectum 1989;32:867–870.
27. Hopping R. Complications of anorectal surgery: cause and treatment (panel discussion). Dis Colon Rectum 1966;9:159–167.
28. Bernstein W. Anorectal surgery: is urinary retention a necessary complication of anorectal surgery? Minn Med 1966;49:463–466.
29. Campbell E. Prevention of urinary retention after anorectal operations. Dis Colon Rectum 1972;15: 69–73.
30. Campbell M. Urologic complications of anorectal and colon surgery. Am J Proctol 1961;12:43–44.
31. Doyle P, Briscoe C. The effects of drugs and anaesthetic agents on the urinary bladder and sphincters. Br J Urol 1976;48:329–335.
32. Dray A. Epidural opiates and urinary retention: new models provide new insights. Anesthesiology 1988;68:323–324.
33. Evron S, Samueloff A, Simon A, et al. Urinary function during epidural analgesia with methadone and

morphine in post cesarean section patients. Pain 1985;23:135–144.

34. Rawal N, Widman B. An experimental study of urodynamic effects of epidural morphine and naloxone reversal. Anesth Analg 1983;62:641–647.

35. Yaksh T. Spinal opiate analgesia: characteristics and principles of action. Pain 1981;11:293–346.

36. Murray K, Feneley R. Endorphins—a role in lower urinary tract function? The effect of opioid blockade on the detrusor and urethral sphincter mechanisms. Br J Urol 1981;54:638–640.

37. Sandyk R, Gillman M. Naloxone causes urinary urgency. Urology 1986;27:79.

38. O'Donovan S, Ferrara A, Larach S, et al. Intraoperative use of Toradol facilitates outpatient hemorrhoidectomy. Dis Colon Rectum 1994;37:793–799.

39. Richman R. Use of Toradol in anorectal surgery. Dis Colon Rectum 1993;36:295–296.

8

Hemorrhoidectomy

Part A: Open Surgical Hemorrhoidectomy

John T. Isler, M.D., F.A.C.S.

Hemorrhoids are a normal feature of human anorectal anatomy. External hemorrhoids arise from the inferior hemorrhoidal plexus and are covered by modified squamous epithelium distal to the dentate line. They may swell or become thrombosed, resulting in pain, or they may ulcerate with subsequent bleeding. Thrombosis can ultimately resolve or may leave a skin tag that may produce itching, burning, or soilage. Internal hemorrhoids originate from the superior hemorrhoidal plexus and are covered by mucosa proximal to the dentate line. Symptomatic internal hemorrhoids may cause bleeding, swelling, itching, protrusion, discharge, pain, and soilage. Internal hemorrhoids are classified as first, second, third, and fourth degree. When these submucosal vascular cushions do not descend below the dentate line on straining, they are considered first-degree hemorrhoids. Second-degree hemorrhoids protrude below the dentate line on straining and can be seen at the anal verge but reduce spontaneously with cessation of straining. Third-degree internal hemorrhoids protrude beyond the anal verge with straining and require manual reduction to return to the anal canal. Fourth-degree internal hemorrhoids lie permanently beyond the anal verge and return to the outside even after they have been manually reduced.

Symptomatic hemorrhoids affect 4.4% of the population in the United States, of whom approximately one-third present to physicians for evalua-tion.[1] It is recognized that over 90% of symptomatic hemorrhoids can be treated with conservative medical and conservative nonsurgical measures and that surgery should be reserved for only the most severe cases.[2] Although practice parameters have been established,[3] the ultimate judgment regarding surgery must be made by the surgeon in light of the patient's complete clinical presentation. A surgical hemorrhoidectomy is intended to restore the anal canal to normal, or nearly normal, functional and anatomical status. There is no question that excellent results are to be expected when a) the appropriate operation is designed for the patient's particular situation, b) the procedure is performed expertly, and c) the appropriate care is delivered preoperatively, perioperatively, and postoperatively.

Over time, a number of different techniques of hemorrhoidectomy have been described. None of them, however, has become accepted as the gold standard. The surgical principles involve eliminating the prolapsing vascular cushions alone or in combination with relocation of the squamous epithelium, thus reconstructing the anal canal. Until the mid-1950s, the Milligan-Morgan hemorrhoidectomy using scissors resection[4] was the most widely performed surgical procedure for hemorrhoids throughout the world. The procedure was relatively simple and easily taught. Although a well-performed operation provided excellent results, it was considered quite painful. (There was also the suggestion that this kind of "everting excision" led to a slightly higher incidence of stenosis.) Sir Alan Parks in 1956[5] described the submucosal hemorrhoidectomy, which reconstructed the anal canal and therefore was expected to better preserve sensory continence and to reduce postoperative pain. In 1959, Ferguson and Heaton[6] described the closed hemorrhoidectomy technique, which has become known as the Ferguson hemorrhoidectomy. As opposed to surgeons in the United Kingdom, more members of the American Society of Colon and Rectal Surgeons report using a closed rather than an open technique when performing a surgical hemorrhoidectomy.[7]

The open and closed techniques each have their proponents and detractors. Roe et al.[8] could demonstrate no differences in postoperative pain between a submucosal and a ligation excisional hemorrhoidectomy. Although the submucosal hemorrhoidectomy preserved better anal sensation, this fact was not reflected in improved function. Interestingly enough, the excision ligation operation described involved ligation of the hemorrhoid tissue above the dentate line rather than at the level originally described by Milligan and Morgan. Watts et al.[9] considered that an individual's reaction to pain was more important than the technique of operation used. On the other hand, Hosch et al.[10] recently reported a randomized prospective study comparing the Parks and Milligan-Morgan hemorrhoidectomy techniques in which the former procedure was preferred on the basis of minimized postoperative discomfort, reduced hospital stay, and shortened time for return to work.

Diathermy hemorrhoidectomy has been advocated as an alternative to traditional scissor dissection. It has been reported that blood loss and postoperative pain are less using the diathermy technique.[11,12] Andrews et al.[13] found that diathermy hemorrhoidectomy offered no significant advantage over the classic Milligan-Morgan hemorrhoidectomy using scissor dissection. On the other hand, in a larger randomized trial, Seow-Choen et al.[14] reported that diathermy excision of hemorrhoids was faster than scissor dissection, involved less bleeding, and resulted in a significant reduction in the requirement for oral analgesics postoperatively. In a prospective randomized trial of open and closed hemorrhoidectomies, both utilizing diathermy for dissection, Ho et al.[15] reported faster and more reliable wound healing with the open technique.

Patient Preparation

Hemorrhoidal symptoms may present as a manifestation of a number of different medical conditions, and therefore careful evaluation of the patient should be conducted to determine the underlying causes of the patient's complaints. (For the purpose of convenience in this subchapter, the patient will be assigned the male gender). A history should include assessment of the patient's coagulation history, the possibility of immunosuppression, and the rare need for antibiotics for prophylaxis. Whenever possible, a complete examination including anoscopy, flexible sigmoidoscopy, and, if indicated, colonoscopy should be performed before surgery. Preoperative counseling, including a complete explanation of the procedure, is important. The patient should be aware that, although complete healing may not occur for several weeks, he will certainly be back at work and participating in his normal activities before that time. The patient is admitted to the ambulatory surgery unit on the day of the procedure. Bowel preparation involves a single disposable sodium phosphate enema administered several hours preoperatively. The patient who has a concomitant fissure or any other extremely painful anorectal condition is spared the enema. No perineal shaving is necessary and no antibiotics are routinely administered. Ideally the patient is already taking a bulk agent of choice prior to the procedure as part of the conservative management of his hemorrhoidal disease. Minimal intravenous fluids should be administered before induction of anesthesia, and the patient should be encouraged to void before entering the operating room.

Anesthesia

Although open hemorrhoidectomy can be performed under a general, spinal, or caudal anesthetic, intravenous sedation and local anesthesia is preferable. Regardless of the type of anesthesia chosen, a local agent with epinephrine to promote hemostasis and aid in postoperative pain management is administered in all cases.

Technique and Equipment

Once in the operating room, the patient is placed in the prone jack-knife position. A roll is placed beneath the iliac crest as well as beneath the feet and thorax to provide proper support for the patient (Figure 8.1). If a general, spinal, or caudal anesthetic is chosen, it is induced before positioning the patient. Intravenous sedation and local anesthesia are administered after the patient has been positioned. Adhesive tape is used to retract the buttocks and provide adequate exposure of the anal verge. Tilting the head downward completes the position, allowing for an unobstructed view of the anus and the anal canal. This position enables the surgeon to work in the "hands-down" position and to be readily assisted by the nurse or assistant surgeon. Furthermore, blood flows away from rather than into the wound. Although some operators use a fiber-optic headlight, properly positioned overhead lighting is usually sufficient. The perineum is prepared with a suitable agent (such as chlorhexidine gluconate 4%).

Once prepared and draped, the patient is sedated with a combination of agents including midazolam, fentanyl, and propofol. A perianal block is achieved using 20 mL of 0.25% bupivacaine with 1:200,000 epinephrine. A 25-gauge needle is used to inject into the perianal and perirectal tissue through a single puncture on each side of the anus. A fan technique to thoroughly infiltrate the perianal tissues is preferred (Figure 8.2). After satisfactory relaxation of the anal canal has been achieved, a thorough examination is performed using a Sawyer or Hill-Ferguson retractor.

It is critical that the anal canal be thoroughly evaluated before beginning the surgical procedure. This evaluation affords the surgeon an opportunity to identify any additional problems that should be addressed during the operative procedure. Although a three-quadrant hemorrhoidectomy involving the right posterior, right anterior, and left lateral regions is most commonly performed, this is by no means the rule. It is important to remember that only excess hemorrhoidal tissue is removed and as much of the anoderm as possible is preserved, within the confines of an appropriate operation. Inspection of the distal rectal mucosa above the anorectal junction determines if a component of rectal mucosal prolapse requires amputation during the dissection.

At this point, submucosal injections of up to 10 mL of 0.25% bupivacaine with 1:200,000 epinephrine are given in the right posterior, right anterior, and left lateral quadrants. This further injection facilitates the submucosal dissection and aids with hemostasis (Figure 8.3).

Initially, the largest hemorrhoidal complex is identified and isolated with the largest retractor that the anal canal will comfortably accommodate. At this point it is critical that the hemorrhoidal tissue is not grasped and prolapsed from the anal canal, as is

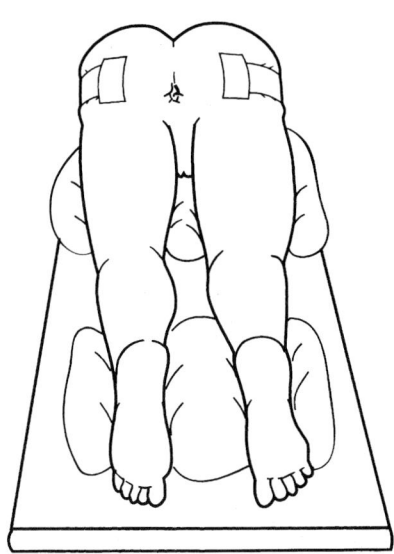

FIGURE 8.1. Prone jack-knife position for open hemorrhoidectomy.

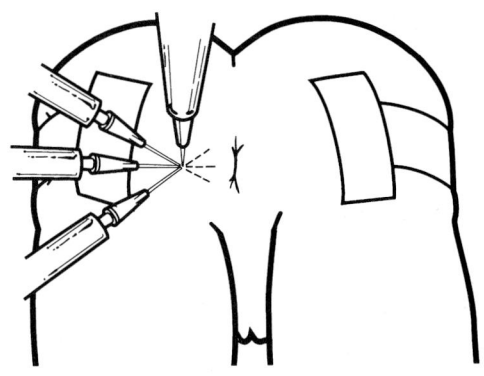

FIGURE 8.2. Fan technique for perianal block using 0.25% bupivacaine with 1:200,000 epinephrine and a 25-gauge needle.

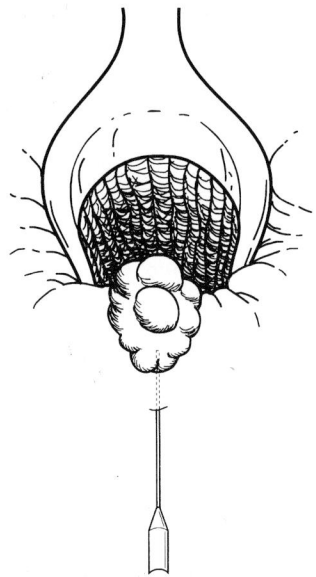

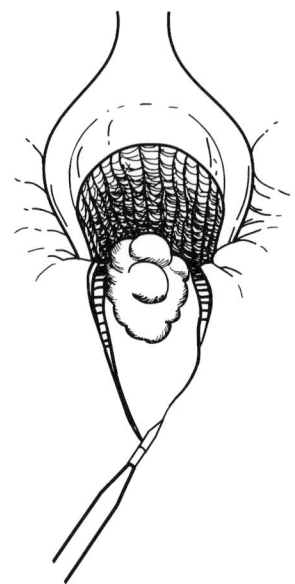

FIGURE 8.3. Submucosal injection of local anesthetic.

FIGURE 8.4. The hemorrhoidal complex is incised to the level of the sphincter and cephalad to the anorectal junction.

often described when performing an open hemorrhoidectomy.[4,8,10,11,13,14] It is important to keep the hemorrhoidal complex in its normal anatomical position. Estimation of the tissue to be excised is gauged by grasping the complex with a forceps or by applying lateral pressure at the edge of the hemorrhoidal complex using the forceps or scalpel handle to demonstrate the mucosal laxity. An elliptical incision is then made around the internal and external hemorrhoidal complex as it lies in its normal anatomical position. For this I use either the scalpel, or more recently, the needlepoint diathermy electrode (in the pure cut mode). The incisions are begun at the anorectal junction and tapered to a V in the perianal skin encompassing the internal hemorrhoids, anoderm, external hemorrhoids, and perianal skin (Figure 8.4). The length of the incision is dependent on the size of the hemorrhoid, with an ideal length-to-width ratio of approximately three to one.

The subsequent dissection is carried out using the needlepoint diathermy electrode (in the pure coagulation mode). The skin, anoderm, hemorrhoidal cushion, and distal rectal mucosa are undermined and excised from the underlying sphincter mechanism and circular muscle of the distal rectum (Figure 8.5). Interestingly enough, the "apical hemor-

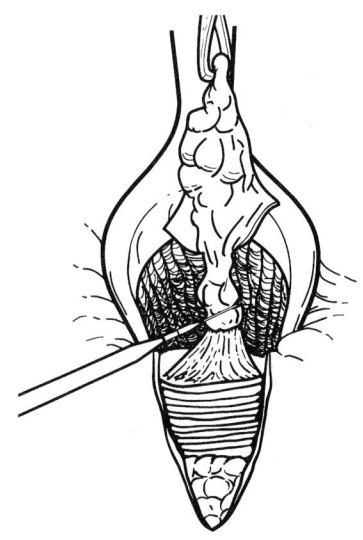

FIGURE 8.5. The hemorrhoidal complex is excised and the "vascular pedicle" amputated with diathermy.

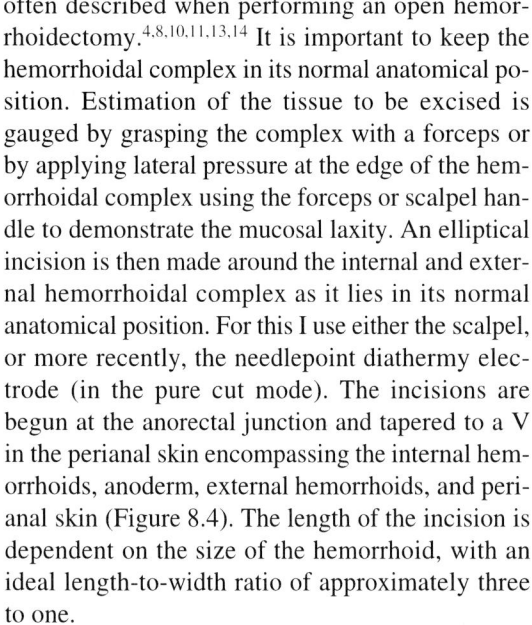

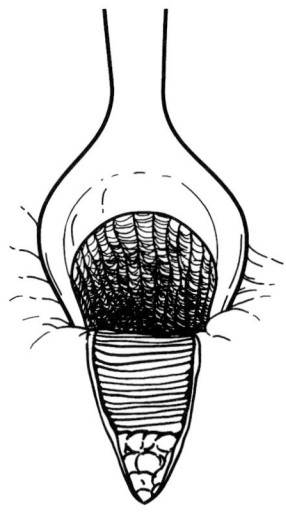

FIGURE 8.6. The open wound.

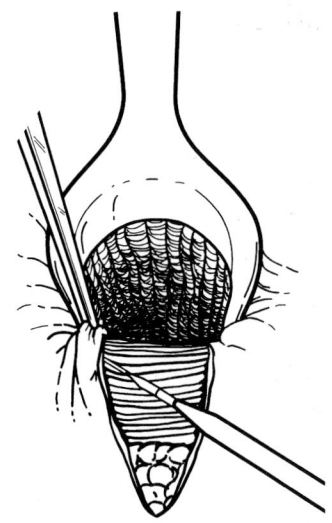

FIGURE 8.7. Accessory hemorrhoidal tissue is excised.

rhoidal pedicle" is often not easily detected as a clear anatomical feature. Routinely, the diathermy electrode is used to transect the "vascular pedicle" without the need of suture ligature. The resulting wound is depicted in Figure 8.6. On rare occasions when hemostasis is not satisfactory, a figure-of-eight ligature of 3–0 polyglycolic acid is used. The ligated tissue lies just above the anorectal junction.

The next largest hemorrhoidal cushion is approached in a similar fashion. Care is always taken to maintain at least 10 mm of anoderm between adjacent hemorrhoidectomy sites. This is facilitated by leaving the hemorrhoidal complex in its anatomical position when gauging the final placement of the incisions.

The same steps are repeated for the third hemorrhoidal complex. At this point, the individual wounds are re-inspected and any accessory hemorrhoidal tissue is excised from the anoderm and the perianal skin. Again, this can be performed with either the scalpel, scissors, or the diathermy electrode (Figure 8.7). It is not necessary to change the size of the retractor to provide exposure, as the surgeon is not narrowing the anal canal with closure of the anoderm.

Sometimes mucosal redundancy is eliminated after a two-quadrant excision and there is no need to perform a three-quadrant hemorrhoidectomy. On these occasions the anoderm is preserved and the diathermy electrode in the coagulation mode is

used to desiccate the hemorrhoidal vessels through the mucosa. Any residual skin tags are removed while carefully avoiding injury to the remaining intervening anoderm. A final inspection of the anal canal is carried out to determine if satisfactory hemostasis has been achieved. A final view of the operative site is shown in Figure 8.8. A small amount of Betadine ointment (Purdue-Frederick, Norwalk, CT) is applied, followed by a gauze pad placed at the anal verge.

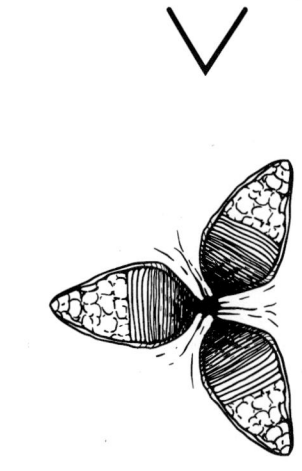

FIGURE 8.8. Final appearance of wounds after open hemorrhoidectomy.

Postoperative Care

When the procedure is performed under a local anesthetic with intravenous sedation, the patient is routinely alert enough to be taken directly back to the ambulatory care unit. In the case of a general or spinal anesthetic which has not worn off, the patient is taken to the postanesthesia care unit first before transfer to the ambulatory care unit. The patient is sent home with a printed instruction sheet specifically addressing his concerns regarding diet, activity, wound care, pain management, and guidelines for calling the office.

The patient is advised to rest for the remainder of the day of surgery but to be up and about without restrictions the following day. The patient is instructed to take ibuprofen regularly (600 mg three times a day) and to use oxycodone with acetaminophen for breakthrough pain. He is encouraged to resume a regular diet and to drink at least three glasses of water daily in addition to his regular beverages. The use of a "bulking agent" such as psyllium, methylcellulose, or calcium polycarbophil is expected. The patient is encouraged to move his bowels and advised to take milk of magnesia if he has not experienced a bowel movement in 2 days. The patient is advised to soak the anal area in a tub of plain warm water for 15 to 20 minutes two to three times a day for the first week and thereafter once or twice a day until complete healing has occurred. If the patient experiences difficulty urinating, voiding in the tub is suggested. The patient is seen in follow-up 3 weeks after surgery and then subsequently in 2 months.

Special Circumstances

When the patient has additional anorectal pathology, the appropriate surgical technique is applied. In the case of an anal fissure, a lateral internal sphincterotomy is performed, and for an anal fistula, a fistulotomy is performed. A transanal rectocele repair can also be included with an open hemorrhoidectomy.

A hemorrhoidal crisis consists of acutely incapacitating prolapsed, thrombosed, and strangulated hemorrhoids involving one, two, or all three primary complexes. I employ an open hemorrhoidec-

tomy in the same fashion as has just been described. An important point to remember is that after injection of the local anesthetic with epinephrine, gentle pressure steadily applied to the hemorrhoidal masses for 5 minutes results in considerable shrinkage of the tissue, usually allowing for reduction of the prolapsing tissue into the anal canal. This permits a more accurate assessment of the amount of tissue and anoderm that can be removed.

The same technique is used for HIV-positive patients. Hewitt et al.[16] reported no significant difference in wound healing time, regardless of HIV status, for wounds that are left open or closed, or between patients who have had one-, two-, or three-quadrant hemorrhoidectomy performed. There was no difference in overall complication rates between HIV-positive and HIV-negative patient groups.

In the rare circumstance when the patient is pregnant, especially when she is in the third trimester, the left lateral decubitus position described by Ferguson and Heaton[6] allows for a comfortable patient, appropriate fetal monitoring, and satisfactory exposure.

Posthemorrhoidectomy Complications

Pain

Although pain is not technically a postoperative complication, it is clearly the single most important reason that people avoid hemorrhoidectomy. Postoperative pain management is dealt with in Chapter 6, but there are a few points that should be emphasized here. It is evident from various studies that the pain experienced after hemorrhoidectomy is extremely patient dependent. Since reflex spasm of the internal sphincter is considered to be the main cause of postoperative pain, several variations of hemorrhoidectomy have been reported. Mortenson et al.[17] combined hemorrhoidectomy with anal dilatation and noted only an increased risk of continence disturbances. Although some report no predisposition to incontinence after the addition of lateral internal sphincterotomy,[18] others have noted decreased resting and squeeze anal canal pressures and slightly increased incontinence.[14] Asfar et al.[19] felt that sphincterotomy was superior to anal stretch in reducing pain after hemorrhoidectomy. There are no studies that clearly demonstrate the utility of an internal anal sphincterotomy concomitant with hemorrhoidectomy unless the patient also has a fissure. The most effective method to manage post-hemorrhoidectomy pain is the frequent administration of narcotic analgesics given in adequate doses.

Early Complications

Postoperative complications after open or closed hemorrhoidectomy are comparable.[2,7,15,16,20] Complications occurring within the first 1 to 2 postoperative days include urinary retention, bleeding, soft fecal impaction, and itching. Urinary retention is discussed in Chapter 7 and will not be addressed here. Despite a well-performed surgical procedure, a finite number of patients will experience bleeding in the immediate postoperative period. The incidence of this after open hemorrhoidectomy approximates 1%. Although perianal itching is often the result of drainage from the open wounds, one should be alert to the frequent overzealous use of petroleum jelly and other ointments by the patient.

Late Complications

Late complications of hemorrhoidectomy include urinary tract infection following catheterization, recurrent fecal impaction, secondary bleeding, superficial wound infection, anal stenosis, formation of skin tags, anal fissure, and incontinence. The incidence of secondary hemorrhage (occurring between the seventh and twelfth post-operative day) after the Milligan-Morgan technique approximates 1.5%. Because open hemorrhoidectomy leaves wide external wounds, superficial wound infections and abscesses are uncommon. Edema of the perianal skin adjacent to hemorrhoidectomy wounds may result in skin tags, which initially can be quite painful. In the more chronic situation, skin tags are rarely painful and can be usually dealt with in the office. This has been reported to occur in up to 4% of patients after excision ligation. Anal fissure and anal stenosis should rarely occur, provided that adequate mucosal and anoderm bridges are maintained between excision sites. There does not appear to be any difference in the incidence of transient incontinence between open and closed techniques. As Roe et al.[8] pointed out in a controlled study comparing submucosal hemorrhoidectomy and excision ligation, although 50% of patients complain of soiling in the early postoperative period, only two patients in each group complained of frank incontinence, and all minor disturbances of continence had resolved in all patients by 6 weeks.

Summary

As many readers will recognize, several of the key features of the open technique we have described are identical to those of the Ferguson closed hemorrhoidectomy. The concept of maintaining the normal anatomical position of the hemorrhoidal cushions, especially when planning the placement of the elliptical incisions, is very important. Secondly, it should be stressed that only excess hemorrhoidal tissue is removed and the anoderm is preserved as much as possible within the confines of an appropriate operation. These points are crucial to restore the anal canal to normal or nearly normal functional and anatomical status. The utility of the needlepoint diathermy electrode for dissection lends itself to this operation. Finally, the importance of preoperative counseling and coordinated postoperative care and support cannot be understated.

References

1. Johanson J, Sonnenberg A. The prevalence of hemorrhoids and chronic constipation, an epidemiologic study. Gastroenterology 1990;98:380–386.
2. Bleday R, Pena J, Rothenberger D, et al. Symptomatic hemorrhoids current incidence and complications of operative therapy. Dis Colon Rectum 1992;35:477–481.
3. American Society of Colon and Rectal Surgeons. Standards taskforce practice parameters for the treatment of hemorrhoids. Dis Colon Rectum 1993;3:1118–1120.
4. Milligan E, Morgan C, Jones L, et al. Surgical anatomy of the anal canal and operative treatment of haemorrhoids. Lancet 1937;1119–1124.
5. Parks A. The surgical treatment of hemorrhoids. Br J Surg 1956;43:337–351.
6. Ferguson J, Heaton J. Closed hemorrhoidectomy. Dis Colon Rectum 1959;2:176–179.
7. Wolf J, Munoz J, Rosin J, et al. Survey of hemorrhoidectomy practices: open versus closed techniques. Dis Colon Rectum 1979; 22:536–538.
8. Roe A, Bartolo D, Vellacott K, et al. Submucosal versus ligation excision haemorrhoidectomy: a comparison of anal sensation, anal sphincter manometry

and post-operative pain function. Br J Surg 1987;74:948–995.

9. Watts J, Bennett R, Duthie H, et al. Healing and pain after haemorrhoidectomy. Br J Surg 1964;51: 808–817.

10. Hosch S, Knoefel W, Pichlmeier U, et al. Surgical treatment of piles. Prospective, randomized study of Parks vs. Milligan-Morgan hemorrhoidectomy. Dis Colon Rectum 1998;41:160–164.

11. Sharif H, Lee L, Alexander-Williams J, et al. How I do it: diathermy haemorrhoidectomy. Int J Colorectal Dis 1991;6:217–219.

12. Lentini J, Leveroni J, Taure C, et al. Twenty five years experience with the high frequency transistorized loop with special reference to haemorrhoidectomy without suture. Coloproctology 1990;4:239–249.

13. Andrews B, Layer G, Jackson B, et al. Randomized trial comparing diathermy hemorrhoidectomy with the scissor dissection Milligan-Morgan operation. Dis Colon Rectum 1993;36:580–583.

14. Seow-Choen F, Ho Y, Ang H, et al. Prospective randomized trial comparing pain and clinical function after conventional scissors excision/ligation vs. diathermy excision without ligation for symptomatic prolapsed hemorrhoids. Dis Colon Rectum 1992;35:1165–1169.

15. Ho Y, Seow-Choen F, Tan M, et al. Randomized controlled trial of open and closed hemorrhoidectomy. Br J Surg 1997;84:1729–1730.

16. Hewitt W, Sohol T, Fleshner P, et al. Should HIV status alter induration for hemorrhoidectomy? Dis Colon Rectum 1996;39:615–618.

17. Mortenson P, Olsen J, Pederson I, et al. A randomized study on hemorrhoidectomy combined with anal dilatation. Dis Colon Rectum 1987;030:755–757.

18. Mathai V, Ong B, Ho Y, et al. Randomized controlled trial of lateral internal sphincterotomy with haemorrhoidectomy. Br J Surg 1996;83:380–382.

19. Asfar S, Juma T, Ala-Edeen T, et al. Hemorrhoidectomy and sphincterotomy: a prospective study comparing the effectiveness of anal stretch and sphincterotomy in reducing pain after hemorrhoidectomy. Dis Colon Rectum 1988;31:181–185.

20. McConnell J, Khubchandani I. Long-term follow-up of closed hemorrhoidectomy. Dis Colon Rectum 1983;26:797–799.

Part B: Closed Hemorrhoidectomy

John M. MacKeigan, M.D., F.R.C.S.(C.), F.A.C.S.

The closed hemorrhoidectomy has been practiced for over 50 years with consistent results.[1,2] The size of hemorrhoids or the degree of their prolapse does not always correlate with the degree of symptoms. Small, actively bleeding hemorrhoids that do not prolapse may be equally or more troublesome than large, prolapsing hemorrhoids that reduce spontaneously. Large internal hemorrhoids with no prolapse, but marked friability may be seen with hypertonic anal sphincters. Small internal hemorrhoids with a large ring of perianal skin tags and significant mucosal prolapse may be seen with anal sphincter hypotonia. Such diversity of anatomy and symptoms requires judgment in choosing the appropriate therapy. A well-conceived, properly executed anatomical operation may correct most forms of hemorrhoidal symptoms but may represent overtreatment and result in significant patient dissatisfaction.

There are few procedures in anorectal surgery that cause more disagreement than the advantages and disadvantages of various forms of surgical therapy for hemorrhoids. The results of different forms of therapy naturally depend on the expertise of the operator. No procedure is comfortably performed by all surgeons. Even comparative studies of techniques are weighted toward the usual procedure performed by the surgeon seeking the result.

The goal of any surgical procedure must be to reestablish normal anatomy in a well-functioning anal canal. This involves completely excising the prominent internal hemorrhoidal tissue while preserving as much of the anal canal lining as possible, thus maintaining pliability and preventing stenosis.

The resulting anus must be skin-lined and pliable to be dry and comfortable. Ectropion of mucosa, such as that seen in an improperly done Whitehead operation, produces a "wet anus" with constant mucus secretion. The wounds should heal in a reasonable time with minimal pain, discomfort, and scar formation. The operative procedures for hemorrhoids are all excisional methods with various ways of addressing the vascular pedicles or different techniques of wound closure.

The closed hemorrhoidectomy was first described in 1959 by Ferguson and Heaton[1] and involves the excision of the hemorrhoidal tissue with total anatomical reconstruction of a normal anal canal. The principles of hemorrhoidal surgery are exemplified in the closed technique.[3] Vascular pads or hemorrhoids are removed with preservation of anal skin and mucosa. All incisions are primarily closed and generally heal quickly, resulting in an anal canal that is smooth and pliable.

Anesthetic

The procedure is usually performed under light, monitored sedation or anesthesia. Various agents are used depending on anesthetic preference. Generally, midazolam and/or droperidol are used as amnestic agents. Induction may be undertaken with propofol or sodium thiopental. The anesthetic agents are synergistic and are given in small doses. They are titrated to provide a level of consciousness with retention of spontaneous ventilation. The procedure is done with an anesthesiologist and appropriate cardiopulmonary monitoring. The surgeon administers local anesthetic, 1% or 2% lidocaine or 0.25% to 0.5% bupivacaine with 1:200,000 epinephrine, into the perianal tissues. Spinal anesthetics may be used according to patient preference or choice of the anesthesia personnel.

Position

We prefer the modified left lateral position (Sims' position) (see Figure 4.6) for most anorectal procedures, but the procedure is equally adaptable to the lithotomy or prone jack-knife position. The patient is placed on the left side, angling the body across the table. The left shoulder is placed near the opposite side of the table, and the hips and buttocks are placed close to the edge of the table. The right shoulder is rolled forward with the arm on a pillow. The hips and buttocks are placed just cephalad of the break in the table near the foot end. The legs are both bent at right angles at the hip and knees and wrapped together in a sheet. The sheet is tucked under the table mattress to maintain position. The right buttock may be taped with wide adhesive to the opposite side of the table to assist exposure of the anus.

The table is placed in a slightly head-down position with a slight lateral roll away from the operator. The foot portion of the table is placed parallel to the floor. The anus is sprayed with povidone iodine and draped in a sterile fashion.

Operation

Excisional hemorrhoidectomy is performed less often in recent years because of improved office treatment of internal hemorrhoids. The operation is well tolerated, and most patients are discharged the same or the next day. Significant distortion of anatomy, failure of elastic banding, extensive mucosal prolapse, or severe acute thrombosis are the most common indications for hemorrhoidectomy. In many instances, one or two hemorrhoids alone may be excised, treating only the symptomatic condition.

The goal of the surgery is to remove the symptomatic disease and leave the anus physiologically normal. Hemorrhoids are operated on in situ with no distortion of the anatomy and no eversion of the lining. A Hill-Ferguson retractor is used to approximate the normal size of the anal canal.

Local anesthetic with epinephrine is injected with a 25-gauge spinal needle. It is injected subcutaneously on either side of the anus, then into the ischioanal fossa in a field pattern. A portion may be injected subcutaneously and submucosally in each of the primary hemorrhoidal sites. Approximately 15 to 20 mL of agent is used, generally 0.25% bupivacaine (Marcaine, Sterling Winthrop, Inc., New York, NY) with 1:200,000 epinephrine. The tissue is compressed with gauze to reduce the swelling of the injection. The use of epinephrine helps reduce swelling and minimizes blood loss. (*Editor's note:* The addition of hyaluronidase to local anesthetic may allow more rapid diffusion of the solution into the tissues with less tissue edema and more rapid onset of the action of the anesthetic.)

The Hill-Ferguson retractor (large) or a lighted version is utilized. The operating lights are brought over the right shoulder of the surgeon. The assistant stands at the end of the table, using the foot portion as a tray to hold the few instruments (curved Mayo scissors, Buie clamp, Allis clamp, suction, and cautery). Another assistant, standing on the opposite side of the table, holds the retractor and the buttock.

The hemorrhoid to be excised is isolated, an elliptical incision is made from the mucocutaneous junction distally, carrying the incision well out into the perianal skin (Figure 8.9 **A** and **B**). The incisions are deepened down to the internal sphincter muscle. If the hemorrhoid is broad, narrow incisions are made over the prominence of the hemorrhoid tissue. The distal apex of the incision is grasped with forceps or Allis clamp. The tissue is excised off the subcutaneous external sphincter and internal sphincter muscles. The incisions are carried proximally above the anorectal junction. The pedicle is amputated or clamped with a Buie clamp and amputated distal to the clamp (Figure 8.9 **C**). All incisions are kept relatively narrow to preserve the squamous epithelium or anoderm. With large circumferential hemorrhoids, the procedure is performed in the same fashion.

A figure-of-eight suture is placed at the proximal apex, or suture is run under the Buie clamp and tied

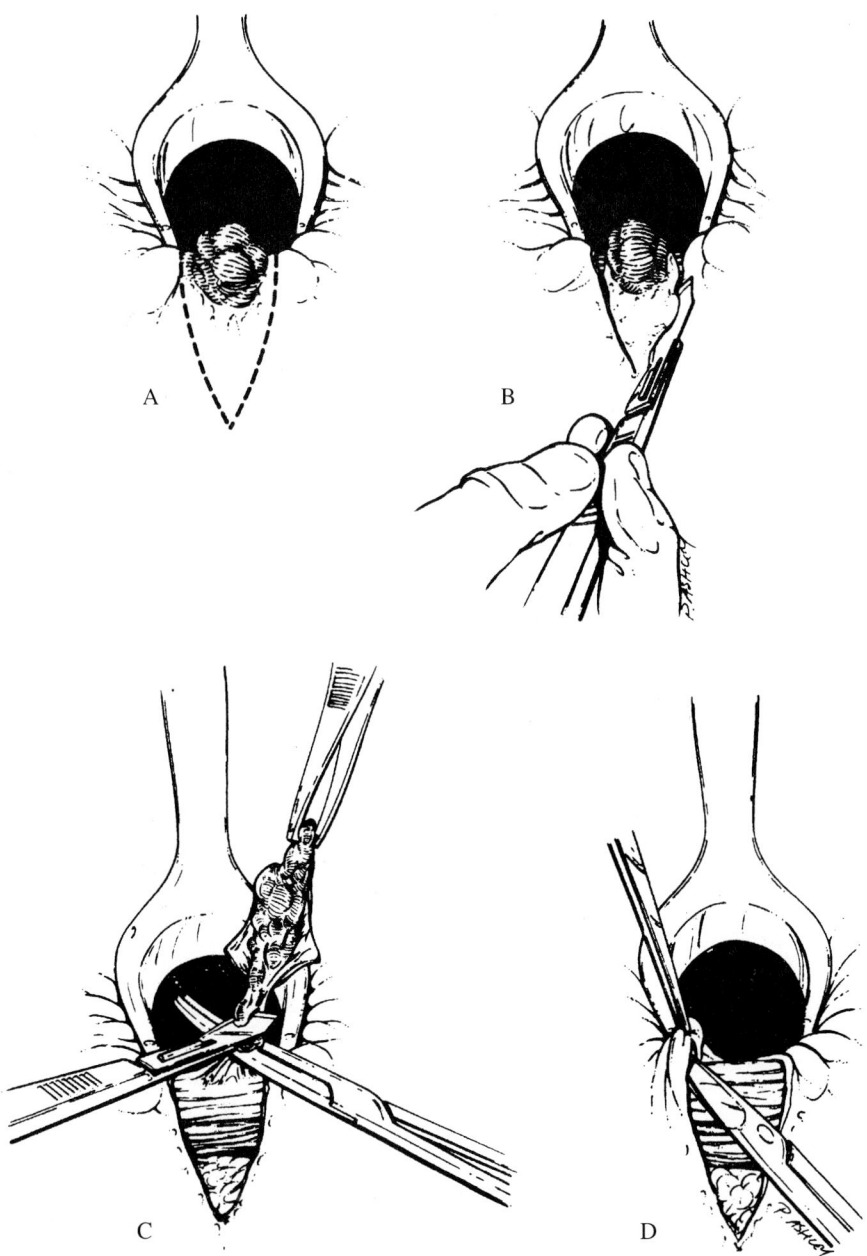

FIGURE 8.9. The Ferguson closed hemorrhoidectomy. **A**, The amount of tissue to be excised is outlined. **B**, The hemorrhoidal complex is incised to the level of the internal sphincter and superiorly to the anorectal ring. **C**, Hemorrhoidal tissue is excised and the pedicle secured. **D**, Anoderm and perianal skin are sharply undermined and accessory hemorrhoidal tissue is excised.

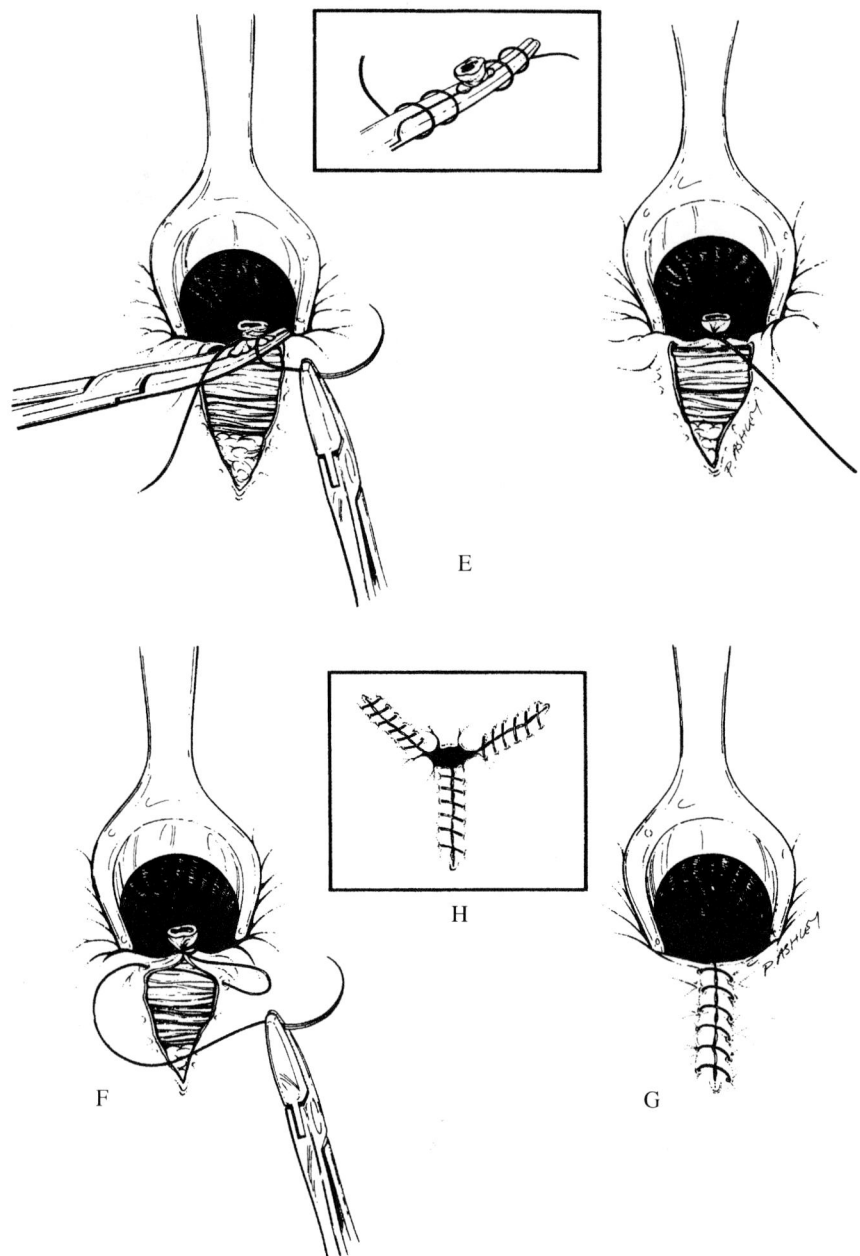

FIGURE 8.9. The Ferguson closed hemorrhoidectomy (*continued*). **E**, The hemorrhoidal pedicle is secured with a suture if necessary. **F**, A running suture closes the wounds. **G**, The wound is secured without excessive tension. **H**, The sutured wounds are properly separated. Reprinted with permission from Mazier WP.[3]

(Figure 8.9 **E**). The suture is generally 4–0 or 5–0 polyglycolic acid. Residual hemorrhoidal tissue on either side of the incised portion is removed. The mucosa and anoderm are elevated off the internal sphincter with scissors while grasping the tissue with forceps (Figure 8.9 **D**). Hemorrhoidal tissue is then trimmed from beneath the skin and mucosa. The incision is closed with a continuous suture. The suture may be tied once or twice further as it is sutured distally for hemostasis. The skin is approximated and the suture line is completed (Figure 8.9 **F** and **G**).

All three incisions are treated in a similar fashion. Care is taken to separate the incisions from one another and to keep the pedicles separated above the anorectal ring. The incisions are inspected closely and re-sutured at sites of residual bleeding. All suturing is done without traction of the pedicle. Forceps are used to push on the sphincter muscle to allow easier access to the pedicle and proximal portion of the wound. Residual skin tags between incisions may be amputated, generally transversely, and closed with suture. During closure of wounds, the anoderm may be moved in or out of the canal to fashion the tissue properly and to approximate the mucocutaneous junction.

The wounds are inspected for bleeding. The anus should comfortably accept the medium or large Hill-Ferguson retractor upon completion of the hemorrhoidectomy. A gauze dressing is applied on the outside. Occasionally, a portion of oxidized cellulose gauze is placed on the suture line in the anal canal for hemostasis. No packing of the anus is performed. In general, the hemorrhoids are excised without distortion, traction, and excessive dilation by retractors.

Combined Hemorrhoid Therapies

It is common to have one or two enlarged hemorrhoids requiring surgical excision, with no treatment or nonresective management optimal for the remaining hemorrhoids. We often combine treatments with excision of some hemorrhoids and rubber band ligation or infrared coagulation of the other hemorrhoids at the same time. Patients receive excisional therapy for only the largest, prolapsing hemorrhoids. Patients have less pain when only one or two excisions are necessary.

Severe Thrombosed Hemorrhoids and Mucosal Prolapse

Large, circumferential, prolapsing thrombosed hemorrhoids or severe circumferential mucosal prolapse without thrombosis are both adaptable to the three-quadrant closed hemorrhoidectomy technique. The principles of narrow elliptical excision of the primary sites is critical. Undermining and excising remaining hemorrhoidal tissue on either side

of the ellipse completes the dissection. The anal lining is preserved and closed as described. If there is tension or inability to approximate the tissue with a medium (and preferably large) Hill-Ferguson retractor in place, then too much tissue may have been elliptically excised. The lining is then sutured and reduced back into the canal in its anatomical position while closing the wounds. Tissue that may appear "gangrenous" is generally only superficially necrotic, and there is almost always good blood supply to the deeper tissue.

Complications

Bleeding in the first 24 hours after the procedure, if not visible externally, is generally from the pedicle. Bleeding also occurs later, most commonly between the fifth and tenth postoperative day. While there are many treatments advocated, the finding of clots or a large volume of blood mandates a return to the operating room with evacuation of clots and oversewing of the pedicle or incisions.

Pain and increased swelling after the first 48 hours is an abscess until proven otherwise. This may require an anesthetic to properly diagnose or drain a submucosal or subcutaneous collection.

Urinary retention is reduced with fluid restriction at the time of surgery and in the immediate postoperative period, along with early discharge and outpatient treatment. Male sex, increased age of the patient, and the need for hospitalization are the most common associated factors for urinary retention. (Urinary retention is discussed in detail in Chapter 7.)

Postoperative Care

Patients may receive ketorolac intravenously at the time of the procedure. In the recovery phase, they generally have no pain for 6 to 8 hours because of the local anesthetic.

Patients are encouraged to take the pain medication (hydrocodone or propoxyphene napsylate) regularly the first few days. Ice packs applied to the perineum are used for the first 2 days. Warm sitz baths for 15 to 20 minutes, twice daily, are begun the first postoperative day. Bowel movement is promoted the first 1 to 2 days by prescribing milk of magnesia or similar medication. Hydrophilic stool softeners (1 Tbsp twice a day) such as psyllium or methylcellulose are also used. Patients are instructed to return early for any problems with voiding, excessive bleeding, or increasing pain.

Summary

The closed hemorrhoidectomy technique as originally described has changed little. Improvements in anesthesia and pain control have allowed most patients to be treated on an outpatient basis or 24-hour stay. The technique is adaptable to most common positions. Some surgeons prefer to leave external wounds open, closing only the anal component. Excision using laser or cautery is possible with this technique but does little to improve healing, pain control, or blood loss. The utility and adaptability of the closed hemorrhoidectomy are the reasons this procedure has stood the test of time.

References

1. Ferguson JA, Heaton JR. Closed hemorrhoidectomy. Dis Colon Rectum 1959;2:176–179.
2. Ferguson JA, Mazier WP, Ganchrow MI, et al. The closed technique of hemorrhoidectomy. Surgery 1971;70:480–484.
3. Mazier WP. Hemorrhoids. In Mazier WP et al. (eds). Surgery of the Colon, Rectum, and Anus. Philadelphia: WB Saunders, 1995, pp 229–254.

9

Anal Fissure

Ernest D. Graves III, M.D., F.A.C.S.

Anal fissure is a common problem and a frequent cause of anal pain. The pain is often severe enough to result in disability far out of proportion to the size of the lesion. The frequency of occurrence of anal fissure and the extent of pain and disability make this lesion a very significant problem indeed.

Anal fissure occurs with equal frequency in both sexes. Although it is more common in young and middle-aged adults, anal fissure occurs in all age groups[1] and is the most common cause of rectal bleeding in infants.[2]

Etiology

Anal fissure has traditionally been attributed to constipation and the passage of hard stool. It is now, however, apparent that the causes are many and complex and that only a minority of patients can in fact recall a causative episode of constipation or straining at hard stool.[3] Anal fissure can be associated with diarrhea, inflammatory bowel disease, and trauma. It has also been noted in association with a number of infectious conditions, including syphilis, genital herpes,[4] and tuberculosis.[5] Accurate diagnosis of the underlying cause of anal fissure resulting from such infections calls for a high index of suspicion. The effect of diet on the etiology of anal fissure has also been studied. For example, when Jensen[6] reviewed the dietary habits of 174 patients with chronic anal fissure and compared them to control subjects, he found that increased risk was associated with a diet characterized by white bread, sauces based on a roux, bacon, and sausage. Conversely, a diet characterized by a high fiber intake (raw fruits, vegetables,

and whole-grain bread) was associated with a decreased risk of anal fissure.[6] Ahmed and Thomson[7] identified an increased risk of anal fissure in those who skip breakfast as opposed to those who do not.[7]

The interest in the relationship between anal canal pressure and anal fissure is reflected by a plethora of reports in the past several years. Keck and associates[8] performed manometry on patients with anal fissure as well as on control patients. The manometric findings were then used to construct computer-generated longitudinal and cross-sectional profiles of the anal canal. The authors found that the mean maximum resting pressure was significantly higher in patients with anal fissure than it was in control subjects and that this hypertonia was unrelated to the presence or absence of pain.[8] Williams and colleagues,[9] performing anal manometry on patients with fissure and control subjects, also found significantly increased mean resting pressure associated with fissure. When manometry was repeated 1 week after lateral sphincterotomy, mean resting pressure had decreased significantly. This decrease was maintained when manometry was repeated 6 weeks after sphincterotomy.[9] When Lund and Scholefield[10] studied anal canal pressures in patients before and after treatment with glyceryl trinitrate applied topically to the anus, treatment resulted in healing of fissures and a significant decrease in the maximum anal resting pressure. Because the decrease was not maintained after cessation of treatment, and some of the treated patients had recurrent symptoms once their anal hypertonicity returned, the investigators concluded that anal hypertonicity may be causative in the pathogenesis of anal fissure.[10]

Ischemia of the anal mucosa is also thought to be involved in the etiology of anal fissure and may explain the lesion's tendency to occur in the posterior midline of the anal canal. To test this hypothesis, Schouten et al.[11] simultaneously studied microvascular perfusion of the anoderm and anal pressures in 27 patients with anal fissure. Compared to controls, mean maximum anal resting pressure in such patients was significantly higher and anodermal blood flow in the posterior anal midline was significantly decreased. Six weeks after sphincterotomy and healing of the fissure, a significant decrease in pressure was noted, along with a consistent rise in blood flow to the former fissure site. These authors concluded that internal sphincter hypertonicity decreases blood flow to the posterior anal midline. They also noted that reduction of anal pressure by sphincterotomy results in healing of the fissure as a result of improving anodermal blood flow to the posterior midline.[11] Work by the same authors, as well as others, has demonstrated that the posterior midline is less richly vascular than other areas of the anus.[12,13]

It is clear, then, that the etiology of anal fissure is far more complex than simple splitting of the mucosa by a hard fecal bolus. Delineation of the various factors described above has led to investigation into new pharmacologic modalities of treatment, which are discussed below.

Symptoms and Clinical Presentation

The hallmark symptoms of anal fissure are pain and bleeding. The pain typically occurs with defecation, gradually subsiding over minutes to hours. The pain is often very severe and may even be temporarily debilitating. It is consistently described as a sharp, stabbing, tearing or ripping sensation. Some patients have rather graphically described the sensation (expletives deleted for publication) as that of evacuating pieces of broken glass. Pain is not inevitably present, however. In a review of 876 patients with anal fissure, Hananel and Gordon[3] found that about 9% of patients had no pain with defecation, and bleeding or pruritus was their presenting complaint.[3]

Bleeding, characterized as bright red and fresh in appearance, is scanty and, like pain, is a frequent but not constant complaint. In the series of patients

described above by Hananel and Gordon, 71.5% of patients presented with bleeding.[3]

The generally discredited theory of constipation as the cause of anal fissure has already been discussed. Frequently, however, patients become constipated after the pain of anal fissure is established. Fear of the pain associated with the fissure can result in refusal to defecate. The ultimate result may be impaction, particularly in children and the elderly.[2]

The large majority of anal fissures occur in the posterior midline of the anal canal, probably related to the relationship between anal hypertonicity and ischemia as described above. The previous conventional wisdom was that this held true for all but about 10% of women and 1% of men.[1,2] However, in their large series of patients, Hananel and Gordon found that 25.1% of women and 7.8% of men had anterior midline anal fissures. Fissures were present both anteriorly and posteriorly in 2.6% of their patients.[3] If fissures are located off the midline, this finding should trigger a high index of suspicion of inflammatory bowel disease, infectious causes, or trauma.

Signs of chronicity of the fissure are development of a skin tag (sentinel pile) at the distal margin of the lesion and a hypertrophic anal papilla at the proximal margin. The circular muscle fibers of the internal anal sphincter may also be visible in the base of the fissure. Once these signs of chronicity are present, operative intervention will frequently be necessary (Figure 9.1).

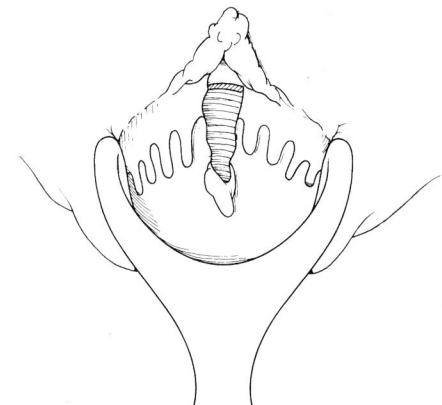

FIGURE 9.1. Appearance of chronic anal fissure with sentinel tag at the distal margin of the fissure and the anal papilla. Note the presence of fibers of the internal sphincter in the base of the chronic fissure. Redrawn from Corman.[2]

Nonoperative Treatment

Acute, superficial fissures of recent onset usually respond well to nonsurgical therapy. Patients are advised to follow a high-fiber diet and to increase their oral fluid intake. Psyllium or methylcellulose fiber supplementation and stool softeners may also be helpful. Patients who are compliant with this advice generally achieve more regular evacuation of formed but soft stool. Patients almost universally appreciate the soothing effect of sitz baths, and compliance with this recommendation is rarely difficult to achieve. A large number of commercially available creams and ointments are available, either by prescription or over-the-counter purchase, for topical application. There is a great deal of controversy regarding the usefulness of these topical agents, but those including local anesthetics may be the most useful.

In the past several years the emerging understanding of the roles of anal sphincter hypertonicity and anal mucosal ischemia has resulted in the treatment of anal fissure with new pharmacologic modalities. That a great deal of interest and investigation have ensued is reflected by the large number of reports in the recent pertinent literature. These new modalities will undoubtedly contribute greatly to the future treatment of anal fissure.

Botulinum Toxin

Infiltration of the internal anal sphincter with botulinum toxin, which prevents the release of acetylcholine from presynaptic nerve terminals,[14] results in temporary paralysis of the muscle for several months and a measurable decrease in anal pressure. To evaluate this effect, Maria et al.[15] carried out a double-blind, placebo-controlled study of 30 patients. The treatment group consisted of 15 patients who underwent infiltration of the internal anal sphincter with botulinum toxin; the 15 patients in the control group were infiltrated with saline. At 2-month follow-up, 11 of the treated patients, compared with only 2 in the control group, had healed ($P = 0.003$). Thirteen of the treated patients, compared with 4 in the control group, had achieved symptomatic relief ($P = 0.003$). Resting and maximum voluntary pressures were measured at baseline and after treatment or saline injection. In both groups the maximum voluntary pressure remained

the same. In patients treated with botulinum toxin, the resting pressure decreased by 25% compared to baseline; this decrease did not occur in the control group. The investigators concluded that infiltration of the internal anal sphincter with botulinum toxin is effective treatment for chronic anal fissure.[15]

Mason and colleagues,[16] measuring anal pressures in 5 patients with anal fissure after infiltration of the internal anal sphincter with botulinum toxin, achieved similar results. They noted a mean decrease in maximum resting anal pressure of 23.3 cm H_2O, with no alteration of maximum voluntary squeeze pressure. Of their patients, 3 had their fissures heal, and the other 2 were symptomatically improved. None of the 5 patients suffered adverse effects.[16]

In another study of botulinum toxin, Jost[17] reported 100 consecutive patients treated with infiltration of botulinum toxin into the internal anal sphincter. Seventy-eight patients were pain free 1 week after injection, and 82 had healed within 3 months. Subsequently, 8 patients had recurrence; 3 of these underwent operative therapy. At 6-month follow-up 79 patients were healed. The remaining 21 patients had operations. None of the patients in this series became incontinent. Jost concluded that internal anal sphincter infiltration with botulinum toxin is effective treatment for anal fissure.[17] In an earlier communication, Jost[18] reported on the complication of perianal thrombosis after infiltration of botulinum toxin in 5 women. These 5 patients had either normal or decreased anal sphincter tone in spite of the presence of fissures. Conversely, none of the patients with anal hypertonicity (including all men in his series at that time) developed thrombosis. Jost concluded that patients with reduced anal sphincter tone in the presence of a fissure, a condition not uncommon in postpartum women,[19] should not undergo treatment with botulinum toxin.[18]

Organic Nitrates

In the last several years, evidence has accumulated that nitric oxide is an inhibitory neurotransmitter in the internal anal sphincter, resulting in relaxation of that muscle.[20,21] As a smooth muscle relaxant, nitric oxide may also increase blood flow to the anal canal. These effects have led to a great deal of clinical investigation into the use of organic nitrates, which are nitric oxide donors, in the treatment of anal fissure.

Watson et al.[22] treated 19 patients with anal fissure with ointment containing increasing concentrations of glyceryl trinitrate (0.2% to 0.8%) to achieve a reduction in mean resting pressure of at least 25%. Nine patients healed, 8 of whom required concentrations of 0.3% or higher. Six patients required sphincterotomy, and 4 were lost to follow-up. Headache caused 2 patients to drop out of the study.[22]

Lund and colleagues,[23] treating patients with 0.2% glyceryl trinitrate ointment, enjoyed more favorable results in three separate series. A report of 21 consecutive patients indicated a significant decrease in maximum anal resting pressure within 20 minutes of application of the ointment. At 6 weeks 18 of the 21 (86%) patients had healed. Mild headache occurred in 4 patients.[23] Lund and Scholefield[24] later reported on 39 consecutive patients similarly treated, with similar favorable results. They concluded that 0.2% glyceryl trinitrate ointment is effective in the management of anal fissure.[24] Next, they embarked on a prospective randomized study of 80 patients, comparing treatment with topical 0.2% glyceryl trinitrate ointment to a placebo. After 8 weeks, 68% of treated patients, but only 8% of controls, were healed ($P = 0.0001$). Maximum anal resting pressure decreased significantly in the treated patients but remained unchanged after administration of placebo. Anodermal blood flow increased significantly after treatment but was not affected by placebo. The authors concluded that topical 0.2% glyceryl trinitrate ointment provided rapid and durable pain relief and that the 68% of patients whose fissures healed would otherwise have required operative intervention.[25]

In 34 consecutive patients treated with topical application of isosorbide dinitrate, Schouten and associates[26] achieved results similar to those of Lund and colleagues. Thirty patients had healed at or before 12 weeks of treatment, with a significant decrease in maximum resting anal pressure and a significant increase in anodermal blood flow. During follow-up, there were only two recurrences in the 30 patients who initially healed.[26]

Further support for the effectiveness of nitrates comes from a prospective, randomized study by Bacher and colleagues[27] of 35 patients with either chronic or acute anal fissure. The 20 treated patients received topical 0.2% glyceryl trinitrate, and the 15 control patients received topical anesthetic gel. At 1-month follow-up 80% of the treated group had healed, compared with only 40% of the patients receiving anesthetic gel. Maximum resting pressure decreased significantly in the treated patients who healed rapidly. However, in patients with chronic fissures who required 28 days to achieve healing, the maximum resting pressure was unchanged. No significant anal pressure reduction was noted in any of the patients receiving anesthetic gel. Four of the 20 treated patients versus none in the control group reported mild, transient headache. The investigators concluded that while topical nitroglycerine is useful in the treatment of acute anal fissure, it does not decrease the need for operative intervention in the treatment of chronic fissure or in patients with acute fissure and persistent anal hypertonia.[27]

Oettle[28] was more enthusiastic regarding the efficacy of glyceryl trinitrate in the treatment of chronic anal fissure. His series included 24 patients with fissures, randomized to undergo sphincterotomy or treatment with topical glyceryl trinitrate. All 12 patients who underwent sphincterotomy healed within 4 weeks. In the 12 patients treated with glyceryl trinitrate, 10 had rapid relief of pain and were healed by 4 weeks. The other 2 patients experienced neither pain relief nor healing; they subsequently underwent sphincterotomy with rapid relief and healing. In neither group were there recurrences during follow-up, and no compromise of continence was reported. Oettle concluded that topical glyceryl trinitrate results in healing of more than 80% of chronic anal fissures, thus greatly reducing the need for sphincterotomy. He observed that patients who did not have rapid relief of pain in response to topical therapy required sphincterotomy, and he suggested that the decision to abandon topical therapy in favor of operative treatment should be made in 1 week or less.[28]

These new pharmacologic modalities show great potential in the evolving management of anal fissure. Clearly, though, there are small but nevertheless persistent failure rates, as noted in each of the reports described above. Patients who fail to respond to the nonoperative treatment described above will obtain relief only by undergoing surgical intervention.

FIGURE 9.2. Technique of anal sphincter stretch. The fingers are inserted one at a time, to a total of four. Males require an anteroposterior stretch rather than a laterally oriented stretch because of the closely placed ischial spines in the male pelvis.[1,2] Redrawn from Corman.[2]

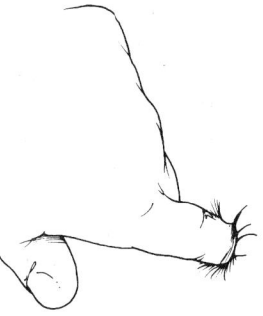 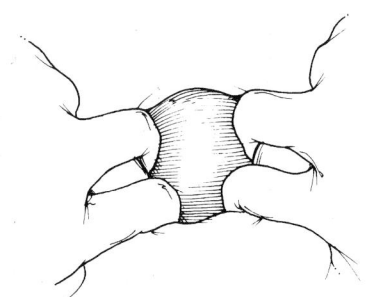

Surgical Therapy

Most of the operations devised for the treatment of anal fissure have been variations of either anal sphincter dilation or division. Both of these techniques decrease anal hypertonicity, setting the stage for improvement in perfusion to the posterior anal midline and subsequent healing. Both variations are effective, with high success rates with regard to healing, and both types of procedures are associated with small failure rates and compromise of continence (thus the extensive interest described above in pharmacologic modalities). The operations currently in greatest favor are variations of lateral internal anal sphincterotomy. Various forms of excision of the fissure, often involving flap coverage and sphincterotomy in the fissure site, have also been employed. (*Editor's note:* Unfortunately, the coding for anal fissure operations is badly conceived, with a significantly larger payment allowable for CPT Code 46200—fissurectomy with or without sphincterotomy than for CPT Code 46080—sphincterotomy.)

Anal Sphincter Stretch

The anal sphincter stretch method of treatment still has enthusiasts who report good results, and therefore the method remains of more than simply historical interest. Ibister and Prasad[29] recently reported their experience with anal dilation as treatment of anal fissure over a 15-year period. During that time, 104 patients underwent 111 anal dilations. Ten patients who were unable to tolerate examination and proctoscopy underwent urgent anal dilation. Those patients able to tolerate examination and proctoscopy were offered an anal dilator and re-evaluated in 4 weeks. Those who remained symptomatic or were unwilling or unable to use the dilator, then underwent elective anal dilation. Gradual dilation of the anal canal to accommodate four fingers was done under general anesthesia (Figure 9.2). The male-to-female ratio in this series was 1.3:1. Seventy-four of the 111 procedures were done on an outpatient basis. Nine patients had simultaneous excision of a sentinel tag. Three patients with anal fissure and Crohn's disease were successfully treated by dilation. Only 5 patients required subsequent dilation due to ongoing symptoms. The authors noted one perianal hematoma, no incontinence, and no mortality in their series. They then proposed gentle anal dilation as the initial management choice in the treatment of anal fissure.[29]

Sohn and associates[30] have reported the successful use of a modification of anal dilation, which they named precise anorectal sphincter dilatation. In patients requiring operative intervention, they performed anal dilation with a Parks' anal retractor opened to exactly 4.8 cm (Figure 9.3), or with a

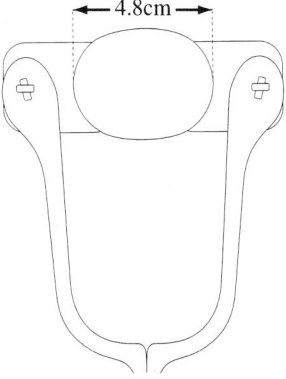

FIGURE 9.3. Depiction of a Parks' retractor opened to exactly 4.8 cm. Note that the removable blade is not attached for this procedure. Redrawn from Sohn et al.[30]

rectosigmoid balloon either 40 or 30 mm in diameter. They first employed Parks' retractor dilation in 105 patients, 30 of whom underwent simultaneous excision of a sentinel tag or hypertrophic anal papilla. At 3-month follow-up, 92% of fissures and associated surgical wounds had healed. In 12 patients with acute or severely painful anal fissures, total or nearly total relief of pain occurred within 12 hours of the procedure. There was late recurrence in 2 of the initially healed patients. Two patients noted incontinence to flatus, which resolved within 3 weeks. Subsequently, Sohn's group changed their method to balloon dilation, believing that use of the Parks' retractor exerted pressure that could vary from patient to patient. A 40-mm rectosigmoid balloon, however, could be inflated to exert a pressure of exactly 20 psi in all patients. (A 30-mm balloon was used in 6 patients, but the associated failure rate was 50%. It was then used only in the occasional patient with marked anal stenosis.) Sixty-six patients were treated by this method, with favorable and similar results compared with those dilated with a Parks' retractor. The fissure and associated wounds healed within 3 months in 94% of the patients. All 10 patients with acute or severely painful anal fissures enjoyed relief of pain within 12 hours of balloon dilation. There was no late recurrence or incontinence during follow-up. After dilation, 1 patient developed a thrombosed hemorrhoid, which resolved spontaneously. The authors concluded that precise anal dilation with either the Parks' retractor or the 40-mm rectosigmoid balloon is safe and effective treatment of anal fissure, and they consider such dilation to be the procedure of choice when operation is necessary.[30]

Fissure Excision With or Without Flap Coverage

The excision procedures have been almost completely replaced by the simpler and equally or more effective variations of anal sphincter stretch and lateral internal anal sphincterotomy. Although favorable results are described, the procedures have disadvantages that have decreased their popularity and usefulness. One frequently used method resulted in a large perianal wound that was quite painful, slow to heal, and difficult to manage on an outpatient basis. Flap coverage eliminates the problem of the open wound, resulting in less pain, less

cumbersome wound care, more rapid wound healing, and decreased postoperative complications. However, these advantages are offset by the more extensive nature of an operation involving dissection and advancement of a flap as opposed to the much simpler options currently available.[31] These techniques receive little space in current texts, and there has been a paucity of reports in the recent literature regarding these procedures.

Sphincterotomy

Sphincterotomy was initially performed in the base of the fissure and was accompanied by fissurectomy. Although a small percentage of fissures occur in the anterior midline, there is scant, if any, mention of anterior midline sphincterotomy in texts or periodic journals. The procedure described was invariably a posterior midline sphincterotomy done simultaneously with fissure excision. Although satisfactory rates of healing were achieved, there were disturbingly high rates of compromised continence, and posterior midline sphincterotomy has, for the most part, fallen into disfavor as an operative option in the treatment of anal fissure.[1,31]

Eisenhammer[32] suggested that lateral sphincterotomy would relieve anal hypertonia with the advantage of a less prominent internal anal sphincter defect, thus resulting in less disturbance of function.[32] Subsequently, variations of lateral internal anal sphincterotomy have become and remain the most common techniques employed in the surgical management of anal fissure. The two techniques in most common use are open and closed lateral internal anal sphincterotomy.

The open technique involves a small, radially oriented incision at the distal tip of the internal anal sphincter laterally, extending over the intersphincteric groove. Alternatively, a partially circumferential incision overlying the intersphincteric groove can be used. The distal tip of the internal anal sphincter and part of the subcutaneous external anal sphincter are exposed. The internal sphincter muscle is grasped with forceps, and its full thickness is divided under direct vision, usually to the level of the dentate line. Definite and immediately evident relaxation of the anus should occur. The surgeon's preference may include dissection of the internal anal sphincter from the anoderm and external anal sphincter. The incision can be closed with rapidly

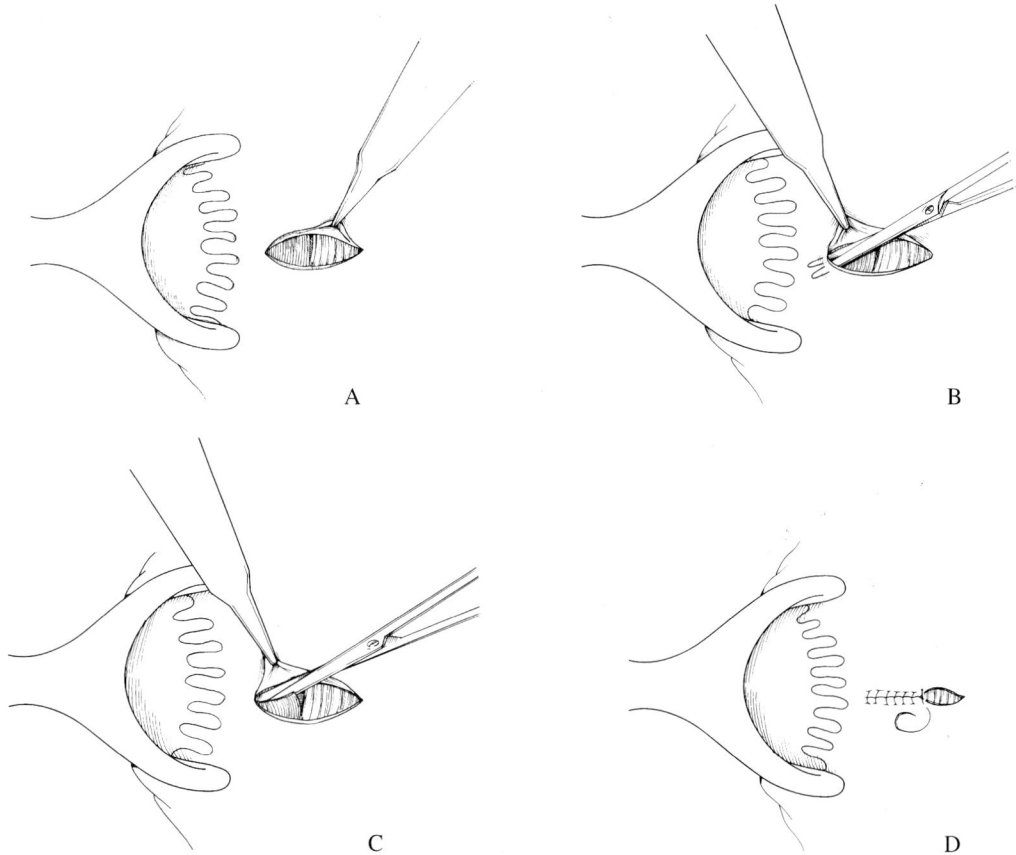

FIGURE 9.4. Technique of open lateral internal anal sphincterotomy. **A**, If the surgeon prefers, a circumferential orientation can be used. **B** and **C**, The internal anal sphincter is isolated and divided. **D**, Depending on the surgeon's preference, the incision can remain open or be closed. Redrawn from Corman.[2]

absorbable suture or be left open, according to the surgeon's preference. (Figure 9.4) Meticulous hemostasis is mandatory. Simultaneous excision of a sentinel tag and/or hypertrophic anal papilla can be performed as necessary.

Notaras[33] first described lateral subcutaneous internal sphincterotomy as an alternative to the open technique, accomplishing sphincter division while leaving a very tiny wound.[33] The technique is now in wide use, although often as a variation of the procedure as initially described. Notaras described insertion of the knife into the submucosal plane, then incision outward through the internal sphincter to the intersphincteric plane (Figure 9.5 **A**). Most contemporary descriptions of the technique involve insertion of the knife into the intersphincteric groove with incision medially toward the mucosa. A Hill-Ferguson or similar anal retractor is

placed into the anal canal to expose the lateral anal wall on either the left or the right side, according to the surgeon's preference and handedness. (*Editor's note:* We perform sphincterotomy in the right lateral position preferentially because of the lesser amount of hemorrhoidal tissue on the right compared to the left. Performing the sphincterotomy on the right side often results in less bleeding.) The exposed intersphincteric groove is easily palpable. A narrow-bladed scalpel (for example, a No. 11 blade or a cataract blade) is inserted into the intersphincteric groove parallel to the muscles. It is then rotated 90°C, so that the sharp edge is toward the internal anal sphincter, which is then divided. As in the open technique, there should be immediately noticeable relaxation of the anus (Figure 9.5 **B**). Also, when the muscle is adequately divided, the knife will be barely visible through the intact anal

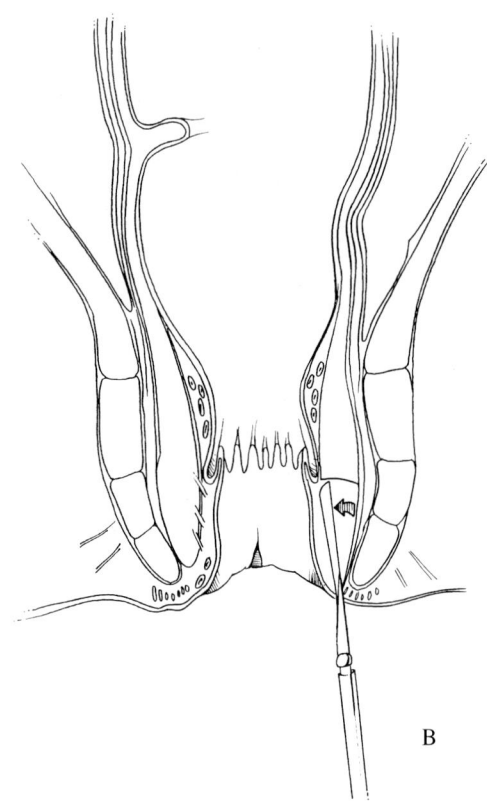

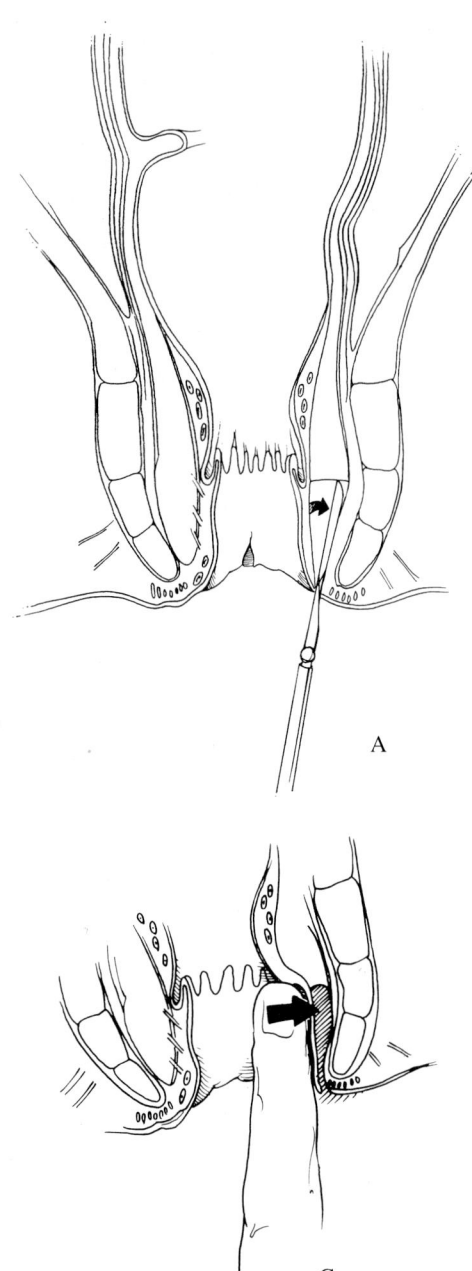

FIGURE 9.5. **A**, Closed lateral internal anal sphincterotomy as originally described by Notaras with blade cutting from the mucosa toward the sphincter. **B**, Knife inserted into the intersphincteric groove with the sharp edge toward the internal anal sphincter and cutting toward the mucosa. **C**, Residual unincised fibers are gently broken up with the side of the finger. Redrawn from Corman.[2105]

mucosa; the knife is then withdrawn. It is crucial that the knife not penetrate the anal mucosa, a complication that can lead to bleeding or postoperative fistula formation. The surgeon's finger can then be used to gently break any residual un-incised fibers (Figure 9.5 **C**). A few moments of direct pressure will usually control bleeding. As in the open technique, meticulous hemostasis is necessary. In rare instances it may be necessary to open the mucosa to achieve hemostasis. Sentinel tags and hypertrophic papillae can be dealt with as necessary. (*Editor's note:* Another technical point to consider in performing sphincterotomy is to locate the sphincterotomy between the crypts. This technique may avoid dividing an anal gland in the base of a crypt, and thus avoid the development of a fistula-in-ano.)

For the brave and daring, Corman[2] describes a variation done with the surgeon's finger, rather than with a retractor, in the anus. The index finger senses the blade as it incises the muscle and approaches the anal mucosa. The side of the finger is then used to break residual internal anal sphincter fibers.[2]

With regard to the facility where sphincterotomy is performed, there is now extensive experience with open and closed sphincterotomy on an outpatient basis. Patients tolerate outpatient sphincterotomy very well, and their admission to the hospital should rarely be necessary. The procedure is easily performed under local, regional, or general anesthesia. Utilizing local anesthesia makes it possible for sphincterotomy to be an office technique.

With regard to the issue of open and closed internal anal sphincterotomy, the periodic journals contain a plethora of articles. A few of the more recent reports are discussed.

Oh and colleagues[34] described their experience with both open and closed techniques over a 20-year period. During that time 1391 patients underwent operations for chronic symptomatic anal fissure. The vast majority of the operations (1313) were internal anal sphincterotomies as treatment of idiopathic fissures. Other operations included C-anoplasty in 36 patients with fissure and anal stricture, débridement and sphincterotomy in 25 patients with nonhealing postoperative wounds, and bilateral excision of the internal sphincter for a protruding condition, which they termed "subluxation." Over 95% of their patients enjoyed prompt relief of pain. Complete wound healing was noted in all but 1.4% of patients, in whom healing was delayed. Early complications included urinary retention (1.4% of patients), bleeding (1.1%), and abscess and fistula (0.7%). Late complications included incontinence to flatus or liquid stool (1.5%), delayed healing, defined as requiring longer than 2 months (1.4%), recurrence (1.3%), and itching and burning (1.1%). The complication rate in this series was higher in the patients who underwent the closed technique. The authors concluded that open lateral internal sphincterotomy is the procedure of choice for the surgical management of chronic anal fissure.[34]

In their report, Garcia-Aguilar et al.[35] expressed a different opinion. They were able to obtain long-term follow-up of 549 patients who underwent

TABLE 9.1. Complications and patient satisfaction of open versus closed sphincterotomy technique.

	Open (%)	Closed (%)	P value
Persistence of symptoms	3.4	5.3	0.27
Fissure recurrence	10.9	11.7	0.77
Need for reoperation	3.4	4	0.70
Lack of control of gas	30.3	23.6	0.06
Soiling underclothing	26.7	16.1	<0.001
Accidental BMs[a]	11.8	3.1	<0.001
Very satisfied	49.7	64.4	NS
Satisfied	40.1	28.0	NS

[a]BMs, bowel movements; NS, not specified.

Data from Garcia-Aguilar et al.[35]

open (324 patients) or closed (225 patients) lateral internal sphincterotomy over a 5-year period by a group of 12 colorectal surgeons. The average length of follow-up was 3 years (range of 1 to 6 years). The results are summarized in Table 9.1. As seen, there were no significant differences between the two groups regarding persistence of symptoms, recurrence, or need for reoperation. However, there were significant differences between the patients undergoing open as opposed to closed sphincterotomies with regard to alterations of anal continence. Although overall patient satisfaction was approximately 90% for both groups, those undergoing closed sphincterotomies had a higher likelihood of being very satisfied. Unlike Oh and colleagues, Garcia-Aguilar et al. concluded that open and closed techniques were equally effective treatments for anal fissure but that closed sphincterotomy resulted in significantly less alteration of anal continence. They recommend closed internal anal sphincterotomy as the preferred technique.[35]

Hoping to decrease the rate of compromise of continence as a consequence of sphincterotomy, Littlejohn and Newstead[36] described a variation of the closed technique, which they termed "tailored lateral sphincterotomy." Their procedure involves division of the internal anal sphincter not to the dentate line, but only to the level of the most proximal extent of the fissure (Figure 9.6). Of 287 patients undergoing the procedure who were available for assessment, there was imperfect control of flatus in 4 (1.4%), minor staining in 1 (0.35%), and urgency in 2 (0.7%). No patients had fecal incontinence or leakage of stool. There were four recurrent fissures and one persistent fissure; those 5 patients underwent a second sphincterotomy. Littlejohn and

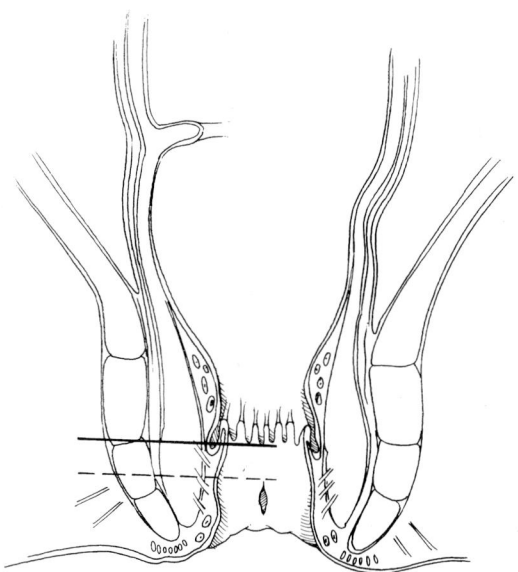

FIGURE 9.6. Tailored sphincterotomy involves division of the muscle only to the proximal extent of the fissure (*dashed line*) rather than to the dentate line (*solid line*). Redrawn from Littlejohn and Newstead.[36]

Newstead concluded that tailored lateral sphincterotomy, with division of less than the traditional amount of internal sphincter, did not compromise the rate of healing or recurrence and resulted in superior preservation of continence.[36]

Unlike Littlejohn and Newstead, Farouk and others[37] found, in a small group of patients, that limited internal anal sphincterotomy corresponded to persistence of anal fissure. They performed endoanal ultrasonography on 13 patients with persistent anal fissure after lateral internal sphincterotomy. Of these patients, 2 had undergone only limited internal anal sphincter division; the others had undergone inadvertent division of the external anal sphincter with no division of the internal anal sphincter. Corrective operations were done, with

extension of the internal sphincterotomy to the dentate line. All patients then experienced early resolution of their symptoms and healing within 8 weeks.[37] In a larger series of patients, Garcia-Granero and associates[38] also used anal endosonography to evaluate the extent of internal anal sphincter division after closed lateral subcutaneous sphincterotomy. Of the 51 patients studied, 10 were symptomatic for anal fissure recurrence. The 41 asymptomatic patients who had undergone sphincterotomy were the control group. As Table 9.2 shows, compared to the patients with recurrence, a significantly higher percentage of the control group had complete sphincter defects. Conversely, a significantly greater percentage of the patients with recurrence had incomplete sphincter division. Of the total series, 10 patients (19.6%) were incontinent for gas and 3 (5.9%) for liquid stool, with no differences between the two groups. Farouk et al. and Garcia-Granero et al. disagreed with Littlejohn and Newstead and concluded that incomplete internal anal sphincterotomy is associated with significant symptomatic anal fissure recurrence. They also found that incomplete division of the internal anal sphincter does not preserve continence.[38]

To assess the rate of complications, Hananel and Gordon[39] retrospectively reviewed their experience with open lateral internal anal sphincterotomy in 265 patients. Unless there were extenuating circumstances (such as allergy to local anesthetics), the operations were done under local anesthesia on an outpatient basis. As shown in Table 9.3, the incidence of complications among these patients was low. The authors concluded that lateral internal sphincterotomy is a good operation for the treatment of chronic anal fissure and can be done successfully and safely on an outpatient basis under local anesthesia.[39]

Neufeld et al.[40] reported follow-up of 108 patients out of 112 who underwent lateral subcuta-

TABLE 9.2. Completeness of internal anal sphincter (IAS) defect versus anal fissure recurrence.

	Recurrence group n (%)	Control group n (%)	P value
Complete IAS defect	1 (10)	31 (75.6)	<0.001
Incomplete IAS defect	9 (90)	10 (24.4)	0.001
Totals	10 (100)	41 (100)	

Data from Garcia-Granero et al.[38]

TABLE 9.3. Complications in 265 patients after lateral internal sphincterotomy (LIS).

	n (%)
Delayed healing (>60 days) of sphincterotomy site	13 (4.9)
Persistent or recurrent fissure	3 (1.1)
Wound infection	2 (0.8)
Impaired control, temporary	1 (0.4)
Impaired control, permanent	1 (0.4)
Fecal soiling, permanent	1 (0.4)
Prolapsed thrombosed hemorrhoids	1 (0.4)
Fecal impaction	1 (0.4)
Total complications	23 (8.7)

Reproduced with permission from Hananel and Gordon.[39]

neous anal sphincterotomy. All patients had failed to respond to nonoperative therapy, and all operations were done under local anesthesia on an outpatient basis in either a clinic or a hospital setting. Patients were observed for a mean of 20 months (range of 2 to 56 months). They were largely satisfied with their operations. Ninety-two patients (85%) considered their result to be excellent, and an additional 8% of the patients had minor complaints and rated their result as good. Postoperative bleeding, which necessitated admission to the hospital, occurred in 4 patients, and another 4 developed abscesses. Initial mild incontinence was noted by 14 patients; this was a temporary condition in all but 1 of the patients. Ten patients reported slight soiling. Three patients reported either no improvement after sphincterotomy or recurrence of fissure. The authors concluded that lateral subcutaneous anal sphincterotomy is the operative treatment of choice for anal fissure and that it can be done effectively and safely under local anesthesia.[40]

Conclusions

Anal fissure is a very common lesion that causes symptoms very much out of proportion to the size of the lesion. The resultant pain is occasionally severe enough to be at least temporarily debilitating. Dietary modification is advised in an attempt to encourage more regular bowel function and to promote soft but formed stool. Topical therapy has traditionally consisted of any number of prescription and over-the-counter preparations, with or without local anesthetics. Acute fissures generally respond very well to these conservative treatments.

With increasing understanding of the etiology of anal fissure, new modalities of nonoperative therapy have been developed. Both botulinum toxin infiltrated into the internal anal sphincter and organic nitrates applied topically have been associated with resolution of anal hypertonicity and fissure healing. In experience already cited, organic nitrates were also noted to cause increased perfusion to the posterior anal midline. These pharmacologic modalities have been useful in the treatment of chronic anal fissures, which have traditionally required operative intervention.

For patients with anal fissure who do not respond to nonoperative therapy, surgical treatment is indicated. Modalities in current use include variations of anal dilation and sphincterotomy by both open and closed techniques. All the techniques described are efficacious with regard to fissure healing, and they all involve complications as discussed. Reports diverge regarding the frequency of complications attributable to the various techniques, and there is no consensus as to which technique is ideal. That being the case, the surgeon should use the technique with which he or she is most familiar and comfortable.

There is consensus regarding the efficacy and safety of operative treatment of anal fissure on an outpatient basis, and it is apparent that admission to the hospital is necessary only infrequently because of extenuating medical circumstances or to deal with complications.

References

1. Goligher J. Anal Fissure. In Goligher J. Surgery of the Anus, Rectum and Colon, 5th edition. London: Bailliere Tindall, 1984:150–166.
2. Corman M. Anal fissure. In Corman M. Colon and Rectal Surgery, 4th edition. Philadelphia: Lippincott-Raven, 1998:206–223.
3. Hananel N, Gordon P. Re-examination of clinical manifestations and response to therapy of fissure-in-ano. Dis Colon Rectum 1997;40:229–233.
4. Winceslaus J, Jones P. Genital herpes masquerading as anal fissure. J R Coll Surg Edinb 1997;42:276–277.
5. Chung C, Choi C, Kwok S, et al. Anal and perianal tuberculosis: a report of three cases in 10 years. J R Coll Surg Edinb 1997;42:189–190.
6. Jensen S. Diet and other risk factors for fissure in ano. Dis Colon Rectum 1988;31:770.

7. Ahmed J, Thomson H. The effect of breakfast on minor anal complaints: a matched case-control study. J R Coll Surg Edinb 1997;42:331–333.

8. Keck J, Staniunas R, Coller J, et al. Computer-generated profiles of the anal canal in patients with anal fissure. Dis Colon Rectum 1995;38:72–79.

9. Williams N, Scott N, Irving M. Effect of lateral sphincterotomy on internal anal sphincter function: a computerized vector manometry study. Dis Colon Rectum 1995;38:700–704.

10. Lund J, Scholefield J. Internal sphincter spasm in anal fissure. Br J Surg 1997;84:1723–1724.

11. Schouten W, Briel J, Auwerda J, et al. Ischaemic nature of anal fissure. Br J Surg 1996;83:63–65.

12. Schouten W, Briel J, Auwerda J. Relationship between anal pressure and anodermal blood flow: the vascular pathogenesis of anal fissures. Dis Colon Rectum 1994;37:664–669.

13. Klosterhalfen B, Vogel P, Rixen H, et al. Topography of the inferior rectal artery: a possible cause of chronic, primary anal fissure. Dis Colon Rectum 1989;32:43–52.

14. Madoff R. Pharmacologic therapy for anal fissure. N Engl J Med 1998;338:257–259.

15. Maria G, Cassetta E, Gui D, et al. A comparison of botulinum toxin and saline for the treatment of chronic anal fissure. N Engl J Med 1998;338:217–220.

16. Mason P, Watkins M, Hall H, et al. The management of chronic fissure-in-ano with botulinum toxin. J R Coll Surg Edinb 1996;41:235–238.

17. Jost W. One hundred cases of anal fissure treated with botulin toxin: early and long-term results. Dis Colon Rectum 1997;40:1029–1032.

18. Jost W. Perianal thrombosis following injection therapy into the external anal sphincter using botulin toxin. Dis Colon Rectum 1995;38:781.

19. Corby H, Donnelly V, O'Herlihy C, et al. Anal canal pressures are low in women with postpartum anal fissure. Br J Surg 1997;84:86–88.

20. O'Kelly T, Brading A, Mortensen N. Nerve mediated relaxation of the human internal anal sphincter: the role of nitric oxide. Gut 1993;34:689–693.

21. O'Kelly T, Davies J, Brading A, et al. Distribution of nitric oxide synthase containing neurons in the rectal myenteric plexus and anal canal: morphologic evidence that nitric oxide mediates the rectoanal inhibitory reflex. Dis Colon Rectum 1994;37:350–357.

22. Watson S, Kamm M, Nicholls R, et al. Topical glyceryl trinitrate in the treatment of chronic anal fissure. Br J Surg 1996;83:771–775.

23. Lund J, Armitage N, Scholefield J. Use of glyceryl trinitrate ointment in the treatment of anal fissure. Br J Surg 1996;83:776–777.

24. Lund J, Scholefield J. Glyceryl trinitrate is an effective treatment for anal fissure. Dis Colon Rectum 1997;40:468–470.

25. Lund J, Scholefield J. A randomized, prospective, double-blind, placebo-controlled trial of glyceryl trinitrate ointment in treatment of anal fissure. Lancet 1997;349:11–14.

26. Schouten W, Briel J, Boerma M, et al. Pathophysiological aspects and clinical outcome of intra-anal application of isosorbide dinitrate in patients with chronic anal fissure. Gut 1996;39:465–469.

27. Bacher H, Mischinger H, Werkgartner G, et al. Local nitroglycerin for treatment of anal fissures: an alternative to lateral sphincterotomy? Dis Colon Rectum 1997;40:840–845.

28. Oettle G. Glyceryl trinitrate *vs.* sphincterotomy for treatment of chronic fissure-in-ano. Dis Colon Rectum 1997;40:1318–1320.

29. Ibister W, Prasad J. Fissure in ano. Aust N Z J Surg 1995;65:107–108.

30. Sohn N, Eisenberg M, Weinstein M, et al. Precise anorectal sphincter dilatation—its role in the therapy of anal fissures. Dis Colon Rectum 1992;35:322–327.

31. Gordon P. Fissure-in-ano. In Gordon P, Nivatvongs S (eds). Principles and Practice of Surgery for the Colon, Rectum, and Anus. St. Louis: Quality Medical Publishing, 1992:199–219.

32. Eisenhammer S. The evaluation of internal anal sphincterotomy operation with special reference to anal fissure. Surg Gynecol Obstet 1959;109:583–590.

33. Notaras M. The treatment of anal fissure by lateral subcutaneous internal sphincterotomy—a technique and results. Br J Surg 1971;58:96.

34. Oh C, Divino C, Steinhagen R. Anal fissure: 20-year experience. Dis Colon Rectum 1995;38:378–382.

35. Garcia-Aguilar J, Belmonte C, Wong W, et al. Open vs. closed sphincterotomy for chronic anal fissure: long-term results. Dis Colon Rectum 1996;39:440–443.

36. Littlejohn D, Newstead G. Tailored lateral sphincterotomy for anal fissure. Dis Colon Rectum 1997;40:1439–1442.

37. Farouk R, Monson J, Duthie G. Technical failure of lateral sphincterotomy for the treatment of chronic anal fissure: a study using endoanal ultrasonography. Br J Surg 1997;84:84–85.

38. Garcia-Granero E, Sanahuja A, Garcia-Armengol J, et al. Anal endosonographic evaluation after closed lateral subcutaneous sphincterotomy. Dis Colon Rectum 1998;41:598–601.

39. Hananel N, Gordon P. Lateral internal sphincterotomy for fissure-in-ano—revisited. Dis Colon Rectum 1997;40:597–602.

40. Neufeld D, Paran H, Bendahan J, et al. Outpatient surgical treatment of anal fissure. Eur J Surg 1995;161:435–438.

10

Anorectal Abscess and Fistula-in-Ano

Scott M. Browning, M.D.

Anorectal sepsis represents a spectrum of disease commonly encountered in surgical practice. The presentation may be acute in the form of anorectal abscess or chronic as fistula-in-ano, an abnormal communication between the perianal skin and the anal canal or rectal mucosa. The majority of anorectal abscesses and fistulae are simple and easily managed. More complex fistulae, however, require a thorough understanding of the etiology and anatomy of anorectal sepsis and a systematic approach to management in order to avoid persistence or recurrence of the fistula or impairment of fecal continence. Though anorectal abscess and fistula-in-ano represent sequential manifestations of a common etiology, their presentation and management differ; for practical purposes, they are discussed separately in this chapter.

Etiology

Anorectal abscess and subsequent fistula-in-ano may arise in association with a variety of specific conditions such as inflammatory bowel disease, malignancy, tuberculosis, actinomycosis, presence of a foreign body, or trauma. However, the vast majority occur in otherwise healthy patients and are believed to be of cryptoglandular origin. The anal canal is invested with multiple (4 to 10) mucin-secreting anal glands with ducts that drain into the anal crypts at the level of the dentate line. Many of these ducts penetrate the internal sphincter, and approximately half of the anal glands originate within the intersphincteric space.[1] Ductal obstruction may lead to stasis, infection, and abscess formation

within the intersphincteric space. Once an abscess develops within the intersphincteric space, spreading may occur in multiple directions along or through the muscular, fascial, or fatty planes surrounding the anus and rectum (Figure 10.1). In addition to spreading vertically along the intersphincteric plane or horizontally through the external sphincter, the abscess may progress in a circumferential manner at any anatomic level (Figure 10.2). Drainage of the abscess, either spontaneous or surgical, through the perianal skin will eventuate in chronic fistula-in-ano in up to two-thirds of cases. According to Parks,[1] "fistula-in-ano is a granulation tissue tract which is kept open by an 'infecting source'—that is, an abscess, deep to the internal sphincter, around a diseased anal gland." This etiology is responsible for approximately 90% of anal fistulae[1] and underlies the rationale for the classification and surgical management of fistula-in-ano.

Anorectal Abscess

Classification

Anorectal abscesses are classified according to the anatomical space in which they reside. From most to least common, the four types of anorectal abscess are perianal, ischiorectal, intersphincteric, and supralevator (Figure 10.3). Perianal abscesses, which account for 43% to 58% of all anorectal abscesses,[4,5] are located superficially, just outside the anal verge, overlying the perineal extent of the intersphincteric space. Ischiorectal abscesses lie within the ischiorectal space. The ischiorectal space appears triangular in the coronal projection

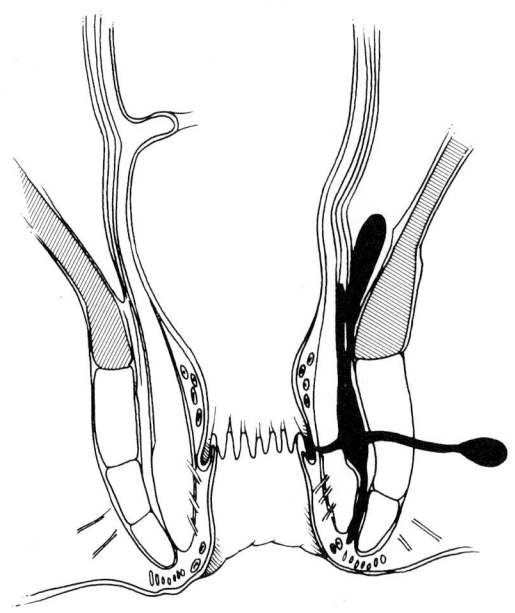

FIGURE 10.1. Routes of spread from the intersphincteric space. Redrawn from Parks et al.[2(p4)]

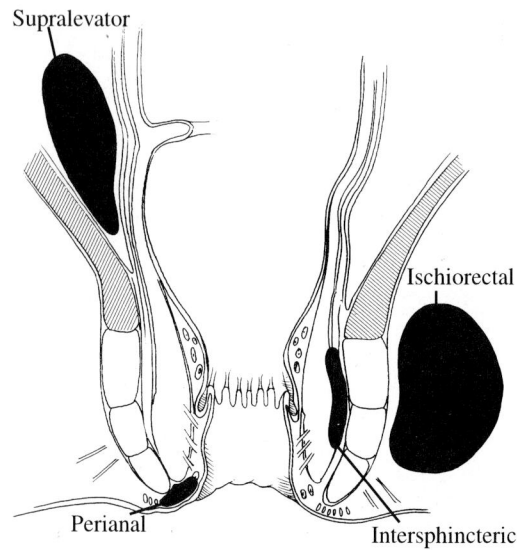

FIGURE 10.3. Classification of anorectal abscess. Redrawn from Vasilevsky.[3(p132)]

and is bordered by the perianal skin inferiorly, the external sphincter and levator muscles medially, and the ischial tuberosity and obturator internus muscle laterally. The left and right ischiorectal fossae communicate posteriorly through the deep postanal space and anteriorly through the deep anterior anal space. The deep postanal space and deep anterior anal space exist in the midline between the superficial external sphincter and the levator muscles. These communications with the ischiorectal fossae allow the potential for abscesses of the deep postanal space or deep anterior anal space to spread into either or both ischiorectal spaces, resulting in horseshoe abscesses.

Intersphincteric abscesses, often erroneously referred to as "submucous" abscesses, are much less common. Lying between the internal and external sphincter muscles, an intersphincteric abscess may also rarely undergo circumferential spread. The rarest of anorectal abscesses are supralevator abscesses, which may arise from either downward extension of pelvic sepsis or the cephalad extension of an intersphincteric or transsphincteric abscess into the supralevator space. Circumferential spread in the supralevator compartment is, fortunately, rare.

Presentation

The patient with an anorectal abscess typically presents with a 2- or 3-day history of progressive, throbbing perianal pain and swelling. The pain of an abscess is constant and may be exacerbated by sitting or walking as well as by bowel movements. The presence of a small amount of bleeding or discharge of pus suggests that partial spontaneous

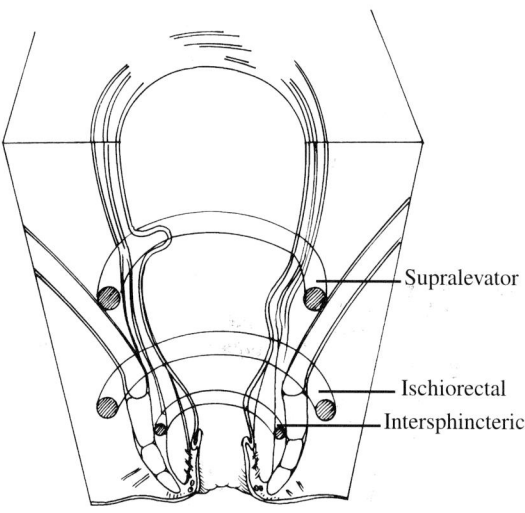

FIGURE 10.2. Routes of circumferential (horseshoe) spread. Redrawn from Parks et al.[2(p11)]

drainage has occurred through either the primary opening or a secondary opening in the perianal skin. Fever, tachycardia, and other systemic manifestations of sepsis are usually absent, but the presence of diabetes, immunosuppression, or delay in treatment can lead to severe sepsis. In the case of perianal abscess, examination is usually straightforward, demonstrating induration, tenderness, and fluctuance to one side of the anus. Cellulitis may or may not be present.

An ischiorectal abscess usually presents as a large, tender fluctuant mass of the buttock but will occasionally demonstrate only unilateral tenderness and asymmetry of the buttocks without focal fluctuance. Needle aspiration may confirm the diagnosis when an abscess is suspected but not obvious. Patients with an intersphincteric or supralevator abscess are more likely to present with fever and may complain of anal pain, rectal pain, gluteal pain, or difficult micturition, yet no obvious abnormality will be found on initial inspection. A tender rectal mass may be noted if digital rectal examination is tolerated. A history suggestive of acute anal fissure (anal pain, exacerbated by bowel movements) with no fissure found on examination should suggest an intersphincteric abscess. With such findings, examination under anesthesia is generally warranted to confirm or exclude the diagnosis, define the nature of the abscess, and effect treatment.

Management

The treatment of anorectal abscess, like abscesses elsewhere, is prompt surgical drainage. When the patient presents with an area of induration and no obvious fluctuance, the surgeon must resist the temptation to postpone surgical treatment in the hope of allowing the abscess to "mature" in order to facilitate drainage. Such management only prolongs the patient's suffering and risks the spread of the infection along or through tissue planes, which may result in a more complex abscess and possible damage to the sphincter muscles. Where focal pain and tenderness suggests an abscess, needle aspiration will confirm the diagnosis and guide drainage. There is little justification for the use of antibiotics in the majority of anorectal abscesses. Exceptions to the avoidance of antibiotics include patients with immunosuppression or diabetes and those with

signs of systemic sepsis, such as significant fever or cellulitis. Antibiotic treatment is also indicated in patients requiring prophylaxis against seeding of prosthetic devices or those with valvular heart disease. Such patients should receive intravenous broad-spectrum antibiotics before drainage of the abscess. Anoscopy and proctoscopy should be performed at some point in the patient's course to exclude inflammatory bowel disease or other rectal disease, but these examinations are best deferred if drainage is to be accomplished under local anesthesia. The method of surgical drainage is dictated by the anatomy of the abscess.

Perianal Abscess

Drainage of a perianal abscess is usually easily accomplished with local anesthetic in the office setting. With the patient in either the prone jack-knife position or Sims' position, the area overlying the point of tenderness and fluctuance is infiltrated with local anesthetic. The scalpel blade or electrocautery is directed straight into the abscess cavity, perpendicular to the plane of the skin. Once the cavity is entered, as evidenced by the return of pus, the skin incision is lengthened in a radial orientation to unroof the entire cavity (Figure 10.4). Once all pus has been drained and the surgeon is satisfied that no loculations or extensions of the cavity have been missed, the skin edges are beveled to prevent premature coaptation. A cruciate extension of the incision and excision of the "corners" may also facilitate this drainage. Such an approach allows adequate drainage and alleviates the need for wound packing. The patient is instructed to perform frequent sitz baths to aid in cleansing the wound. Office follow-up in several weeks will demonstrate either complete healing of the wound or the presence of fistula-in-ano. Anoscopic and proctoscopic examinations may be performed at the time of follow-up without undue patient discomfort.

Ischiorectal Abscess

Most ischiorectal abscesses can also be managed in the office setting under local anesthesia. Exceptions to office drainage include patients who refuse or cannot withstand the manipulation associated with drainage under local anesthesia, those with evidence of systemic sepsis, or those who are suspected to have a deep postanal space or horseshoe

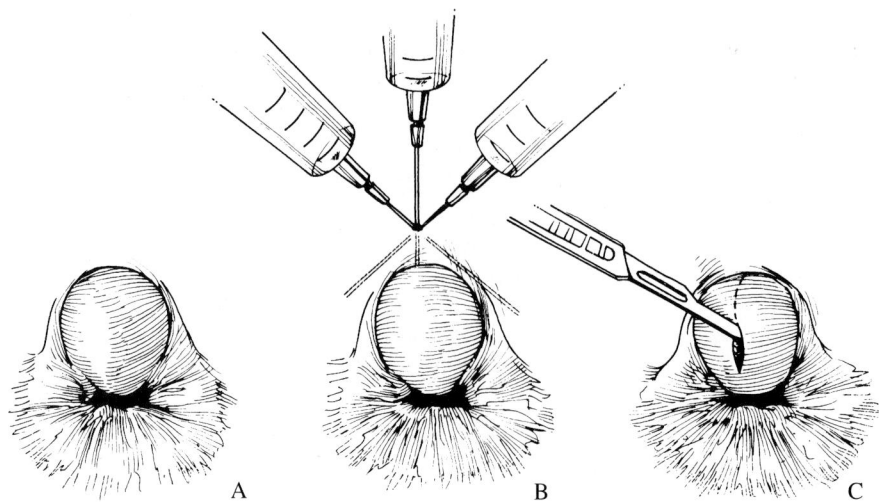

FIGURE 10.4. Technique of incision and drainage of perianal abscess. **A**, Abscess. **B**, Infiltration of local anesthetic. **C**, Drainage of abscess. Redrawn from Marti.[6]

abscess. Again, anoscopic or proctoscopic examination is poorly tolerated acutely under local anesthesia and is best deferred until the abscess has resolved. Drainage is accomplished in the prone jack-knife position. As the patient with an ischiorectal abscess is at considerable risk for development of fistula-in-ano, the drainage incision should be placed as close as possible to the anal canal to minimize the length of any subsequent fistula tract and fistulotomy wound. If the examination reveals a small abscess, it may be drained in the manner described for perianal abscesses. However, ischiorectal abscesses may be quite large, and simple incision and drainage can result in a considerable wound. Therefore, catheter drainage may be preferable. Once the medial site for drainage is chosen, a 1- to 2-cm area is infiltrated with local anesthetic and the incision is made into the abscess cavity. Once the purulent material has been expressed and all loculations have been broken down, the cavity is irrigated with saline. A small (10 to 16 French) soft mushroom catheter may then be inserted into the cavity over a probe. The head of the catheter should be of sufficient size, relative to the size of the wound and the abscess cavity, to secure the catheter within the cavity without the need for suture. The catheter is then amputated leaving enough length (2 to 3 cm) outside the cavity to eliminate the possibility of the catheter falling into the cavity (Figure 10.5). A dressing is put in place,

and the patient is advised to keep the area clean. After approximately 1 week, the patient is reexamined. If the cavity has closed around the catheter head and drainage has ceased or become serous, the catheter may be removed. Anoscopy and proctoscopy may be performed at that time. If, on the other hand, a significant cavity remains, the catheter is left in place and the patient is examined

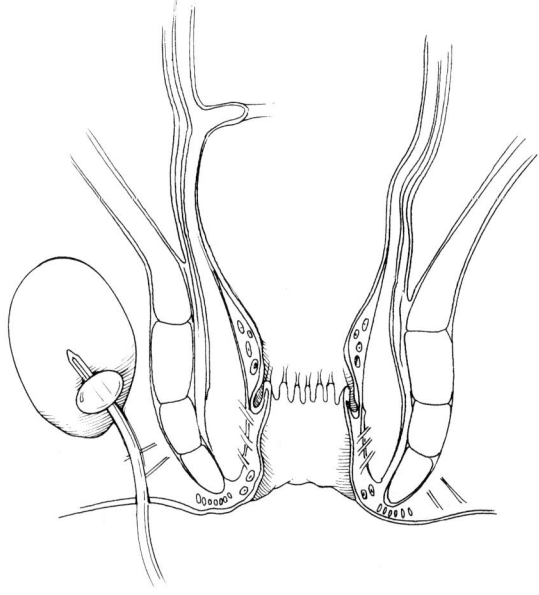

FIGURE 10.5. Technique of catheter drainage of ischiorectal abscess.

at weekly intervals until healing has occurred. If a large catheter was used initially, it may need to be replaced with a smaller catheter. The patient is observed until the cavity has healed and is then reexamined for the presence of fistula-in-ano. If the cavity is so large as to be inadequately drained by a single catheter, the use of counter incisions is preferable to the creation of a single large wound.

Abscess of the deep postanal space, with or without horseshoe extension, should be suspected in a patient with posterior rectal pain, fever, and exquisite posterior tenderness on rectal examination. Examination and drainage under anesthesia are indicated when the diagnosis is apparent or strongly suspected. Under either regional or general anesthesia, the patient is examined in the prone jack-knife position. Bimanual palpation of the deep postanal space and ischiorectal fossae may demonstrate the extent of the abscess. When the abscess is compressed, anoscopy will nearly always reveal pus draining from the internal opening in the posterior midline at the level of the dentate line. If the abscess is confined to the deep postanal space without horseshoe extension, primary fistulotomy is the most appropriate treatment. This management method has a reported recurrence rate of 7.7% and no incontinence.[7] A malleable probe is passed from the primary opening into the deep postanal space abscess. A midline fistulotomy incision is carried out over the probe from the primary opening toward the coccyx, separating the fibers of the superficial external sphincter and unroofing the deep postanal space. The wound is packed loosely. The patient is instructed to remove the packing the following day and to take frequent sitz baths. Office follow-up should be frequent, as periodic digital separation of the wound edges may be necessary to prevent premature closure of the deep postanal space.

When horseshoe extension of the deep postanal space abscess is present, primary fistulotomy and counter drainage of the ischiorectal space(s), as described by Hanley,[8] yields a recurrence rate of 28.6%.[7] Abscess recurrence and wound morbidity following treatment of deep postanal space horseshoe abscess can be reduced by the performance of seton fistulotomy and counter drainage.[9] With the primary opening identified by anoscopy, a malleable probe is directed through this opening into the deep postanal space abscess and the tip palpated

through the skin. An incision is then made in the posterior midline, outside of the subcutaneous external sphincter, and deepened through and parallel to the fibers of the superficial external sphincter until the deep postanal space cavity is entered. The cavity is then explored for extension into either ischiorectal space. Counter drainage wounds are made at the anterior extent of each side of the horseshoe (determined by digital or probe examination through the posterior wound), and curettage of all cavities and fistula tracts is performed. With the probe passed through the primary opening into the now open deep postanal space, the perianal skin and anoderm between the primary opening and deep postanal space wound are incised. A rubber seton (vessel loop) is then drawn through the fistula tract around the distal internal and external sphincters and secured loosely to itself with several heavy silk ligatures. Penrose drains are then looped between each counter drainage wound and the posterior midline wound and secured to themselves with heavy silk ligatures (Figure 10.6). No packing is necessary. Once the acute infection has resolved, the lateral Penrose drains are removed, and their respective tracts are allowed to heal. Sitz baths are encouraged, and the wound is examined at weekly intervals. Once healing is complete, the patient is left with a chronic posterior fistula-in-ano around a seton. Beginning several weeks after the initial procedure the seton is then tightened slightly at weekly intervals until the deep postanal space is obliterated

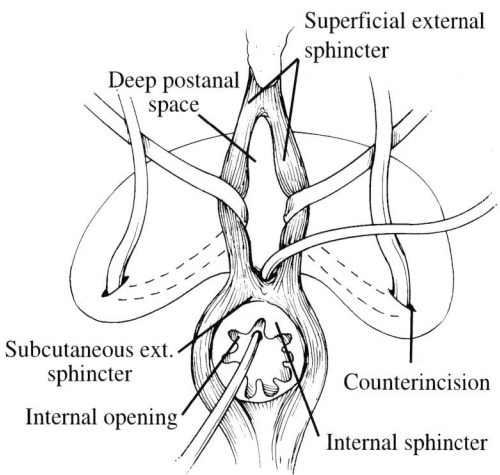

FIGURE 10.6. Drainage of posterior horseshoe abscess. Redrawn from Ustynoski et al.[9]

(see "Seton Fistulotomy [Cutting Seton]," p. 122). Alternatively, if the patient does not tolerate tightening of the seton, a staged fistulotomy can be performed. This more conservative approach to the deep postanal space abscess yields a recurrence rate of 18.1%[9] and should result in less sphincter separation than is seen with the simple laying-open procedure.

The management of deep anterior anal space abscess is similar to that of deep postanal space abscess, with the exception that, especially in women, incontinence is much more likely to occur if primary fistulotomy is performed. Therefore, seton drainage of the deep anterior anal space abscess is the preferred treatment.[10] This is accomplished by opening the deep anterior anal space in the anterior midline over a probe inserted through the primary opening, being careful to stay outside of the subcutaneous external sphincter. The rubber band seton is then drawn around the anterior sphincter complex and secured loosely to itself. Again, any horseshoe extensions are drained with counter incisions bridged by Penrose drains. Subsequent management is as already described for seton drainage of deep postanal space abscess.

Intersphincteric Abscess

As mentioned previously, the diagnosis of intersphincteric abscess is difficult to establish in the office. With the exception of anorectal tenderness precluding digital examination, physical findings are often lacking. Therefore, general or regional anesthesia is frequently required to allow the surgeon to make the diagnosis and obtain adequate exposure to effect treatment. With anesthesia accomplished in the prone jack-knife position, digital examination will reveal the location and extent of the abscess. Although intersphincteric abscesses are usually oriented vertically (along the long axis of the anal canal), they may occasionally demonstrate circumferential spread. Proctoscopy is performed to evaluate the rectum. Anoscopy may reveal purulent discharge from the offending crypt at the level of the dentate line. To avoid recurrence, the entire extent of the abscess cavity must be unroofed, crossing the dentate line to eliminate the diseased gland (dividing the anoderm, rectal mucosa, and internal sphincter fibers overlying the abscess). After débridement of the cavity, the wound edges are marsupialized to ensure adequate drainage. Failure to unroof the entire abscess cavity is likely to result in recurrence.[11]

Supralevator Abscess

The proper method of drainage for a supralevator abscess is dependent on the source of the abscess. A supralevator abscess may result from upward extension of an intersphincteric abscess, extension of an ischiorectal abscess upward through the levator muscle, or from downward extension of a pelvic septic process (appendicitis, diverticulitis, Crohn's disease, etc.). The management of each of the three possible scenarios is different. Therefore, the origin of the abscess must be determined before treatment is undertaken. In the case of a supralevator abscess resulting from pelvic sepsis, management involves drainage of the abscess (through the rectum, perineum, vagina, or abdominal wall, depending on the location of the abscess and the overall state of the patient) and treatment of the underlying disease. For either of the other two scenarios, drainage should be performed in the operating room with either regional or general anesthesia.

For a supralevator abscess that arises as an upward extension of an intersphincteric abscess, internal drainage should be directed into the rectum. If drainage were to be attempted through the ischiorectal fossa, and therefore through the levator muscle, a suprasphincteric fistula would likely result (Figure 10.7). This is a situation to avoid. Positioning of the patient depends on the location of the abscess; if the abscess is more posterior, the lithotomy position is used. If more anterior, the prone jack-knife position is preferred. The area of the abscess is identified by transanal palpation and by advancing a needle through an anal speculum into the mass to confirm the abscess location. A knife is then passed along the needle into the abscess cavity. If technically feasible, the cavity is unroofed and débrided. The wound edges are then marsupialized with an absorbable suture to maintain adequate drainage. If the position of the abscess or the anatomy of the patient would render this approach to drainage unduly difficult, an alternative is to make only a small opening into the cavity, through which is passed a mushroom catheter for drainage. Again, the head of the catheter should be of sufficient size to hold it within the cavity without the

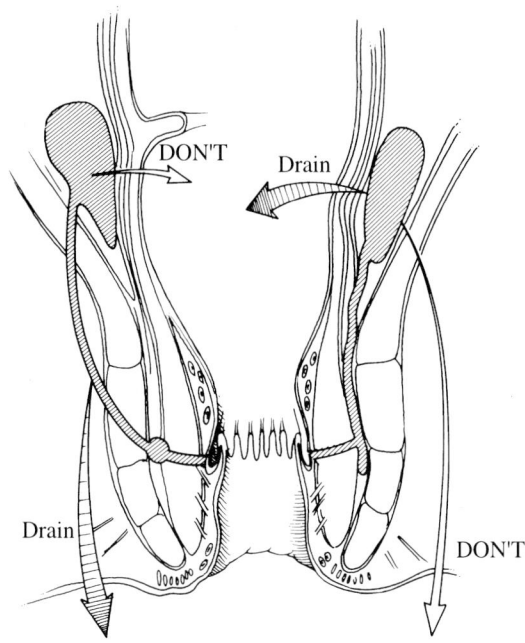

FIGURE 10.7. Drainage of a supralevator abscess. Redrawn from Gordon.[12(p230)]

need for suture, and the catheter should be just long enough to exit the anal verge. The drain catheter may be removed after 48 hours, though a longer duration may be advisable if the abscess cavity is particularly large.

If, on the other hand, the supralevator abscess has resulted from extension of an ischiorectal abscess upward through the levator muscle (a very rare situation), external drainage should be effected through the ischiorectal fossa. Drainage of this kind of abscess internally into the rectum would potentially result in an extrasphincteric fistula, another situation to avoid (Figure 10.7). External drainage of this type of supralevator abscess is most easily performed with the patient in the prone jack-knife position. The ischiorectal fossa is entered through a medially placed perianal wound. The tract leading through the levator muscle to the supralevator component of the abscess is identified, enlarged, and curetted. A mushroom catheter is placed through this tract into the supralevator abscess and secured at the skin. The duration of catheter drainage is tailored to the size of the abscess cavity, but in most cases the catheter can be safely removed after 48 hours. The patient is seen in follow-up within 2 weeks of removal of the catheter and is instructed to return sooner if the original symptoms return.

The Role of Primary Fistulotomy

If anorectal abscess and fistula-in-ano are manifestations of the same underlying abnormality—an infected anal gland within the intersphincteric space—then it would seem reasonable that the treatment should be the same. This is the rationale underlying the argument for primary fistulotomy at the time of abscess drainage. Primary fistulotomy, by eradicating the underlying infected gland, should, in theory, eliminate recurrence of the abscess and the development of fistula-in-ano. Proponents of primary fistulotomy report large series of patients with rates of recurrence (abscess or fistula) of 1.8%[4] and 3.6%[13]—rates considerably lower than those published for incision and drainage alone.

However, recurrent abscess or fistula-in-ano are not inevitable consequences of simple drainage of anorectal abscess. Retrospective studies examining the incidence of abscess recurrence or the development of fistula-in-ano following incision and drainage of anorectal abscesses demonstrate that only 32% to 48% of such patients will require a second procedure.[5,14] Therefore, primary fistulotomy would expose between one-half and two-thirds of abscess patients to the unnecessary division of sphincter muscle with the attendant risks of fecal incontinence and delayed wound healing. Furthermore, the internal opening cannot be demonstrated at the time of abscess drainage in 65% of cases where it is sought.[4] Vigorous probing in an attempt to accomplish fistulotomy at the time of abscess drainage may lead to the creation of false passages and neglect of the source of infection. An additional practical concern is the matter of anesthesia. Simple incision and drainage of anorectal abscesses can be accomplished under local anesthesia in the vast majority of cases. Anoscopy, probing of the abscess wound, and the performance of fistulotomy, on the other hand, usually require either regional or general anesthesia. Despite the theoretical advantages and low recurrence rates associated with primary fistulotomy, the majority of anorectal abscess patients will not benefit from this approach for the reasons outlined above. If, however, abscess drainage is performed under regional or general anesthesia for other reasons and the internal opening is obvious and low, primary fistulotomy may be reasonable. This is especially true for the drainage of a recurrent anorectal abscess. Under any circumstance, only a surgeon experienced in anorectal sepsis and who is well acquainted with the anatomy should perform primary fistulotomy.

Fistula-in-Ano

Fistula-in-ano is defined as an abnormal communication between the perianal skin and the anal canal or rectal lumen. As discussed previously, 90% of anal fistulae are of cryptoglandular origin,[1] and most are preceded by surgical or spontaneous drainage of an anorectal abscess. The remainder can be related to specific conditions such as inflammatory bowel disease, tuberculosis or fungal infections, anal malignancy, anal fissure, previous anorectal surgery, or perineal or rectal trauma. In a series of 233 consecutive patients requiring operations for anorectal sepsis, Winslett and colleagues found 11.6% to harbor occult rectal or systemic disease;[5] this finding emphasizes the importance of evaluating patients thoroughly before performing definitive fistula surgery.

Classification

Of the many classification systems published for fistula-in-ano, the most practical, comprehensive, and widely used is that proposed by Parks, Gordon, and Hardcastle in 1976.[2] The Parks classification (Figure 10.8) categorizes fistulae anatomically into intersphincteric (Type 1), transsphincteric (Type 2), suprasphincteric (Type 3), and extrasphincteric (Type 4) fistulae. Subtypes are defined based on the amount of muscle encompassed by the fistula and on the presence or absence of secondary tracts (Table 10.1). A reasonable estimate of the distribution within the general population is as follows: intersphincteric fistulae, 70%; transsphincteric, 23%; suprasphincteric, 5%; and extrasphincteric, 2%.[2] The following discussion summarizes the most important aspects of the Parks classification of fistula-in-ano.[2]

Intersphincteric Fistula

As described under "Etiology" above, fistula-in-ano of cryptoglandular origin begins with an infection within the intersphincteric space. It is not sur-

prising, then, that intersphincteric fistula, in which the fistula ramifies only within the intersphincteric plane, is the most common of anal fistulae. Intersphincteric fistula (Figure 10.8**A**) may present as a simple fistula (Type 1a) in which the fistula tract proceeds directly from the internal opening at the dentate line, within the intersphincteric space, to an opening at the anal verge. In the acute setting this presents as a perianal abscess. Treatment of this simple fistula involves elimination of its source (infected anal gland within the intersphincteric space) by simple fistulotomy. Disturbance of continence is distinctly unlikely. In addition to this simple fistula tract, a high blind extension (Type 1b) may be present between the internal sphincter and the longitudinal muscle of the upper anal canal and rectal wall. Treatment is by fistulotomy from the external opening to the most cephalad extension of the blind tract. Though a long segment of internal sphincter is divided, little disturbance of continence will result, as the edges of the divided sphincter are held together by fibrosis from the fistula. When the high extension penetrates the rectal lumen (Type 1c), care must be taken to differentiate this long intersphincteric fistula from an extrasphincteric fistula. Although management of the latter is complex, intersphincteric fistula with a high opening in the rectal wall is treated by fistulotomy from the external opening, through the primary source in the mid-anal canal, to the high rectal opening. Again, significant impairment of continence is unlikely.

The initial intersphincteric infection may spread in a cephalad direction with no perineal opening (Type 1d) to form an intersphincteric abscess, which may then discharge into the rectal ampulla. In either case, the entire tract should be opened into the rectum, being certain to incise the primary source at the level of the dentate line. High intersphincteric fistula with a pelvic extension (Type 1e) actually describes a supralevator abscess arising from cephalad extension of an intersphincteric abscess. As described previously, correct treatment is drainage into the rectum. Intersphincteric fistula from pelvic disease (Type 1f) is not a true anal fistula, but rather a downward extension of pelvic sepsis through the intersphincteric space. Treatment is directed at the pelvic disease process; the fistula will heal once the source is addressed.

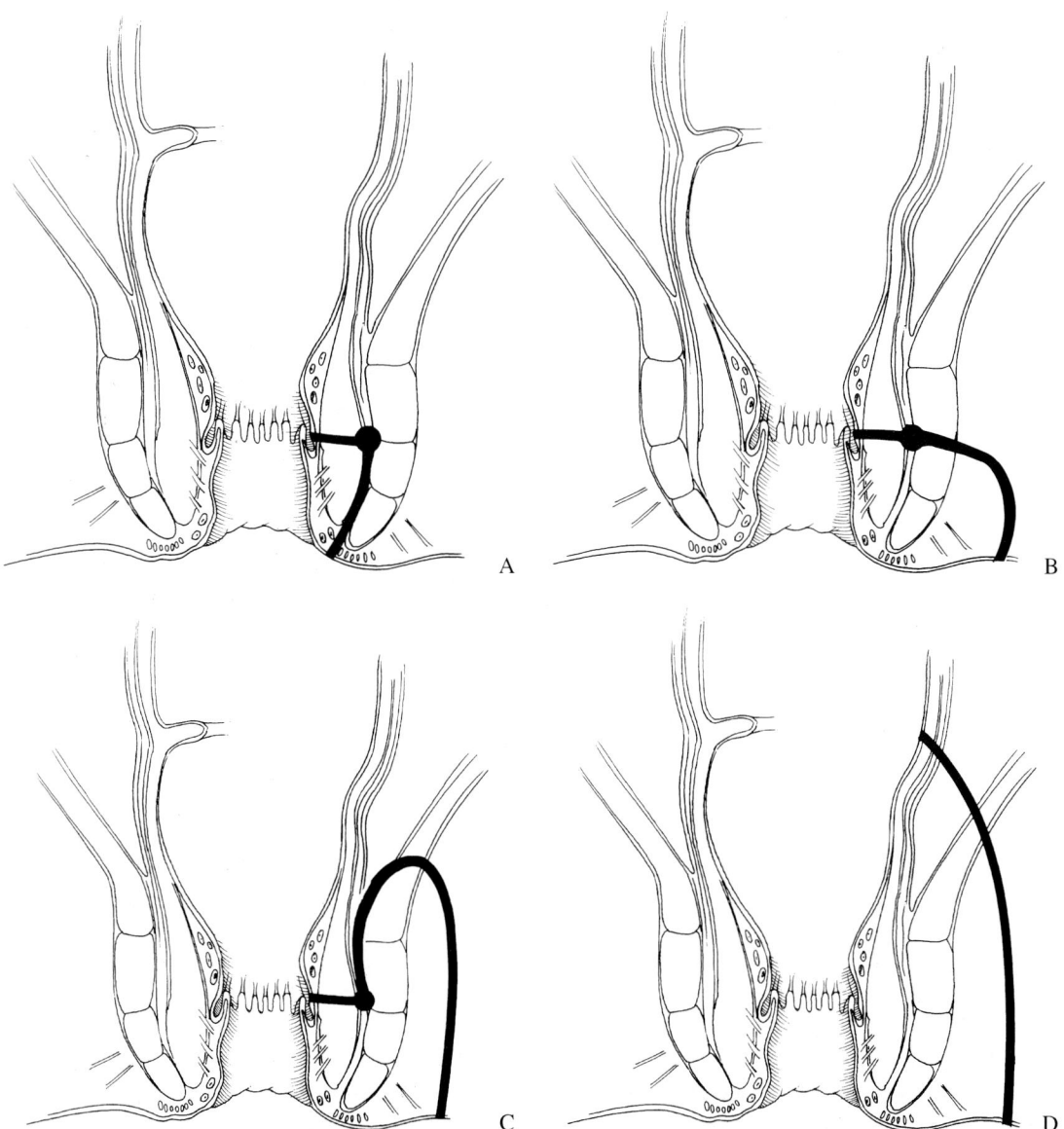

FIGURE 10.8. Classification of fistula-in-ano. **A**, Type 1. **B**, Type 2. **C**, Type 3. **D**, Type 4. Redrawn from Parks et al.[2(p5)]

Transsphincteric Fistula

Uncomplicated transsphincteric fistula (Type 2a) consists of a fistula tract that passes from its source in the intersphincteric space of the mid-anal canal, through the external sphincter into the ischiorectal space, and finally to the perineal skin (Figure 10.8**B**).

The acute presentation is usually that of an is-chiorectal abscess. The level at which the fistula tract crosses the external sphincter and the resulting amount of muscle that would be cut if fistulotomy were to be performed varies considerably. Fortunately, most are low enough that simple fistu-lotomy is unlikely to have a permanent impact on

TABLE 10.1. Parks classification of fistula-in-ano.

Type 1. Intersphincteric fistula
  a. Simple intersphincteric fistula
  b. Intersphincteric fistula with a high blind tract
  c. Intersphincteric fistula with a high tract opening into the
     lower rectum
  d. High intersphincteric fistula without a perineal opening
  e. High intersphincteric fistula with a pelvic extension
  f. Intersphincteric fistula from pelvic disease
Type 2. Transsphincteric fistula
  a. Uncomplicated
  b. Transsphincteric fistula with a high blind tract
Type 3. Suprasphincteric fistula
Type 4. Extrasphincteric fistula
  a. Extrasphincteric fistula secondary to a transsphincteric
     fistula
  b. Extrasphincteric fistula due to trauma
  c. Extrasphincteric fistula due to specific anorectal disease
  d. Extrasphincteric fistula due to pelvic inflammation

Data from Parks et al. [11]

continence. It has been reported that division of the entire external sphincter (as would be done for fistulotomy of a high transsphincteric fistula) has only minimal impact on continence as long as the puborectalis muscle is preserved.[2] More conservative techniques such as the use of a seton or endorectal advancement flap may, however, be advisable in the management of high transsphincteric fistulae.

An uncommon but important variant of the transsphincteric fistula is the presence of a high blind tract (Type 2b). In this variant the fistula tract crosses from the intersphincteric space, through the external sphincter, into the ischiorectal space. There it gives off two branches, one heading to an opening in the perineal skin and the other as a blind tract reaching the top of the ischiorectal fossae or even penetrating the levator muscle to reach the supralevator space. Thus, a probe passed from the external opening may appear to follow a direct path to the supralevator space, where it is palpated just outside the rectal wall. The primary fistula, branching off this long tract at a right angle, may not be noticed. In this situation, the examiner may believe the patient to have an extrasphincteric fistula, or worse, may create one by penetrating the rectal wall while probing. The true source of the fistula in the mid-anal canal can usually be felt as focal induration at the level of the dentate line. Treatment consists of management of the primary (transsphincteric) fistula and drainage of the high blind tract.

Suprasphincteric Fistula

Suprasphincteric fistula (Type 3) develops when an intersphincteric abscess extends cephalad in this plane to reach the supralevator space, passes over the puborectalis muscle, and then descends between the puborectalis and levator muscles to reach the ischiorectal space and finally the perineal skin (Figure 10.8C). The path of the fistula therefore surrounds the entire sphincter mechanism. (*Editor's note:* It is my opinion that this type of fistula rarely occurs spontaneously and that the vast majority of these complex fistulae are the result of injudicious probing of simpler fistulae and creation of abnormal communications—i.e., iatrogenic fistulae.) Treatment is complex, requiring a staged approach that allows fibrosis around the tract to limit muscle separation as successive portions of muscle are divided by partial fistulotomy or seton. Blind extensions within the supralevator space may occur.

Extrasphincteric Fistula

An extrasphincteric fistula is a tract passing from the rectal lumen through the levator muscle and ischiorectal space to the perineal skin, entirely outside of the sphincter complex. This may occur via several mechanisms. As described above, the high blind tract of a transsphincteric fistula (Type 2b) may penetrate the rectum (spontaneously or due to overzealous probing of the tract) and thus lead to an extrasphincteric fistula (Type 4a). In this setting, the fistula is perpetuated by the infected anal gland within the intersphincteric space as well as continual contamination from the high-pressure rectal lumen. Treatment may require a diverting ostomy in addition to fistulotomy of the primary (transsphincteric) fistula and closure of the high rectal opening. Perineal or rectal trauma may also result in extrasphincteric fistula (Type 4b). (Figure 10.8D) Temporary colostomy, closure of the internal opening, and drainage of the fistula tract without muscle division may be sufficient, as the anal canal is not the source of the fistula. Finally, extrasphincteric fistula may result from inflammatory bowel disease (Type 4c) or other pelvic inflammatory process (Type 4d). Treatment in these situations is directed at the underlying pathology. Management of these complex fistulae may require long-term drainage of the tract using either a vessel loop seton or a mushroom catheter, as discussed under "Anorectal Fistula in Crohn's Disease" below (see Figure 10.14).

Not included within the Parks classification,[2] because it is not of cryptoglandular etiology, is the superficial or submucosal fistula. This fistula is associated either with bridging of anal fissure edges in the posterior midline or with a hemorrhoidectomy wound. As there is no muscle involved, treatment is simple fistulotomy or excision and primary closure.

Presentation

The majority of patients presenting with fistula-in-ano will have an antecedent history of abscess, either surgically or spontaneously drained. The most common symptoms are discharge (65%), pain (34%), swelling (24%), bleeding (12%), and diarrhea (5%).[15] Discharge may be constant or intermittent and may be purulent, serosanguinous, or feculent. Pain and swelling suggest intermittent obstruction of the fistula tract by temporary closure of the external opening or the presence of an inadequately drained secondary tract. When no suppuration is present, the fistula is painless and the patient may complain only of skin irritation from chronic drainage. When present, bleeding is likely the result of granulation tissue at the external opening. The complaint of diarrhea should raise suspicion for inflammatory bowel disease.

Assessment

Success in the surgical management of fistula-in-ano is highly dependent on accurate assessment of the cause and anatomy of the fistula tract as well as the medical status of the patient. Goodsall[16] defined the five essentials of fistula evaluation as identification of 1) the internal opening, 2) the external opening, 3) the course of the primary tract, 4) the presence and course of any secondary tracts, and 5) the existence of any other medical or surgical conditions that might complicate the fistula. Of these factors, success rests most singularly on identification of the internal opening. Most of the necessary information can usually be gained from the office examination, with the remainder obtained during examination under anesthesia immediately before

definitive therapy. However, certain complex or recurrent fistulae may warrant more sophisticated preoperative evaluation to improve the likelihood of surgical success.

Office Evaluation

When interviewing the patient with suspected fistula-in-ano, certain historical information may help guide proper treatment: What is the history and chronicity of the fistula? The surgeon's approach to the acute fistula and the chronic, recurrent fistula will differ. Are there any symptoms to suggest an inadequately drained abscess (pain, swelling)? Has the patient had prior procedures for this fistula, for other fistulae, or other previous anal surgery? What is the patient's continence status? The knowledge that sphincter muscle has been previously divided or that the patient's continence is marginal may alter the surgeon's choice of procedures. Are there any complicating medical conditions (diabetes, HIV infection, blood dyscrasias, or immunosuppression)? Is there any suggestion of inflammatory bowel disease (abdominal pain, diarrhea, rectal bleeding)? The management of fistula-in-ano in the patient with Crohn's disease is discussed under "Anorectal Fistula in Crohn's Disease," below.

Once the history has been obtained, the perineum is carefully examined. The secondary opening may appear as an obvious raised papule or, occasionally, as a subtle opening that is demonstrated only by drainage expressed on palpation of the tract. The location of the internal opening can be predicted with reasonable accuracy in accordance with Goodsall's rule[16] (Figure 10.9). External openings anterior to an imaginary transverse line through the center of the anus correspond to an internal opening in the same radial position. Fistulae with external openings posterior to this line usually originate from a crypt in the posterior midline. Exceptions include the following situations: an anterior opening more than 3 cm from the anal verge, which is likely to be the anterior extension of a posterior horseshoe fistula; the presence of multiple openings; and the existence of Crohn's disease or anorectal malignancy. Fifty-eight percent of internal openings are located in either anterior or posterior quadrants of the anal canal.[15] As a rule of thumb, an external opening near the anal verge

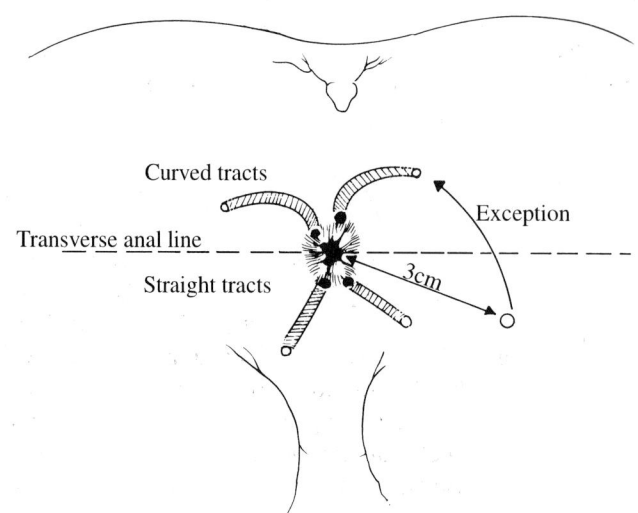

FIGURE 10.9. Goodsall's rule. Redrawn from Vasilevsky.[3(p139)]

suggests an intersphincteric tract, whereas a more peripheral opening suggests a transsphincteric fistula. The farther the external opening lies from the anal verge, the greater is the likelihood of a complex upward extension. The presence of more than one external opening suggests a single complex fistula (horseshoe fistula if the openings are bilateral). Simultaneous independent fistulae are rare. The examiner should also search for other conditions that may simulate the appearance of fistula-in-ano, such as hidradenitis suppurativa, Bartholin's gland abscess, pilonidal sinus, or presacral dermoid cyst.

Attention is then turned to the primary fistula tract. Palpation of the skin over the predicted fistula course may detect a cord of induration, suggesting a superficial tract that may lead the examiner to the internal opening. Digital examination will allow bimanual palpation of the tract and assessment of the supralevator space. Induration at the level of the levator muscles suggests either a high secondary tract from a transsphincteric fistula, upward extension of an intersphincteric fistula, or, rarely, a suprasphincteric fistula. The site of the internal opening, most likely at the dentate line, may be detectable as focal induration, retraction of the crypt, or an enlarged papilla. An entirely normal anal canal with a lateral opening raises concern for an extrasphincteric fistula. Assessment is made of sphincter tone and any preexisting sphincter defects. Anoscopy, performed in further search of the internal opening, may demonstrate discharge when the tract is compressed. However, the internal "opening" is not always patent at the time of examination. Proctoscopy should also be performed to exclude coexisting rectal disease such as proctitis or inflammatory bowel disease. Although the examination will be repeated in the operating room, the information obtained from the office examination will aid in surgical planning and patient counseling. Manipulation of the tract via probe, injection, or otherwise is best left for examination under anesthesia.

Preoperative Studies

Although no further studies are necessary prior to examination under anesthesia and definitive treatment in the majority of anal fistulae, the presence of a recurrent fistula, previous anal surgery with resultant deformity, multiple or extensive tracts, or suspicion of inflammatory bowel disease may indicate the need for further assessment. If symptoms suggest the possibility of inflammatory bowel disease, either barium enema or colonoscopy and an upper gastrointestinal study (small bowel follow-through) are indicated. There are several modalities available to attempt to image the fistula itself.

The simplest and historically most widely used investigation is fistulography. Water-soluble contrast material is injected into the external opening under fluoroscopy in an attempt to identify the location of the internal opening, the course of the primary tract, and any secondary extensions. Fistulography is most helpful in the setting of a suspected extrasphincteric fistula, because contrast material may be seen entering the rectum, sigmoid colon, or small bowel. Despite the occasional usefulness of this easily performed study, published results have been disappointing.[17] Fistulography may fail to demonstrate the internal opening and may identify false-positive high extensions. Fistulography may have a role in the evaluation of a recurrent fistula when the internal opening was not identified at the initial procedure. Computed tomographic (CT) scanning lacks sufficient resolution to delineate the anatomy of an anal fistula, and CT fistulography rarely adds information that is not apparent on two-dimensional fistulography.

Endorectal ultrasonography (ERUS) is able to make visible the details of the internal and external anal sphincter muscles, and it may therefore have a role in the evaluation of complex fistula-in-ano.[18] Though ERUS is safe and images most anal fistulae well,[19] it is less accurate than clinical assessment by an experienced examiner and does not image suprasphincteric or extrasphincteric tracts well.[20] For the patient with prior anal surgery or trauma, ERUS may be helpful in the identification of sphincter defects that may influence the surgeon's choice of procedure. The use of hydrogen peroxide in the fistula tract at the time of the ERUS may increase the accuracy of identification of the tract and its internal opening.

Magnetic resonance imaging (MRI) is noninvasive, involves no ionizing radiation, allows imaging in any plane, allows sufficient resolution to image the anal canal, and can differentiate inflammation from scar tissue. A prospective study has shown that MRI is accurate, demonstrates pathology missed at surgery by an experienced surgeon, and is superior to endorectal ultrasound.[21] Although it is expensive, MRI may represent the most accurate assessment of fistula-in-ano available. Because fistula-in-ano is usually managed successfully without preoperative imaging, MRI should be reserved for difficult or recurrent fistulae.

Examination Under Anesthesia

Before proceeding with definitive fistula surgery, examination under regional or general anesthesia is performed. The maneuvers outlined under "Office

Evaluation" above are repeated with the goal of identifying the external opening, the internal (primary) opening, the course of the primary tract, the presence of secondary extensions, and the presence of other rectal disease.[16] If not previously completed, proctoscopy should be performed to evaluate the rectum.

With an anal speculum placed in such a way as to view the known or predicted location of the internal opening, a curved blunt-tipped probe is gently introduced through the external opening and guided to the internal opening. Great care must be taken to avoid the creation of false passages. If passage from the external opening is difficult and the internal opening is visible, a malleable probe may be passed from the internal to the external opening. (*Editor's note:* Occasionally, the presence of the anal retractor distorts the tract sufficiently to prevent easy passage of the probe. Removal of the retractor and insertion of the examining finger at the site of the expected internal opening will often facilitate passage of the probe through the tract.) Persistent difficulty suggests the presence of a secondary tract (as in transsphincteric fistula with a high blind tract), and simultaneous passage of probes from internal and external openings may identify the course of the primary and secondary tracts. Additional measures to aid in the identification of the internal opening include manipulation of the anoderm away from the predicted internal opening or traction on the external opening and tract away from the anal canal, both of which may produce dimpling at the internal opening due to inflammatory tethering. Alternatively, the external opening is cannulated with a small catheter and the tract injected with hydrogen peroxide, sterile milk, saline, or air to demonstrate the internal opening at anoscopy. Methylene blue may also be used but tends to cause excessive tissue staining, interfering with the remainder of the procedure. Mazier[22] was able to demonstrate the internal opening in 86.2% of 1000 fistula-in-ano cases. Once the anatomy of the fistula is delineated, the surgeon may proceed with treatment.

Fistula Management

Principles

The surgeon's goals in the treatment of fistula-in-ano include abolition of the primary fistula and all secondary tracts, prevention of fistula recurrence, and preservation of continence (the division of as little sphincter muscle as possible). The procedures described below differ in how they accomplish these goals, but they share a common theme. If one accepts Parks' assertion that anal fistulae are maintained by a diseased anal gland within the intersphincteric space,[1] the prevention of recurrence depends on elimination of this gland via excision, curettage, or laying open of the intersphincteric space. The likelihood of recurrence, as a practical matter, is most related to the surgeon's success in identifying the internal opening, as this is the key to the anatomy of the fistula and the location of the diseased anal gland. Even in experienced hands, the internal opening cannot always be identified and the tract cannulated during the examination under anesthesia. In this case the internal opening is assumed to have healed, if only temporarily.

Management depends on the anatomy of the fistula. If it is apparent that the fistula is simple, straight, and low and the location of the internal opening can be inferred by probing from the external opening, fistulotomy may be performed over the probe through the predicted site of the internal opening at the dentate line.[12] If the primary fistula tract can be only partially navigated, whether or not the internal opening has been identified via injection techniques, dissection along the tract can be carefully performed from the external opening following the granulation tissue tract with the probe and scissors.[23] (*Editor's note:* We prefer to use electrocautery for the fistulotomy in order to maintain the hemostasis that is needed to accurately follow the granulation tissue.) The tract is thus followed until the internal opening is reached. If the tract is lost before the intersphincteric space is reached, the procedure should be terminated and attempted another day when the (now shortened) fistula tract is more apparent.[24]

Simple fistulae without secondary tracts or active sepsis are definitively treated at the initial procedure. Fistulae with secondary tracts or undrained sepsis may be best managed with a two-stage approach wherein the secondary tracts are drained and a marking seton is placed. Once sepsis has resolved and all secondary tracts have healed, the simple primary fistula may be addressed. Patient preparation for most fistulae consists of enemas the morning of the procedure. When a sphincter-

preserving procedure is contemplated, the patient should undergo mechanical and antibiotic bowel preparation and receive perioperative intravenous antibiotics. A very short intersphincteric fistula can be treated in the office setting with local anesthetic if the anatomy of the fistula can be clearly defined. The vast majority of fistula procedures, however, should be performed in the operating room. This is usually done in the ambulatory setting, but complex fistulae for which sphincter-preserving procedures are planned may be best managed in an inpatient setting (or a 23-hour postoperative stay). Though a simple low fistula can be adequately treated under local anesthetic with sedation, most fistula procedures should be performed under either regional or general anesthetic to allow adequate exploration of the tract(s). Positioning depends on the preference of the surgeon, and most prefer the prone-jack-knife position over the lithotomy position.

Fistulotomy

The procedure of choice for most anal fistulae is fistulotomy. This includes submucosal, intersphincteric, and most low transsphincteric fistulae (those involving less than one-third of the external sphincter). With the patient positioned and adequate anesthesia established, 0.5% lidocaine with 1:200,000 epinephrine is injected along the fistula tract to improve hemostasis. (*Editor's note:* We prefer to use a local anesthetic solution of 0.25% bupivacaine with epinephrine 1:200,000 with 150 units of hyaluronidase added to each 25 mL of local anesthetic. Bupivacaine has a significantly longer duration of action than lidocaine. Hyaluronidase allows rapid diffusion of the solution into the tissues and minimizes the distortion of the tissues and anatomy of the fistula tract.) With an anal speculum in place, the fistula probe is gently passed from the external to the internal opening. The primary fistula tract is then laid open and all granulation tissue is curetted. This tissue may be sent for histologic examination. Focal persistence of granulation tissue suggests the take-off of a secondary tract that should be sought with the probe. Secondary tracts are managed by either open or catheter drainage. Hemostasis is obtained with electrocautery. Any redundant skin is trimmed, and the wound edges are marsupialized to the fistula tract with ab-

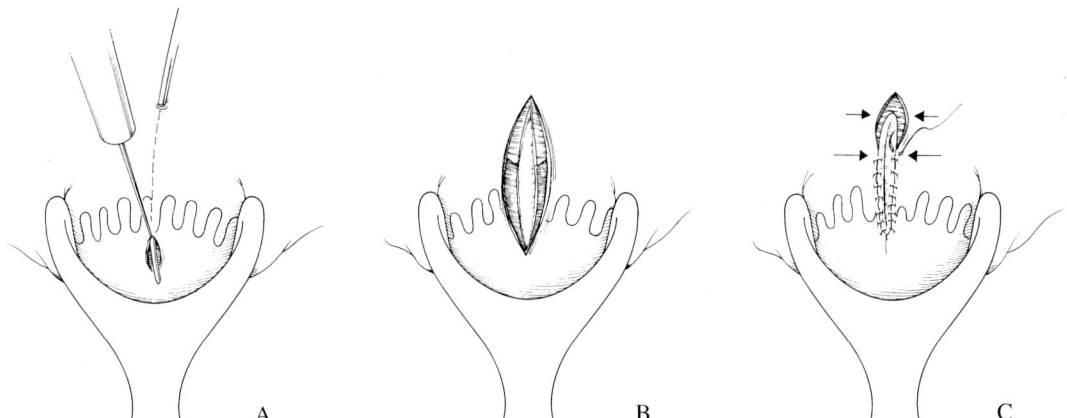

FIGURE 10.10. Simple fistulotomy and marsupialization. **A**, Probe in fistula tract unroofed with electro-cautery. **B**, Fistula after unroofing showing division of portion of internal sphincter and intact base of fistula tract. **C**, Skin edges marsupialized to base of fistula. Redrawn from Vasilevsky.[3(p141)]

sorbable suture to reduce wound healing time and potentially improve postoperative continence[25] (Figure 10.10). (*Editor's note:* We rarely utilize marsupialization of the tracts. It has been our experience that the marsupialized edges rarely remain in apposition for healing and that the sutures produce significant discomfort in the postoperative period.)

Fistulectomy, in which the fistula tract and surrounding fibrotic tissue is completely excised from external to internal opening, results in a larger wound, prolonged healing time, and an increased risk of incontinence without improving the recurrence rate. In earlier years, some surgeons may have used the term *fistulectomy* because of the higher reimbursement rate for such procedures. Today, there is no separate code for fistulectomy. Therefore, fistulectomy is strongly discouraged. Exceptions include cases in which pathologic examination of the entire tract is desired and in conjunction with sphincter-preserving procedures. If the tract is completely epithelialized, either curettage or superficial electrocautery may remove the epithelium.

Anal fistulae that involve a significant amount of external sphincter (high transsphincteric or suprasphincteric), anterior transsphincteric fistulae presenting on the perineal body in women, multiple simultaneous fistulae, and fistulae in patients with inflammatory bowel disease or impaired preoperative continence are considered complex. This re-flects the complexity of management rather than the anatomy of the fistula per se. By definition, simple fistulotomy of a complex fistula would likely result in impairment of continence. Management of such fistulae may involve the use of seton sutures or sphincter-preserving procedures (closure of the internal opening with or without endorectal advancement flap).

Use of Seton Sutures

Seton sutures may be used in a variety of ways in the management of complex fistulae. The loose seton may be used as a marker or drain. It can also be used in either staged division of the fistula or as a cutting seton.

Loose Seton

It is often difficult to assess the position of the primary fistula tract relative to the sphincter mechanism while the patient is anesthetized. If during examination under anesthesia the surgeon cannot determine with confidence whether or not sufficient muscle will remain above the fistula tract if fistulotomy is performed, a marking seton may be placed allowing later assessment of the fistula and sphincter while the patient is awake. In general, if the surgeon encounters unexpected findings or is uncertain how best to manage a fistula, it is safer to place a loose seton and return another day than to divide an inappropriate amount of muscle. When a fistula is found to have associated local sepsis or secondary tracts, opening the primary tract outside the sphincter, draining the secondary tracts, and placing a loose draining seton around the intact lower anal canal will allow resolution of sepsis before the performance of a definitive procedure. This approach is most applicable if a sphincter-preserving procedure is intended. The sphincter-preserving procedures should not be attempted in the presence of active sepsis or multiple secondary tracts. The loose seton has also been used in a curative manner without division of the external sphincter. During the initial procedure, secondary tracts are drained. The primary tract outside the sphincter is laid open. The remaining skin and anoderm over the primary tract are opened and the internal sphincter is divided distal to the internal opening. The seton is placed loosely around the external sphincter and is left in place, without tightening, for 2 to 3 months. If the wounds have healed and inflammation has resolved, the seton is simply removed. Success (defined as complete healing without subsequent need to divide the external sphincter) has been reported in 44% to 78% of transsphincteric and suprasphincteric fistulae so managed.[26,27]

Staged Fistulotomy

Staged fistulotomy may be performed in the patient whose fistula involves too much sphincter muscle to allow safe division in a single stage. With the fistula probe in the tract, the amount of muscle present above and below the probe is assessed. In the setting of a transsphincteric fistula, fistulotomy is begun at the external opening and is carried medially along the probe until the external sphincter is encountered with no division of the external sphincter. The skin and anoderm between this wound and the internal opening are opened and the internal sphincter is divided distal to the internal opening (Figure 10.11A and B). A seton of either heavy nonabsorbable suture or a vessel loop is tied over the end of the probe and drawn back through the fistula tract. At this point only the external sphincter is contained within the seton. If a heavy suture is used, it is loosely tied to itself with multiple knots, creating a handle for manipulation. If a vessel loop is used, the two ends are secured together with multiple nonabsorbable suture ties (Figure 10.12). After an interval of several weeks,

during which the external wound and any secondary tracts are allowed to heal, the primary tract is laid open over the seton dividing the enclosed muscle (Figure 10.11C and D). The purpose of the staged approach is to allow fibrosis to occur around the seton tract (the result of soft tissue division at the initial procedure rather than cutting by the seton itself), preventing gaping of the enclosed muscle when it is divided at the second stage. If the entire external sphincter is confined within the seton at initial placement, which may become apparent during office follow-up before the second stage, consideration should be given to dividing only half of the enclosed muscle at each of two further stages. (*Editor's note:* In this situation, we prefer to divide the remaining sphincter from its deepest portion outward using a curved scalpel blade that cuts from its inside edge [No. 12 scalpel blade].)

Suprasphincteric fistulae, which surround both the external sphincter and puborectalis muscles, may also be managed via staged fistulotomy. With the probe across the entire primary tract, the skin and anoderm between the internal and external openings are incised and the internal sphincter below the internal opening is divided. The lower half of the external sphincter is also divided. A seton is placed around the remaining muscle (puborectalis and upper half of external sphincter) in the manner described above. After a period of months, the remaining muscle is divided in stages. Parks and Sitz[28] reported on 80 patients with suprasphincteric and high transsphincteric fistulae treated in this manner. If all wounds and secondary tracts healed before performance of the second stage, the seton was removed without further muscle division. These authors were able to achieve healing without division of the upper sphincter in 62.5% of their patients. Ramanujam et al.[29] reported a series of 45 patients with suprasphincteric fistulae treated by division of the puborectalis and upper external sphincter with placement of a seton around the distal sphincter during the first procedure and division of the distal sphincter 1 to 2 months later. They found that only one patient developed recurrence of the fistula and one patient experienced incontinence to flatus.

Seton Fistulotomy (Cutting Seton)

Seton fistulotomy is another alternative for the complex anal fistula. With this technique, fistu-

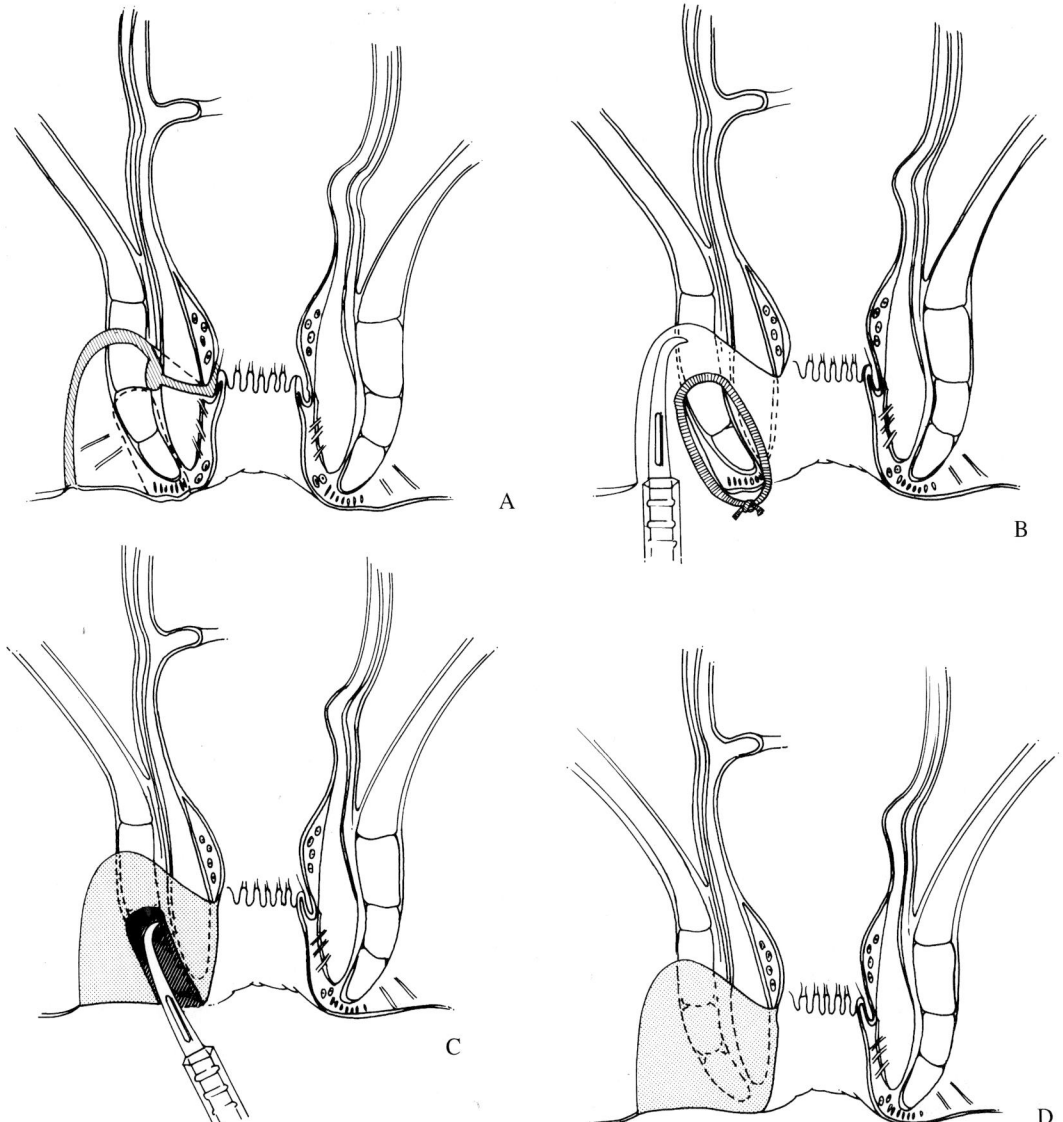

FIGURE 10.11. Seton placement for staged (seton) fistulotomy. See text for detailed explanation.

lotomy is accomplished gradually. In theory, the muscle contained within the seton is slowly divided due to pressure necrosis, with the divided muscle ends separating only minimally because of the fibrosis that develops behind the seton. This is analogous to pulling a steel wire through a block of ice; the ice melts ahead of the wire and freezes behind it. In this manner, the muscle within the seton is divided, curing the fistula, without significant separa-

tion of the muscle ends. The technique is quite simple. As described above for staged fistulotomy, the portion of the fistula tract outside the external sphincter and the internal sphincter distal to the internal opening are unroofed (to eradicate the source of the fistula). An elastic seton (vessel loop) is then drawn back through the tract and loosely secured to itself. It is important that all skin and anoderm within the seton be divided to minimize patient

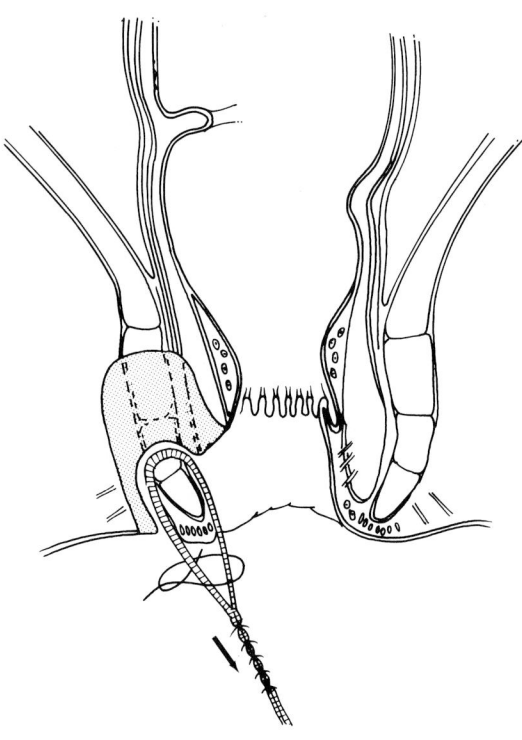

FIGURE 10.12. Technique of elastic seton tightening.

Seton as a Permanent Drain

A final use of the seton is as a permanent drain. In certain cases such as in a patient with Crohn's disease and multiple fistulae, an elderly patient with marginal continence and a high fistula, or a patient with multiple previous fistula procedures, it may desirable to leave a loose seton (without division of perineal skin, sphincter muscle, or anoderm) indefinitely. This is usually successful in preventing recurrent abscess formation and relieving symptoms without affecting continence.

Sphincter-Preserving Procedures

An alternative to the procedures described above is direct closure of the internal opening without division of sphincter muscle. Although they are more technically demanding than the other options, sphincter-preserving procedures are especially attractive for high fistulae and fistulae in patients with inflammatory bowel disease or less than perfect continence. The internal opening may be closed by endorectal advancement flap or by direct suture. The fistula tract is managed either by curettage with open or catheter drainage or by fistulectomy. These procedures should not be performed in the presence of active sepsis and are best performed as a second stage if secondary tracts are initially present.

Mechanical and antibiotic bowel preparation is utilized, and perioperative intravenous antibiotics are given. With the patient under regional or general anesthesia, in the prone jack-knife or lithotomy position (depending on the location of the internal opening), the anatomy of the fistula tract is defined. With an anal retractor in place, a flap of the lower rectal wall is raised including mucosa, submucosa, and the underlying circular muscle. The base of the flap should be twice as wide as the tip and the tip should extend 1 cm below the internal opening. The fistula tract is curetted and the internal opening in the muscle is closed with absorbable sutures. Next the tip of the flap, containing the internal opening, is excised and the flap advanced over the muscular closure and sutured in place so that the site of muscular closure and the flap suture line do not overlap (Figure 10.13). The external opening may be managed by wide external drainage, placement of a catheter for drainage, or fistulectomy (performed before creation of the endorectal flap). Results of

discomfort when the seton is later tightened (Figure 10.12). Once all suppuration has resolved, usually 3 to 6 weeks postoperatively, the seton is tightened in the office. Traction is applied to the seton to stretch the elastic. A silk tie is then secured around the two limbs of the seton near the enclosed muscle (Figure 10.12). When released, the seton should be snug but not overly tight. The likelihood of subsequent impairment of continence may be proportional to the speed with which the muscle is divided. This routine is repeated every 2 weeks until division of the muscle is complete. (*Editor's note:* We strongly prefer the staged fistulotomy over the cutting seton. As the seton is tightened, it cuts into the muscle in a circumferential fashion, burying itself in the muscle instead of gradually transposing the tract more superficially. [Try putting the elastic seton around an ice cube and observe the results.] If the cutting pressure of the seton is downward as a result of a small weight or elastic attached to the patient's leg, then the effect is the same as in the staged fistulotomy.)

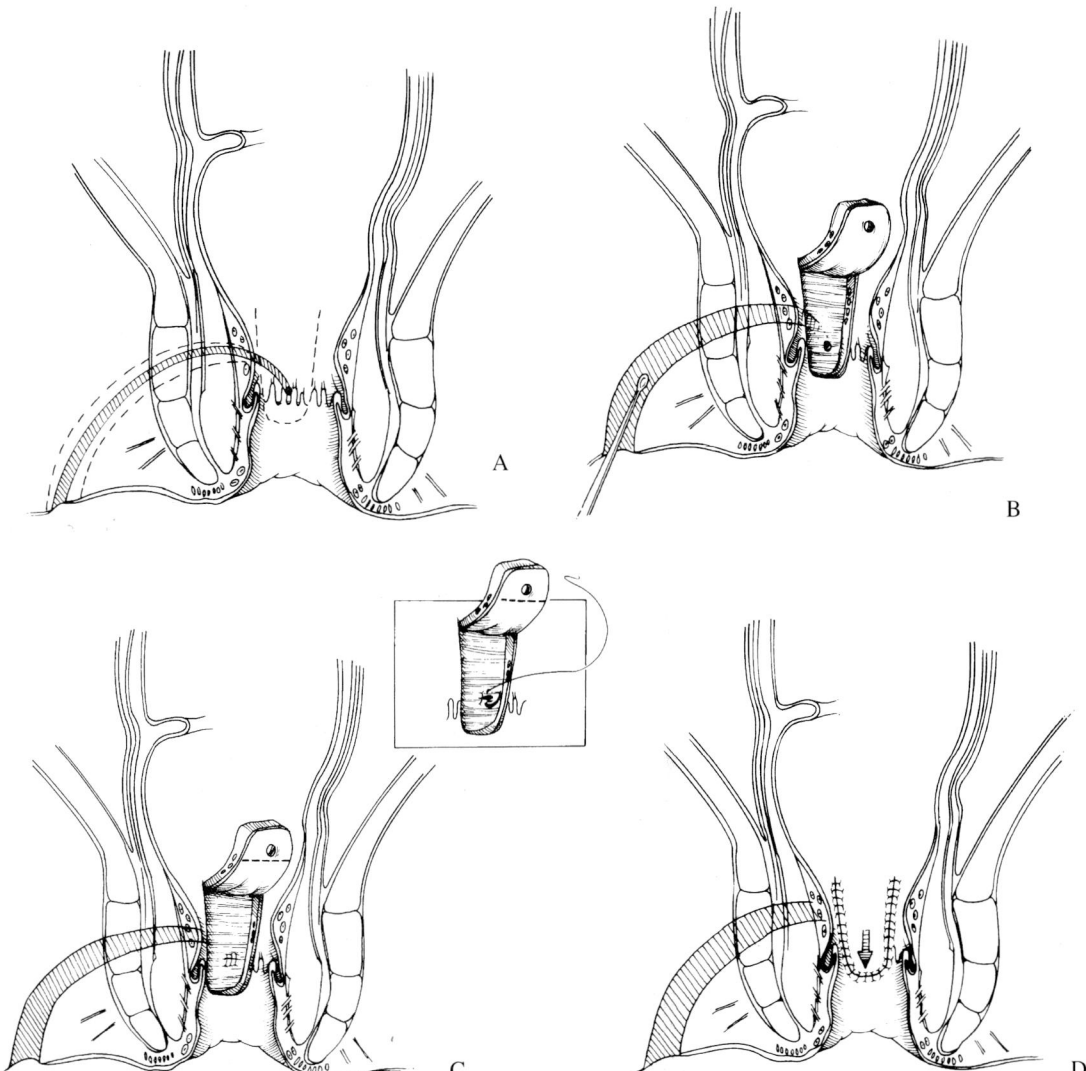

FIGURE 10.13. Endorectal advancement flap procedure. **A**, Flap outlined and extent of tract excision shown. **B**, Flap (including internal sphincter) elevated and tract curetted. **C**, Muscle wall closed and tip of flap excised. **D**, Flap sutured in place with tract open for drainage. Redrawn from Reznick and Bailey.[31]

the advancement flap procedure have been encouraging in most series, with reports of cure rates above 85%[30-32] and excellent physiologic and functional results.[33] The procedure has also been associated with success in patients with Crohn's disease,[32] as long as concomitant rectal disease is absent.[34] Because of fibrosis from previous procedures or anorectal sepsis it is not always possible to raise a satisfactory flap. In such cases, the internal opening may be excised and the muscular opening closed with interrupted sutures. Though preferring to close the internal opening with an advancement flap, Reznick and Bailey[31] achieved success with direct suture closure alone when necessary.

Fibrin glue has been used successfully in the treatment of complex fistula-in-ano. Following mechanical and antibiotic bowel preparation and the administration of preoperative intravenous antibiotics, the fistula tract is thoroughly curetted with a strip of gauze. The thrombin and fibrinogen are simultaneously introduced through the external opening to fill the tract. The internal opening is usually closed by simple suture technique after the glue is injected. Over time, the fibrin clot is replaced with scar tissue, permanently sealing off the fistula tract. The ability to cure complex fistulae by a simple procedure without division of sphincter muscle or perineal tissue makes the success reported in the small series published most encouraging.[35,36] Favorable results from larger series and standardization of the production of fibrin glue may some day make this the first line of treatment for many anal fistulae.

Special Circumstances

Horseshoe Fistula

Horseshoe fistula, involving either the deep postanal space or the deep anterior anal space with extension into one or both ischiorectal fossae, is the chronic form of horseshoe abscess discussed under "Ischiorectal Abscess," above. Management is similar. In the chronic setting, it may be worthwhile to obtain a preoperative fistulogram if the anatomy of the fistula is not apparent. Once the internal opening (usually in the posterior midline at the dentate line) and lateral extension have been identified, the deep postanal space is opened in the midline. This is facilitated by passing a probe from either the internal opening or one of the external openings into the deep postanal space (or deep anterior anal space, as the case may be). Definitive treatment involves opening the deep postanal space (or deep anterior anal space) curettage and draining the primary and all secondary tracts (see Figure 10.6). The fistula into the deep postanal space may be managed by primary fistulotomy or the use of a seton (see "Staged Fistulotomy" and "Seton Fistulotomy [Cutting Seton]," above). Success was achieved in 9 of 11 patients managed with seton fistulotomy by Ustynoski et al.[9] An alternative to the seton fistulotomy portion of this approach is to perform internal sphincterotomy distal to the inter-

nal opening during the initial procedure, to eradicate the diseased anal gland, and to remove the seton when all wounds have healed, as discussed above under "Loose Seton."

Extrasphincteric Fistula

As described in the fistula classification section, the management of an extrasphincteric fistula is dependent on its etiology. The extrasphincteric fistula may be an upward extension of a transsphincteric fistula that has penetrated the rectal wall. It is distinctly uncommon for this to occur spontaneously. Penetration of the rectal wall is more likely the result of overzealous probing from the external opening along what was a high blind tract. In either case, appropriate treatment requires addressing both the transsphincteric fistula and the extrasphincteric fistula. The former is accomplished with any of the techniques previously described for transsphincteric fistulae (fistulotomy, staged fistulotomy, seton fistulotomy, etc.) depending on the anatomy of the fistula and the status of the patient. The latter is addressed by curettage of the extrasphincteric tract and suture closure of the internal opening. To improve the likelihood of healing of the internal opening, this closure should be performed after mechanical and antibiotic bowel preparation. Restriction of oral intake postoperatively, including the use of antidiarrheals to produce a "medical colostomy" for a period of several days may also be advisable. If the fistula is large or recurrent, it may be best to perform a diverting stoma before addressing the fistula.

An extrasphincteric fistula may also be due to trauma, from either the perianal area into the rectum or from the rectal lumen into the ischiorectal space and onto the perianum (as may be seen with a swallowed foreign body). In this setting the tract is drained and any foreign body removed, the internal opening is closed, and a diverting ostomy is performed. As the anal canal is not involved in the fistula, no sphincter division is necessary. Another source of extrasphincteric fistula is intrinsic rectal disease, such as Crohn's disease or carcinoma. Management of such a fistula is directed at the underlying pathology, often by proctectomy. Finally, an extrasphincteric fistula may result from downward extension of pelvic sepsis, such as diverticulitis. Management is directed at the source of pelvic sepsis. The fistula will heal once the source is appropriately treated and the external tract is drained.

Anorectal Fistula in Crohn's Disease

Patients with Crohn's disease and fistula-in-ano require special consideration for several reasons. The fistula may be due to intrinsic rectal disease (proctitis). Wound healing may be delayed in patients with active Crohn's disease, and such patients are likely to develop additional fistulae in the future and potentially undergo additional fistula procedures. Finally, patients with Crohn's disease are prone to significant diarrhea that will magnify the impact of any impairment of anal continence. With these points in mind, the surgeon should proceed cautiously. Most anal fistulae in patients with Crohn's disease are of cryptoglandular origin. If the tract is low (intersphincteric or very low transsphincteric), continence is normal, and no active disease is present in the rectum, fistulotomy is safe and effective. If the tract is high or continence is impaired, closure of the internal opening with an endorectal advancement flap may prove optimal. If active proctitis or multiple fistulae are present, a loose seton (Figure 10.14) may reduce or eliminate symptoms and delay the need for proctectomy.[37]

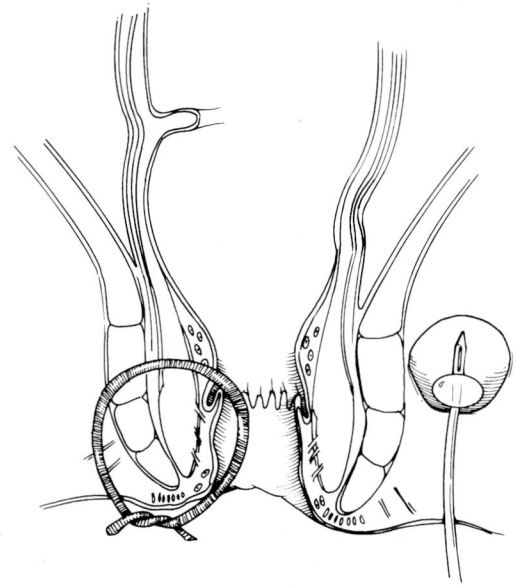

FIGURE 10.14. Techniques for loose seton drainage (*left*) and catheter drainage (*right*) for anal fistula or abscess in a patient with Crohn's disease.

When secondary tracts or abscesses require drainage, long-term catheter drainage may be preferable to wide incision because of delayed wound healing (Figure 10.14).

Postoperative Care

Postoperative patient care varies with the nature of the fistula and the procedure performed. If fistulotomy is performed, a regular diet, nonnarcotic analgesics, and a bulk laxative are prescribed. No packing is used and the patient is instructed to take sitz baths at least twice daily and after each bowel movement. The postoperative follow-up interval is determined by the nature of the wound; if the wound is simple and shallow, the patient is seen after 2 weeks; if deep or complex, the patient is seen within a week to ensure that healing is occurring from the depths toward the surface. If the wound edges heal prematurely, digital opening of the wound may be necessary. Patients having a seton placed are managed similarly. Patients undergoing an endorectal advancement flap procedure are maintained on intravenous fluids only for the first few days after the procedure to improve healing of the flap. Subsequent to this, a regular diet with bulk laxative is initiated and the patient is seen after 2 weeks. (*Editor's note:* We do not "confine" the bowels of patients undergoing endorectal advancement flap procedures. Many of these patients are now discharged the day of surgery and are given an oral, broad-spectrum antibiotic such as trovafloxacin.) After any fistula operation the patient should be reassured that some temporary mild impairment of continence is common in the immediate postoperative period and that this will likely improve within a week to 10 days. The patient should also have realistic expectations for the duration of wound healing. Simple wounds will heal completely in as little as 4 to 5 weeks, and most fistula wounds will heal within 12 weeks.[15]

Complications

Early complications after fistula surgery occur in less than 6% of patients[22] and include fecal impaction, thrombosed external hemorrhoids, and urinary retention. Long-term complications include delayed wound healing, fistula recurrence, and incontinence. The published rates for each of these vary widely due to differences in the complexity of fistulae and the thoroughness of follow-up. The duration of wound healing is related to the amount of soft tissue divided and the successful drainage of sepsis. Recurrence is related to failure to identify and manage the internal opening or secondary tracts and occurs in 0% to 17% of patients.[12] Impairment of continence after fistula surgery is related to the amount of muscle divided, injury to the inferior rectal nerves, or the use of prolonged packing. Impaired continence has been reported to occur in 0% to 45.5% of patients.[12]

Specific Concerns for Ambulatory Surgery

Outpatient management of anorectal abscess and fistula-in-ano is safe and cost-effective[38] and may be appropriate for approximately 90% of anal fistulae.[39] Exceptions include patients in whom systemic signs of sepsis dictate admission for intravenous antibiotic therapy (in addition to surgical drainage) and patients undergoing procedures for which postoperative restriction of oral intake, close observation of wounds, or extensive wound care are required. Although most anorectal abscesses can be drained in the office, nearly all anal fistulae will benefit from the anesthesia support and facilities of an ambulatory surgery center.

References

1. Parks AG. Pathogenesis and treatment of fistula-in-ano. BMJ 1961;1:463–469.
2. Parks AG, Gordon PH, Hardcastle JD. A classification of fistula-in-ano. Br J Surg 1976;63:1–12.
3. Vasilevsky CA. Fistula in ano and abscess. In Beck DE, Wexner SD (eds). Fundamentals of Anorectal Surgery. New York: McGraw Hill, 1992, pp 132–141.
4. Ramanujam PS, Prasad ML, Abcarian H, et al. Perianal abscesses and fistulas. A study of 1023 patients. Dis Colon Rectum 1984;24:593–597.
5. Winslett MC, Allan A, Ambrose NS. Anorectal sepsis as a presentation of occult rectal and systemic disease. Dis Colon Rectum 1988;31:597–600.
6. Marti MC. Anorectal abscesses and fistulas. In Marti MC, Givel JC (eds). Surgery of Anorectal Diseases with Pre- and Postoperative Management. New York: Springer-Verlag, 1990, p 87.
7. Held D, Khubchandani I, Sheets J, et al. Management of anorectal horseshoe abscess and fistula. Dis Colon Rectum 1986;29:793–797.
8. Hanley PH. Conservative surgical correction of horseshoe abscess and fistula. Dis Colon Rectum 1965;8:364–368.
9. Ustynoski K, Rosen L, Stasik J, et al. Horseshoe abscess fistula: Seton Treatment. Dis Colon Rectum 1990;33:602–605.
10. Hanley PH. Rubber band seton in the management of abscess and anal fistula. Ann Surg 1978;187:435–437.
11. Chrabot CM, Prasad ML, Abcarian H. Recurrent anorectal abscesses. Dis Colon Rectum 1981;26:105–108.
12. Gordon PH. Anorectal abscesses and fistula-in-ano. In Gordon PH, Nivatvongs S (eds). Principles and Practice of Surgery for the Colon, Rectum and Anus. St. Louis: Quality Medical Publishing, 1992, pp 221–265.
13. McElwain JW, Maclean MD, Alexander RM, et al. Experience with primary fistulectomy for anorectal abscess: A report of 1000 cases. Dis Colon Rectum 1975;18:646–649.
14. Vasilevsky CA, Gordon PH. The incidence of recurrent abscess or fistula-in-ano following anorectal suppuration. Dis Colon Rectum 1984;27:126–130.
15. Vasilevsky CA, Gordon PH. Results of treatment of fistula-in-ano. Dis Colon Rectum 1985;28:225–231.
16. Goodsall DH. Anorectal fistula. In Goodsall DH, Miles WE (eds). Diseases of the Anus and Rectum, Part I. London: Longmans Green, 1900.
17. Kuijpers HC, Schulpen T. Fistulography for fistula-in-ano. Is it useful? Dis Colon Rectum 1985;28:103–104.
18. Deen KI, Williams JG, Hutchinson R, et al. Fistula-in-ano: endoanal ultrasonographic assessment assists decision making for surgery. Gut 1994;35:391–394.
19. Law PJ, Talbot RW, Bartram CI, et al. Anal endosonography in the evaluation of perianal sepsis and fistula-in-ano. Br J Surg 1989;76:752–755.
20. Choen S, Burnett S, Bartram CI, et al. Comparison between anal ultrasonography and digital examination in the evaluation of anal fistulae. Br J Surg 1991;78:445–447.
21. Lunniss PJ, Barker PG, Sultan AH, et al. Magnetic resonance imaging of fistula-in-ano. Dis Colon Rectum 1994;37:708–718.
22. Mazier WP. The treatment and care of anal fistulas: A study of 1000 patients. Dis Colon Rectum 1971;14:134–144.
23. Corman ML. Anorectal abscess and anal fistula. In Corman ML (ed). Colon & Rectal Surgery, 3rd edition. Philadelphia: JB Lippincott, 1993, pp 133–187.
24. Phillips RK, Lunnis PJ. Anorectal sepsis. In Nicholls RJ, Dozois RR (eds). Surgery of the Colon

& Rectum. New York: Churchill Livingstone, 1997, pp 255–284.

25. Ho YH, Tan M, Leong AF, et al. Marsupialization of fistulotomy wounds improves healing: a randomized controlled trial. Br J Surg 1998;85:105–107.

26. Thompson JP, Ross AH. Can the external sphincter be preserved in the treatment of transsphincteric fistula-in-ano? Int J Colorectal Dis 1989;4:247–250.

27. Kennedy HL, Zegarra JP. Fistulotomy without external sphincter division for high anal fistula. Br J Surg 1990;77:898–901.

28. Parks AG, Sitz RW. The treatment of high fistula-in-ano. Dis Colon Rectum 1976;19:487–499.

29. Ramanujam PS, Prasad ML, Abcarian H. The role of seton in fistulotomy of the anus. Surg Gynecol Obstet 1983;157:419–422.

30. Aguilar PS, Plasencia G, Hardy TG, et al. Mucosal advancement in the treatment of anal fistula. Dis Colon Rectum 1985;28:496–498.

31. Reznick RK, Bailey HR. Closure of the internal opening for treatment of complex fistula-in-ano. Dis Colon Rectum 1988;31:116–118.

32. Kodner IJ, Mazor A, Shemesh EL, et al. Endorectal advancement flap repair of rectovaginal and other complicated anorectal fistulae. Surgery 1993;114:682–690.

33. Kreis ME, Jehle EC, Ohlemann M, et al. Functional results after transanal rectal advancement flap repair of transsphincteric fistula. Br J Surg 1998;85:240–242.

34. Joo JS, Weiss EG, Nogueras JJ, et al. Endorectal advancement flap in perianal Crohn's disease. Am Surg 1998;64:147–150.

35. Hjortrup A, Moesgaard F, Kjaergard J. Fibrin adhesive in the treatment of perineal fistulas. Dis Colon Rectum 1991;34:752–754.

36. Abel ME, Chiu YS, Russell TR, et al. Autologous fibrin glue in the treatment of rectovaginal and complex fistulas. Dis Colon Rectum 1993;36:447–449.

37. White RA, Eisenstat TE, Rubin RJ, et al. Seton management of complex anorectal fistulas in patients with Crohn's disease. Dis Colon Rectum 1990;33:587–589.

38. Medwell SJ, Friend WG. Outpatient anorectal surgery. Dis Colon Rectum 1979;22:480–482.

39. Smith LE. Ambulatory surgery for anorectal diseases: An update. South Med J 1986;79:163–166.

11

Management of Rectovaginal Fistulae

Andrew A. Shelton, M.D.
Ann C. Lowry, M.D., F.A.C.S.

A rectovaginal fistula is an abnormal communication between the epithelial lined surface of the vagina and the rectum, whereas an anovaginal fistula joins the vagina and the anal canal. Fistulae between the anorectum and vagina are relatively uncommon, accounting for less than 5% of all anorectal fistulae. The symptoms due to the fistula and the management problems it poses can be vexing to both the patient and the surgeon.

Etiology

A rectovaginal fistula can be the common end point of a variety of disease states. Fistulae can be congenital or acquired. Most acquired rectovaginal fistulae are caused by obstetric injury, inflammatory bowel disease, infection, or trauma, although unusual causes have also been reported. The reported frequency of each etiology is strongly influenced by referral patterns. However, in many reported series, obstetric trauma accounts for the majority of fistulae (50% to 90%).[1-4] Obstetric rectovaginal fistulae are most commonly seen after an inadequately repaired or unrecognized fourth-degree perineal laceration or a repair that breaks down due to infection. Necrosis of the rectovaginal septum due to prolonged or stalled second stage of labor has also been reported to result in rectovaginal fistula.[5,6] Fortunately, rectovaginal fistula is rare, complicating less than 0.1% of vaginal deliveries.[7]

Obstetric injury is just one traumatic cause of rectovaginal fistula. Complications of transanal or transvaginal surgery can result in rectovaginal fistula, as can complications of hysterectomy, anterior resection, and ileal pouch anal anastomosis.[8-10] Sexual abuse and forceful sexual intercourse have also been reported as etiologic factors for rectovaginal fistulae.

Rectovaginal fistulae are seen in patients with both ulcerative colitis and Crohn's disease. Although the transmural nature of Crohn's disease results in a higher rate of fistulization, rectovaginal fistula is still a relatively rare complication, occurring in from 0.91% to 18% of women with Crohn's disease.[11] In a series of 886 women with Crohn's disease at St. Mark's Hospital, 90 (10.2%) developed some form of anovaginal or rectovaginal fistula.[12] Rectovaginal fistula and other forms of perianal disease may precede intestinal symptoms.[2] In general, the more distal the location of intestinal disease, the higher the risk of rectovaginal fistula. Fewer than 25% of patients with Crohn's disease confined to the small bowel have anal disease, compared with more than 50% with colorectal disease.[13,14] Although the incidence of rectovaginal fistula complicating Crohn's disease may be low, this may be the only significant manifestation of disease.

Any infectious process that involves the rectovaginal septum can result in a rectovaginal fistula. The most common infectious cause is a cryptoglandular abscess that drains through the rectovaginal septum into the vagina. Drainage of a diverticular abscess through the rectovaginal septum can result in a high rectovaginal fistula. Less common infectious causes include tuberculosis, lymphogranuloma venereum, schistosomiasis, and human immunodeficiency virus.[15,16]

Primary or recurrent cancers in the anogenital region may present as rectovaginal fistulae either from local extension of disease or as a complication of therapy. Adjuvant radiation therapy plays an increasing role in the management of many cancers and is a primary therapy for squamous cell carcinoma of the cervix and the anal canal. Rectovaginal fistula is a well-described complication of pelvic radiation therapy. It can occur as a result of a deeply eroding radiation-induced ulcer on the anterior rectal wall or from necrosis of a carcinoma involving the rectovaginal septum. The incidence of rectovaginal fistula following pelvic radiotherapy varies from 0.3% to 6% and is related to the dose of radiation therapy and the technique employed.[17-19] Most fistulae develop between 6 months and 2 years after therapy. Prior hysterectomy increases the risk of fistula formation.[20]

Unusual causes of rectovaginal fistula include fecal impaction, retained rectal foreign bodies, drugs, and graft versus host disease after bone marrow transplantation.[21-24]

Symptoms

The most common symptoms of a rectovaginal fistula are the passage of stool and/or gas through the vagina. With a small fistula the only symptom may be a malodorous vaginal discharge or recurrent vaginitis. Sometimes a rectovaginal fistula is asymptomatic. At other times, symptoms related to the underlying disease might predominate. Tenesmus, diarrhea, and rectal bleeding are prominent symptoms in patients with inflammatory bowel disease. Incontinence from obstetric disruption of the anal sphincters may be difficult to distinguish from vaginal discharge and may be the most troublesome symptom to the patient.

Clinical Evaluation

The diagnosis of a rectovaginal fistula is usually straightforward. The goals of examination of the patient are to locate the fistula, determine its cause, and assess the extent of any underlying disorder or associated injury. A directed history usually suggests the likely underlying cause. If the cause is not readily apparent, careful questioning about intestinal symptoms is important. Failure to recognize an underlying condition such as inflammatory

bowel disease can lead to repeated failure of corrective procedures.

Most often, the fistula is felt as a midline pit in the anterior midline on rectal examination and is easily visible on anoscopic examination. If the fistula is small, it may only appear as a depression or pit-like defect. In the case of obstetric injury, the perineal body may be attenuated and a sphincter defect may be palpated anteriorly. Multiple perianal fistulae should raise the suspicion of Crohn's disease. On vaginal examination, the dark red color of the granulation tissue or mucosa of the fistula tract contrasts with the light pink of the vaginal mucosa. Stool or signs of vaginitis may be present in the vagina.

Sigmoidoscopy completes the examination when perineal infection or trauma is thought to be the cause of the fistula. If other causes, such as inflammatory bowel disease, are suspected, colonoscopy, barium enema, or small bowel contrast studies may be necessary. Biopsy should be performed on any abnormal mucosa, ulcers, or mass lesions. Biopsy should also be performed on all rectovaginal fistulae occurring after radiation therapy, as up to one-third of these will harbor recurrent carcinoma.[19]

Occasionally, the diagnosis of a rectovaginal fistula remains elusive despite highly suggestive symptoms. A number of techniques have been used to establish the diagnosis. Dilute methylene blue can be instilled into the rectum and retained for 20 minutes with a vaginal tampon in place. Staining of the tampon confirms the diagnosis. Alternatively, a radiograph may be made of a tampon after the performance of a barium enema. At times a careful examination under anesthesia may be necessary. Detection of air bubbles in a saline-filled vagina upon insufflation of the rectum can help localize an occult fistula. Evaluation with endoanal ultrasound may be useful for detecting an occult rectovaginal fistula, but the primary role of ultrasonography is in the evaluation of an associated anterior sphincter defect.

Classification

A number of classification schemes have been proposed for rectovaginal fistulae. Size, location, and cause are used to classify fistulae as simple or complex (Table 11.1).

TABLE 11.1. Classification of rectovaginal fistulae.

Simple
Low or mid-vaginal septum
<2.5 cm in diameter
Trauma or infection
Complex
High vaginal septum
>2.5 cm in diameter
Inflammatory bowel disease, radiation, or neoplasm
Multiple failed repairs

Operative Techniques

Numerous techniques are available for the management of rectovaginal fistulae, attesting to the often difficult nature of this condition and the lack of a single clearly superior technique. The choice of technique depends on the nature of the fistula and any previous attempts at repair, as well as the experience and preferences of the surgeon. Procedures that can be performed on an outpatient or short-stay basis are the major focus of this chapter.

There are some general principles that apply to most of the techniques discussed below. A full mechanical and antibiotic bowel preparation is used. Perioperative prophylactic antibiotics covering Gram-negative and anaerobic organisms are given. The administration of antibiotics should not extended beyond 24 hours after the operation. Procedures done via the transanal or transperineal route should be done in the prone jack-knife position. This position affords the best exposure for both the surgeon and the first assistant. A headlight is very helpful in illuminating the operative field. When using a transanal approach, the buttocks are taped apart and a Lone Star Retractor™ (Lone Star Medical Products Co., Houston, TX) can be used to efface the anal canal. Low-lying fistulae can be easily exposed with a Pratt bivalve anoscope. For higher fistulae, Wylie renal vein retractors, narrow Deaver retractors, or narrow malleable retractors can be used. Procedures

performed transvaginally are done in the lithotomy position. General anesthesia or regional techniques, such as epidural or spinal, are usually used, although local anesthesia and conscious sedation may be appropriate in certain cases. Although some of the following procedures can be done on an ambulatory or outpatient basis, our preference is to admit the patient for one to several days after most repairs. The purposes of the admission are to control pain and ensure normal bowel function.

Transanal Techniques

Layered Closure

A layered closure can be performed through a transanal, transvaginal, or transperineal approach. A longitudinal or elliptical incision is made around the fistula site and mucosal flaps are raised for 2.0 to 3.0 cm. The fistula is then excised and the vaginal mucosa, rectovaginal septum, and rectal mucosa are closed in sequential order.[25] The reported rate of successful fistula closure after the layered technique ranges from 88% to 100% (Table 11.2).

Endorectal Advancement Flap

A Pratt bivalve anoscope is inserted into the anus and the fistula site is identified. A trapezoid-shaped flap of mucosa, submucosa, and partial thickness of the inner circular muscle (internal anal sphincter) is then raised. The apex of the flap should be 1.0 cm distal to the fistula. The base of the flap should extend at least 4.0 cm proximal (craniad) to the fistula and should be at least twice as wide as the apex to ensure an adequate blood supply. The fistula tract is then curetted. Next, the circular smooth muscle is mobilized laterally from the submucosa and reapproximated in the midline with interrupted absorbable sutures. The distal portion of the flap, including the rectal opening of the fistula, is excised and the flap is sutured in place. The vaginal side of the fistula is left open for drainage[30] (Figure 11.1).

TABLE 11.2. Layered closure.

Author	Year	Patients (n)	Success (%)	Technique
Ayhan[27]	1995	36	88	Transvaginal
Wiskind[26]	1992	21	100	Transperineal
Tancer[28]	1990	19	100	Transvaginal
Hoexter[29]	1985	15	100	Transanal

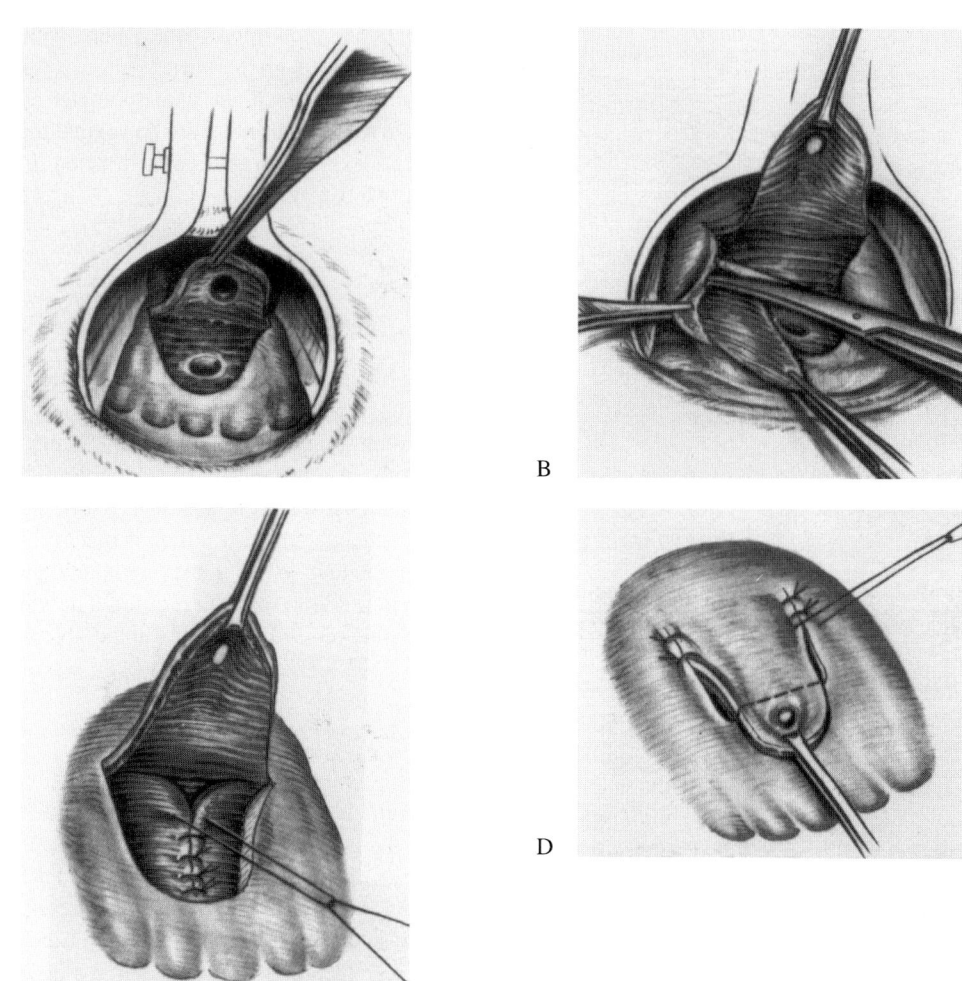

A

B

C

D

E

FIGURE 11.1. Endorectal advancement flap technique. **A**, After identifying the fistula, a flap consisting of mucosa, submucosa, and circular muscle fibers is raised. **B**, The rectal mucosa is elevated off the internal sphincter. **C**, The internal sphincter is approximated over the fistula site. **D**, The tip of the flap is excised and the flap is sutured into place. **E**, The completed operation with flap in place.

TABLE 11.3. Endorectal advancement flap.

Author	Year	Patients (n)	Success (%)
Joo[31]	1998	26	75
Tsang[32]	1998	27	41
Hull[33]	1997	35	54
Ozuner[34]	1996	101	71
Watson[35]	1995	12	58
Makowiec[36]	1995	32	58
Mazier[37]	1995	19	97
MacRae[4]	1995	17	29
Khanduja[38]	1994	16	100
Kodner[2]	1993	71	88
Wise[39]	1991	25	92
Lowry[3]	1988	85	78
Stern[40]	1988	8	88
Jones[41]	1987	39	70
Hoexter[29]	1985	35	100

Successful closure after endorectal advancement flap has been reported in 54% to 100% of cases. Results of several large series are shown in Table 11.3. The reasons for the wide variation in results are not completely clear. It is, in part, an issue of how results are reported. Many series combine the results of endorectal flaps with and without sphincteroplasty. Including patients who underwent a sphincteroplasty would be expected to improve the results. In addition, it is often unclear whether primary or ultimate success (after multiple procedures) is being reported. Finally, because most series include patients with fistulae secondary to varying etiologies, the patient mix may affect the results. Patients with fistulae resulting from obstetrical injuries might be expected to have a higher incidence of concomitant sphincter defect, which might therefore reduce the success rate.

Anocutaneous Advancement Flap

The patient is placed in the prone jack-knife position. A Pratt bivalve anoscope is used to identify the fistula opening in the anal canal. The anoderm or mucosa around the fistula is excised and, beginning at the level of the fistula, an anocutaneous flap with a wide base at the perineum is created. The scarred, fibrotic apex of the flap is excised to provide a fresh flap with a good blood supply. The fistula tract is excised and the defect in the internal sphincter is closed with interrupted absorbable suture. The anocutaneous flap is then advanced and the apex anastomosed to the rectal

mucosa with interrupted absorbable suture, including fibers of the internal anal sphincter with every stitch. The opening in the external anal sphincter can be closed from the vaginal side, but the vaginal mucosa is left open for drainage. One series reported success in both of two patients.[42]

Transvaginal Techniques

Fistula Inversion

Inversion of the fistula is one of the simpler techniques. The patient is placed in the lithotomy position. A circumferential incision is made in the vaginal mucosa around the fistula opening and a circular mucosal flap is raised. The fistula tract is cored out and a purse-string suture is placed around the fistula opening. When the suture is tied, the fistula tract is inverted into the rectum. The vaginal mucosa is then closed with interrupted absorbable sutures.[43] A 72% success rate has been reported.[44]

Vaginal Advancement Flap

The patient is placed in the lithotomy position and the site of the fistula is identified. A vaginal flap is raised with a broad base and is mobilized cephalad and laterally. The fistula site is excised and the rectal opening is closed with absorbable sutures. The levator muscles are then approximated in the midline without tension. The excess vaginal mucosa including the vaginal opening of the fistula is excised and the flap is sutured in place with absorbable suture. It is believed that the levatoroplasty is an essential step in the operation, as it interposes healthy, well-vascularized muscle between the rectal and vaginal suture lines[11] (Figure 11.2). This technique is essentially a variation of the endorectal advancement flap performed transvaginally. In one series of 14 patients with Crohn's disease, closure of the fistula occurred in 93% of those treated with the vaginal advancement flap. All patients in this series had a temporary diverting stoma.[11]

Transperineal Techniques

Perineoproctotomy

Perineoproctotomy is one of the most common surgical approaches employed by gynecologists for the

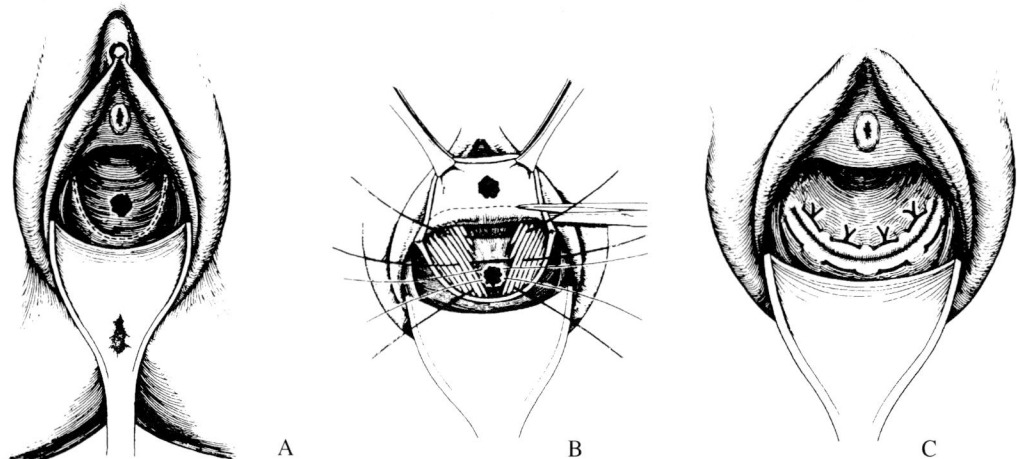

FIGURE 11.2. Vaginal advancement flap technique. **A**, After identifying the fistula, a vaginal flap is raised. **B**, The levator muscles are approximated in the midline and the distal vaginal flap is resected. **C**, The vaginal flap is advanced and sutured in place with interrupted absorbable sutures.

repair of low-lying rectovaginal fistulae. Standard mechanical and antibiotic bowel preparation is employed and the patient is placed in the lithotomy position. The fistula is identified and the perineal bridge—including the skin, subcutaneous tissue, perineal body, sphincter muscle, and anal and vaginal mucosa—is divided, thus converting the fistula to a fourth-degree laceration. The fibrous fistula tract is excised and the laceration is closed in layers; the surgeon must take care to reconstruct the sphincter muscles and perineal body.[1] Results are generally good, with reported success rates ranging from 88% to 100% (Table 11.4).

Overlapping Sphincteroplasty

A curvilinear incision is made in the perineum and flaps are raised consisting of skin and anoderm distally and mucosa and submucosa proximally. The fistula is divided and any granulation tissue is curetted. The divided ends of the internal and external anal sphincters are identified and mobilized

TABLE 11.4. Perineoproctotomy.

Author	Year	Patients (n)	Success (%)
Watson[35]	1995	8	88
Mazier[37]	1995	38	97
Tancer[28]	1990	42	100
Pepe[45]	1987	9	100

posterolaterally. Care must be taken not to injure branches of the pudendal nerves. The muscle ends are then overlapped and sutured with interrupted horizontal mattress absorbable sutures. A levatoroplasty can also be performed by approximating the levator muscles in the midline. The flap of anoderm is then sutured to the muscle, and the perineal skin and subcutaneous tissue are partially closed. The perineal body is thus reconstructed and a bulk of healthy muscle is interposed between the rectal and vaginal openings of the fistula (Figure 11.3). Success rates of 86% to 100% are reported (Table 11.5).

Tissue Interposition

Martius Procedure (Bulbocavernosus Interposition)

A full mechanical and antibiotic bowel preparation is employed and the patient is placed in the lithotomy position. A generous mediolateral episiotomy is made and carried up to the inferior margin of the fistula. The vaginal wall is sharply incised 0.5 to 1.0 cm from the fistula margin. The rectovaginal septum is then opened and mobilized superiorly, inferiorly, and laterally by careful sharp dissection. The fistula tract is then excised and the freshened rectal wall is re-approximated with full-thickness

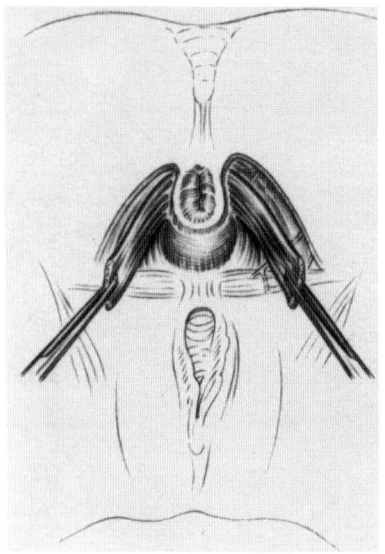

A

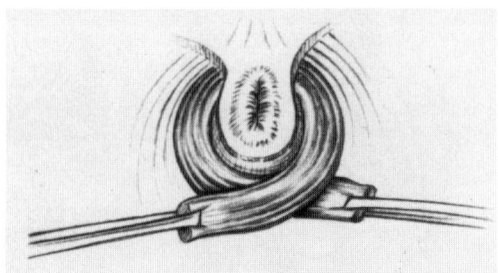

B

FIGURE 11.3. Overlapping sphincteroplasty technique. **A**, After the dissection is complete, the levator muscles are in the midline. **B**, An overlapping sphincteroplasty is performed with mattress sutures.

TABLE 11.5. Overlapping sphincteroplasty.

Author	Year	Patients (*n*)	Success (%)
Mazier[37]	1995	38	97
MacRae[4]	1995	7	86
Khanduja[38]	1994	32	100
Wise[39]	1991	15	100
Lowry[3]	1988	29	93

absorbable suture material. The sutures are left long with needles attached for later use in positioning the labial fat pad. An incision is then made centrally over the labium majus from the level of the mons pubis to the level of the posterior fourchette. By the use of thin skin flaps, the fat and fibromuscular content of the labium are freed. The pedicle graft should not be divided until it has been determined that adequate length has been developed. The graft is usually based posteriorly on the perineal branch of the internal pudendal artery. A subcutaneous tunnel is the made between the episiotomy and the labial incision. The bulbocavernosus fat pad is then drawn through the tunnel into the vagina, with care being taken not to twist the graft. The fat pad is then placed over the site of fistula closure and excess tissue is excised. The retained sutures are then used to secure the pedicle graft in place well over the suture line of the fistula closure. The widely mobilized vaginal mucosa is then carefully reapproximated with absorbable su-ture. Defects in the vaginal closure are preferable to undue tension on the wound. The labial defect and episiotomy are then closed. The considerable labial dead space often requires drainage.[46] Alternatively, a curvilinear perineal incision can be made and the rectovaginal septum dissected up to the fistula site. The bulbocavernosus fat pad is mobilized in the previously described manner and is brought through a subcutaneous tunnel into the perineal wound and sutured in place above the fistula. The skin and subcutaneous tissue of the perineal wound are reapproximated, and the labial incision is closed as previously described (Figure 11.4). Success rates of 71% to 100% are reported with the Martius flap for repair of rectovaginal fistula (Table 11.6).

Graciloplasty

A number of other interposition techniques utilizing normal, well-vascularized muscle—including rectus abdominus, gluteus maximus, and gracilis—have been described. Only the technique utilizing gracilis muscle will be described here. The operation can be performed entirely in the lithotomy position. Alternatively, the gracilis muscle can be harvested with the patient supine and the patient can then be moved into the prone position for the remainder of the operation. The gracilis muscle has its origin from the pubis and has a tendinous insertion

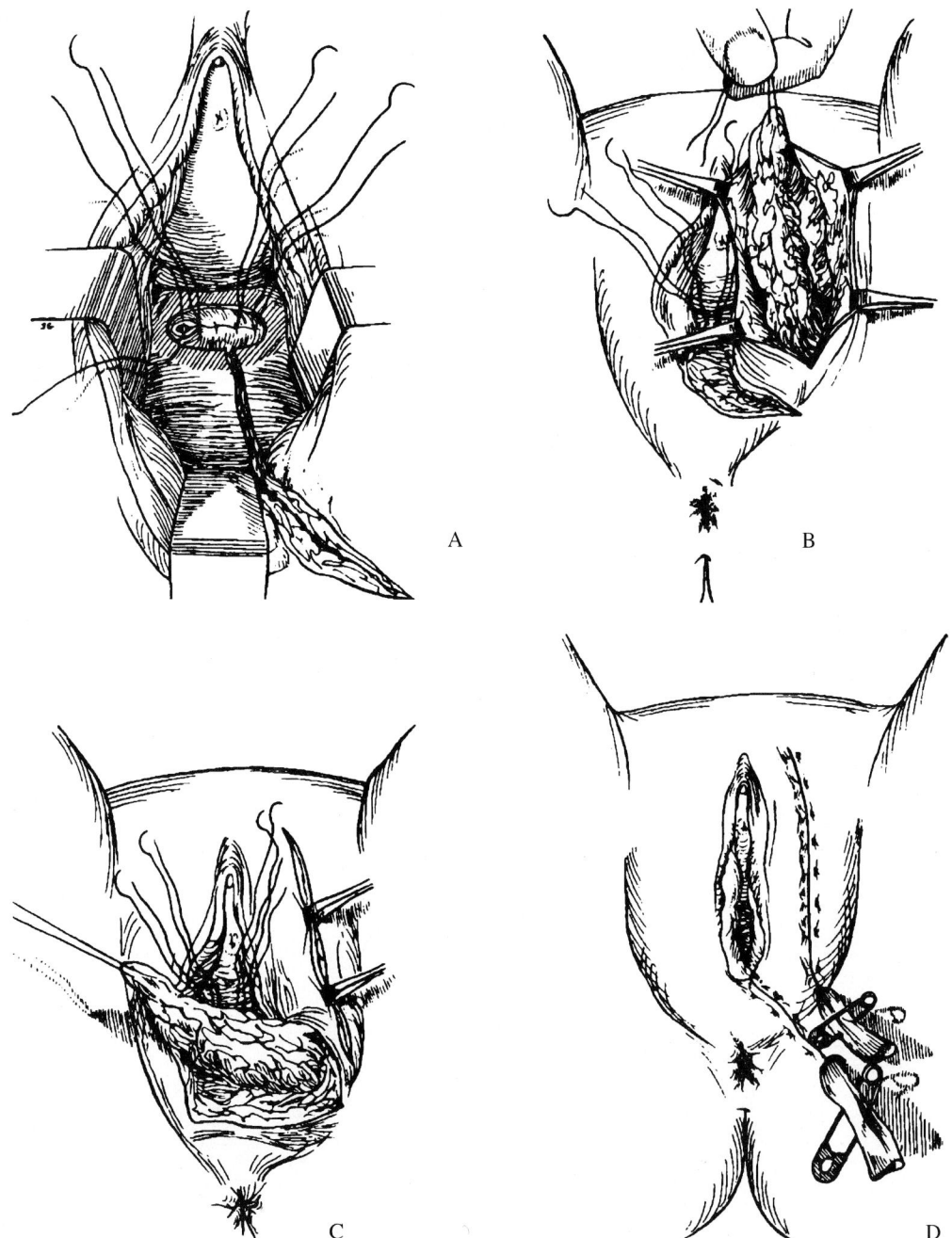

FIGURE 11.4. Martius flap procedure for repair of rectovaginal fistula. **A**, The fistula is excised and the rectal wall closed. The sutures are left long for securing the bulbocavernosus fat pad. A mediolateral episiotomy is made. (Alternatively, a perineal dissection can be used, dividing and extending above the fistula.) **B**, An incision is made in the skin of the labium majus and the posteriorly based bulbocavernosus fat pad is mobilized. **C**, The fat pad is brought through a subcutaneous tunnel between the incisions and sutured into place over the fistula. **D**, After the vaginal mucosa is closed, the skin wounds are closed and drained.

TABLE 11.6. Martius procedure (bulbocavernosus flap).

Author	Year	Patients (n)	Success (%)
Elkins[47]	1990	7	71
Aartsen[48]	1988	14	100
Boronow[46]	1986	19	84

on the tibial tuberosity. The primary neurovascular bundle is proximally based, making it suitable for mobilization and transposition. The gracilis muscle is innervated by a discrete branch of the obturator nerve that has a relatively consistent course along the anterior surface of the adductor brevis muscle, entering the gracilis muscle at the junction of the proximal and middle thirds of the muscle.[49] A large artery enters the gracilis muscle proximally along with the nerve. However, in addition to this, there are two or three smaller vessels that enter the muscle more distally. These distal vessels must be divided during mobilization of the muscle, making it susceptible to ischemic necrosis or fibrosis. The gracilis muscle is mobilized through several small incisions in the thigh, and its tendinous insertion on the tibial tuberosity is detached. A curvilinear incision is made in the perineum, and the rectovaginal septum is dissected in a plane anterior to the external anal sphincter proximal to the level of the fistula. The fistula is divided and débrided. The gracilis muscle is then brought through a subcutaneous

tunnel into the perineal wound and is sutured to the apex of the vagina. The perineal wound is then closed. Two small series with a total of four patients demonstrated fistula closure in 100% of patients.[4,50]

Infragluteal Skin Flap

The patient is placed in the prone jack-knife position. A mediolateral episiotomy is made and extended around the vaginal opening of the fistula. The edges of the incision are widely undermined and the fistula tract is excised. The rectal opening is then closed with absorbable suture. The length of the episiotomy incision determines the length of the gluteal skin flap. A triangular flap consisting of skin, subcutaneous fat, and the membranous layer of the superficial perineal fascia is raised in the infragluteal fold. This preserves the branches of the internal pudendal artery supplying the flap. The incision of the flap is in continuity with the intravaginal incision, allowing the flap to be rotated to cover the rectovaginal fistula. The vaginal incision is then sutured to the edges of the flap and the donor defect is closed[51] (Figure 11.5).

Nonoperative Techniques

A number of nonoperative techniques have been reported for the management of rectovaginal fistulae.

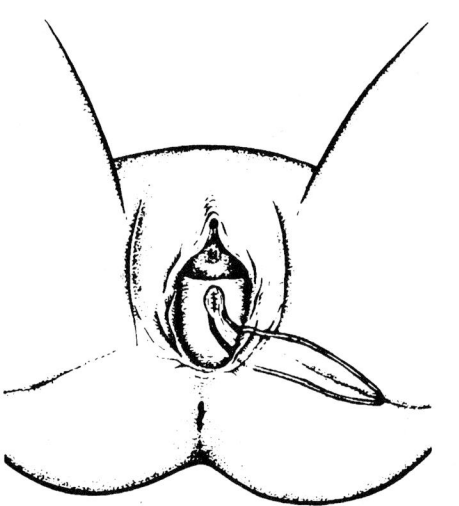 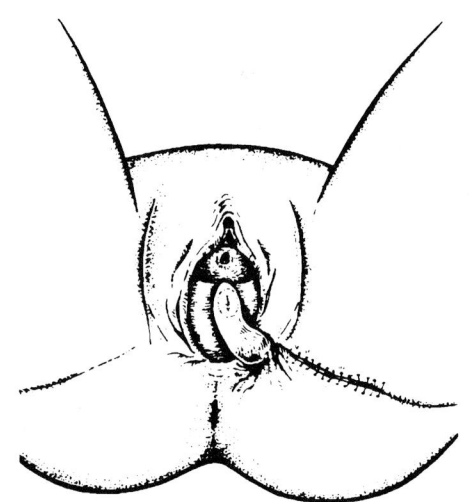

FIGURE 11.5. Infragluteal skin flap procedure. **A**, A flap of skin and subcutaneous tissue is raised in the infragluteal fold in continuity with the incision in the vagina. **B**, The flap is proximally based and rotated to cover the site of the fistula. It is sutured to the vaginal incision with interrupted absorbable sutures.

These include the use of antibiotics and immuno-suppressive medications such as metronidazole, cyclosporine, and mercaptopurine in the management of fistulae in patients with Crohn's disease.[40,52] Autologous fibrin glue has been used to "plug" a fistula tract, with some success in achieving closure.[53] (*Editor's note:* It has been our experience that the fibrin glue works best in fistulae greater than 1.5 cm in length. It is rare for a rectovaginal fistula to reach this length, and for that reason, our results with this technique in these fistulae have been poor.) Several new prosthetic devices for occlusion of rectovaginal fistulae have shown early clinical promise.[54,55]

Specific Considerations

Obstetrical Trauma

Repair of fistulae due to obstetrical trauma should be deferred until most local inflammation has subsided. The surrounding tissue must be soft and pliable to maximize the chance for successful repair. During the period of waiting for resolution of the inflammation, as many as 50% of fistulae will close spontaneously. Timing of surgical repair is also dependent on the patient's desire for future children. If the patient is only minimally symptomatic, repair should be delayed until childbearing is complete. If immediate repair is warranted and is performed because of intolerable symptoms from the fistula or associated incontinence, future children should be delivered by cesarean section.

An important consideration when planning surgery for a fistula caused by obstetrical trauma is the status of the anal sphincters. A fistula can be present with or without a persistent defect of the anterior internal and external anal sphincter muscles. Suspicion of a sphincter defect, whether based on the findings of a physical examination or symptoms of incontinence, should prompt a thorough investigation of the sphincter mechanism. This investigation may include anal manometry, endoanal ultrasonography, and measurement of pudendal nerve terminal motor latency. In a patient with a rectovaginal fistula and incontinence due to a sphincter defect, an overlapping sphincteroplasty should be performed in addition to the fistula repair, because postoperative continence is a critical issue in judging the success of an operation for rectovaginal fistula. In a recent review, only 58% of patients with a healed rectovaginal fistula were satisfied, 19% were partly satisfied, and 23% were not satisfied at all. Of the dissatisfied patients, all were incontinent.[32] Improvement or maintenance of continence is as important as fistula closure in determining patient satisfaction and should be addressed when selecting the operative technique.

In the absence of an associated sphincter defect, an endoanal advancement flap is recommended, although the true success rate of this operation in carefully selected patients without sphincter defects is not yet known. Reasonable alternatives include transvaginal flaps or layered closures. The rectal approach has been preferred because the rectal aspect of the fistula is the high-pressure side, but no comparative study of the endorectal and vaginal approaches exists to date.

Radiation-Induced Fistulae

Most radiation-induced fistulae are not amenable to treatment on an ambulatory basis because of the complexity of the surgery required and the frequent need for fecal diversion. A number of factors play a role in the decision making regarding the appropriate operative procedure for a patient with a radiation-induced rectovaginal fistula. Of paramount importance is the cancer status of the patient, as recurrent cancer can present as a rectovaginal fistula. Therefore, biopsies of the margin of the fistula are imperative. Careful endoscopic examination of the vagina and rectosigmoid are important to identify the height and size of the fistula as well as to assess the degree of surrounding inflammation and infection.

Preoperative fecal diversion plays an important role in the operative management of radiation-induced rectovaginal fistulae. Diversion allows the inflammatory reaction around the fistula to subside, thus improving the chance of future technical success. The choice of site for fecal diversion is also important. Adequate blood supply of the proximal colon is essential. During performance or closure of a left-sided colostomy, the marginal artery may be injured or divided, thus decreasing the crucial blood supply to the descending colon, which may be used in future repairs. Therefore, a loop ileostomy or right-sided transverse colostomy is preferred for temporary diversion. After local inflammation has subsided, definitive therapy can be undertaken.

The only local procedures that are appropriate for radiation-induced fistulae are techniques that bring well-vascularized nonirradiated tissue between the rectum and vagina, thus separating the fistula and improving the blood supply in the area. Because the tissues are poorly vascularized and fibrotic, direct closure of these fistulae is doomed to failure. The Martius procedure has been utilized for radiation-induced fistulae and is one operation that can be done with only a short hospital stay.

Crohn's Disease

Crohn's disease is a chronic, relapsing condition that may involve the rectum and anal canal. Anorectal suppuration related to Crohn's disease can cause disabling symptoms. In the past, local repair of rectovaginal fistulae associated with Crohn's disease has been strongly discouraged and proctectomy advised instead. Many authors claimed that unsuccessful local repair would worsen the problem and leave the patient with a larger defect than before. Recent experience has challenged the pessimistic attitude regarding local repair of Crohn's disease–related rectovaginal fistulae and has shown that a reasonable success rate can be expected. Careful patient selection is obviously important. Women with active proctitis are rarely candidates for repair. Medical therapy is the first line of treatment. Placement of a loose draining seton may reduce the need for proctectomy by limiting perianal sepsis and providing symptomatic relief. Local repair should be considered only in patients who do not have active rectal disease and who are not taking high-dose steroids. A variety of repairs have been reported with reasonable success rates.[11,12,41] The transvaginal route of repair is preferred by some authors, who believe that minimizing dissection of the rectal wall improves the chance of successful repair.[11] The choice of repair ultimately depends on the exact clinical situation and the surgeon's judgment. The need for temporary fecal diversion is controversial. Diversion may decrease the chance of perianal sepsis and may thus have a beneficial effect on healing. If the repair does fail and the resulting

defect is larger, mucus, but not stool, will be discharged through the vaginal opening.

Conclusion

Rectovaginal fistulae can result from a number of causes and disease states. These fistulae can test the patient's patience and the surgeon's skill. A number of local techniques are available for their treatment, and the operative procedure should be tailored to the specific clinical situation. With careful patient selection, success can be achieved.

References

1. Hibbard LT. Surgical management of rectovaginal fistulas and complete perineal lacerations. Am J Obstet Gynecol 1978;130:139–140.
2. Kodner IJ, Mazor A, Shemesh EI, et al. Endorectal advancement flap repair of rectovaginal and other complicated anorectal fistulas. Surgery 1993;114:682–690.
3. Lowry AC, Thorson AG, Rothenberger DA, et al. Repair of simple rectovaginal fistulas. Influence of previous repairs. Dis Colon Rectum 1988;31:676–678.
4. MacRae HM, McLeod RS, Cohen Z, et al. Treatment of rectovaginal fistulas that has failed previous repair attempts. Dis Colon Rectum 1995;38:921–925.
5. Arrowsmith S, Hamlin EC, Wall LL. Obstructed labor injury complex: obstetric fistula formation and the multifaceted morbidity of maternal birth trauma in the developing world. Obstet Gynecol Surv 1996;51:568–574.
6. Lawson J. Rectovaginal fistula following difficult labour. Proceedings of the Royal Society of Medicine, 1972; 65:283–288
7. Venkatesh KS, Ramanujam PS, Larson DM, et al. Anorectal complications of vaginal delivery. Dis Colon Rectum 1989;32:1039–1041.
8. Sugarbaker PH. Rectovaginal fistula following low circular stapled anastomosis in women with rectal cancer. J Surg Oncol 1996;61:155–158.
9. Rex JC, Khubchandani IT. Rectovaginal fistula: complication of low anterior resection. Dis Colon Rectum 1992;35:354–356.
10. Fazio VW, Tjandra JJ. Pouch advancement and neoileoanal anastomosis for anastomotic stricture and anovaginal fistula complicating restorative proctocolectomy. Br J Surg 1992;79:694–696.
11. Sher ME, Bauer JJ, Gelernt I. Surgical repair of rectovaginal fistulas in patients with Crohn's disease. Dis Colon Rectum 1991;34:641–648.

12. Radcliffe AG, Ritchie JK, Hawley PR, et al. Anovaginal and rectovaginal fistulas in Crohn's disease. Dis Colon Rectum 1988;31:91–94.

13. Homan WP, Tang C, Thorgjarnarson B. Anal lesions complicating Crohn's disease. Arch Surg 1976;111: 1333–1335.

14. Rankin GB, Watts HD, Melnyk CS, et al. National cooperative Crohn's study: extraintestinal manifestations and perianal complications. Gastroenterology 1979;4:914.

15. Kunin J, Bejar J, Eldar S. Schistosomiasis as a cause of rectovaginal fistula: a brief case report. Isr J Med Sci 1996;32:1109–1111.

16. Borgstein ES, Broadhead RL. Acquired rectovaginal fistula. Arch Dis Child 1994;71:165–166.

17. Graham JB. Vaginal fistulas following radiotherapy. Surgery, Gynecology, and Obstetrics 1965;1019–1030.

18. Cooke SA, Wellsted MD. The surgical treatment of the radiation damaged rectum. Br J Surg 1981;68: 488–492.

19. Allen-Mersh TG, Wilson EJ, Hope-Stone HF, et al. The management of late radiation induced rectal injury after treatment of carcinoma of the uterus. Surg Gynecol Obstet 1987;164:521–524.

20. Perez CA, Breaux S, Bedwinek JM, et al. Radiotherapy alone in treatment of carcinoma of the uterine cervix. II. Analysis of complications. Cancer 1985; 54:235–246.

21. Pfeifer J, Reissman P, Wexner SD. Ergotamine-induced complex rectovaginal fistula. Report of a case. Dis Colon Rectum 1995;38:1224–1226.

22. Anderson PG, Anderson M. An unusual cause of rectovaginal fistula. Aust N Z J Surg 1993;63:148–149.

23. Houdart R, Salmeron M. Rectovaginal fistula following fecal impaction. Gastroenterol Clin Biol 1987;11:98.

24. Kessler BH, Cochran WJ, Wagner ML, et al. Graft-versus-host disease: gastrointestinal involvement with a rectovaginal fistula. J Pediatr Gastroenterol Nutr 1988;7:288–292.

25. Greenwald JC, Hoexter B. Repair of rectovaginal fistulas. Surg Gynecol Obstet 1978;146:443.

26. Wiskind AK, Thompson JD. Transverse perineal repair of rectovaginal fistulas in the lower vagina. Am J Obstet Gynecol 1992; 167:694–699.

27. Ayhan A, Tuncer ZS, Dogan L, et al. Results of treatment in 182 consecutive patients with genital fistulas. Int J Gynaecol Obstet 1995;48:43–47.

28. Tancer ML, Lasser D, Rosenblum N. Rectovaginal fistula or perineal and anal sphincter disruption or both after vaginal delivery. Surg Gynecol Obstet 1990;171:43–46.

29. Hoexter B, Labow SB, Moseson MD. Transanal rectovaginal fistula repair. Dis Colon Rectum 1985;28: 572–575.

30. Rothenberger DA, Christenson CE, Balcos EG, et al. Endorectal advancement flap for treatment of simple rectovaginal fistulas. Dis Colon Rectum 1982;25:297–300.

31. Joo JS, Weiss EG, Nogneras JJ, et al. Endorectal advancement flap in perianal Crohn's disease. Am Surg 1998;64:147–150.

32. Tsang CB, Madoff RD, Wong WD, et al. Anal sphincter integrity and function influences outcome in rectovaginal fistula repair. Dis Colon Rectum 1998;41:1141–1146.

33. Hull TL, Fazio VW. Surgical approach to low anovaginal fistula in Crohn's disease. Am J Surg 1997;173:95–98.

34. Ozuner G, Hull TL, Cartmill J, et al. Long-term analysis of the use of transanal advancement flaps for complicated anorectal/vaginal fistulas. Dis Colon Rectum 1996;39:10–14.

35. Watson SJ, Phillips RK. Non-inflammatory rectovaginal fistula. Br J Surg 1995;82:1641–1643.

36. Makowiec F, Jehle EC, Becker HD, Starlinger M. Clinical course after transanal advancement flap repair of rectovaginal fistula. Br J Surg 1995;82:603–606.

37. Mazier WP, Senagore AJ, Schiesel EC. Operative repair of anovaginal and rectovaginal fistulas. Dis Colon Rectum 1995;38:4–6

38. Khanduja KS, Yamashita HJ, Wise WE Jr, et al. Delayed repair of obstetric injuries of the anorectum and vagina. A stratified surgical approach. Dis Colon Rectum 1994;37:344–349.

39. Wise WE Jr, Aguilar PS, Padmanabhan A, et al. Surgical treatment of low rectovaginal fistulas. Dis Colon Rectum 1991;34:271–274.

40. Stern H, Gamliel Z, Ross T, et al. Rectovaginal fistula: initial experience. Can J Surg 1988;31:359–362.

41. Jones IT, Fazio VW, Jagelman DG. The use of transanal rectal advancement flaps in the management of fistulas involving the anorectum. Dis Colon Rectum 1987;30:919–923.

42. Hesterberg R, Schmidt WU, Muller F, et al. Treatment of anovaginal fistulas with an anocutaneous flap in patients with Crohn's disease. Int J Colorectal Dis 1993;8:51–54.

43. Mattingly RF. Anal incontinence and rectovaginal fistulas. In Mattingly RF (ed). TeLinde's Operative Gynecology, 5th edition. Philadelphia: JB Lippincott, 1977, pp 618–626.

44. Given FT. Rectovaginal fistula. A review of 20 years experience in a community hospital. Am J Obstet Gynecol 1970;108:41–46.

45. Pepe F, Panella M, Arikan S, et al. Low rectovaginal fistulas. Aust N Z J Surg 1987;27:61–63.

46. Boronow BC. Repair of the radiation-induced rectovaginal fistula utilizing the Martius technique. World J Surg 1986;10:237–248.

47. Elkins TF, DeLancey JO, McGuire EJ. The use of modified Martius graft as an adjunctive technique in vesicovaginal and rectovaginal fistula repair. Obstet Gynecol 1990;75:727–733.

48. Aartsen EJ, Sindram IS. Repair of radiation induced rectovaginal fistulas without or with interposition of the bulbocavernosus muscle (Martius procedure). Eur J Surg Oncol 1988;14:171–177.

49. Patel J, Shanahan D, Williams NS, et al. The arterial anatomy and surgical relevance of the human gracilis muscle. Clin Anat 1991;176:270–272.

50. Gorenstein L, Boyd JB, Ross TM. Gracilis muscle repair of rectovaginal fistula after restorative procto-colectomy. Report of two cases. Dis Colon Rectum 1988;31:730–734.

51. Knol AC, Hage JJ. The infragluteal skin flap: a new option for reconstruction in the perineogenital area. Plast Reconstr Surg 1997;99:1954–1959.

52. Present DH, Lichtiger S. Efficacy of cyclosporine in treatment of fistula of Crohn's disease. Dig Dis Sci 1994;39:374–380.

53. Abel ME, Chiu YS, Russell TR, et al. Autologous fibrin glue in the treatment of rectovaginal and com-plex fistulas. Dis Colon Rectum 1993;36:447–449.

54. Lee BH, Choe DH, Lee JH, et al. Device for occlu-sion of rectovaginal fistula: clinical trials. Radiology 1997;203:65–69.

55. McGovern R, Weinstein MB, Barkin JS. Balloon tamponade prosthesis for rectovaginal fistula. Gas-trointest Endosc 1991;37:82–83.

12

Miscellaneous Surgical Procedures: Treatments for Condyloma Acuminatum, Sacrococcygeal Pilonidal Disease, and Fecal Impaction; Examination Under Anesthesia; and Minor Revision of Intestinal Stomas

Debra Holly Ford, M.D., F.A.C.S.

Condyloma Acuminatum

Anogenital warts (vulvar, vaginal, perineal, anal, penile) are among the most frequently diagnosed sexually transmitted diseases (STDs) in the United States. Condyloma acuminatum is one of several manifestations of human papillomavirus (HPV) infection. It is common within all races and socioeconomic groups and is prevalent in sexually active men and women. An estimated 24 million Americans are infected with this virus, with 1 million new infections occurring annually.[1] The incidence of anal condyloma is difficult to determine, but it is the most common STD referred to surgeons for treatment. The economic burden of HPV infection in the United States exceeded $3.8 billion in 1994. This figure represented over one-third of the approximately $10 billion spent annually on common STDs and related syndromes.[1] The cost of care for condyloma management would be even higher if not for the fact that the overwhelming majority of treatment for this disease are carried out in an ambulatory setting.

Etiology

Condyloma acuminatum is caused by the human papillomavirus (HPV), a member of the papovavirus family. HPV is a double-stranded DNA virus with more than 70 types identified by DNA probe analysis and enzymatic restriction methods.[2] Types 6 and 11 are typically associated with anogenital benign warts. There is a strong epidemiological association between infection with many HPV types and the development of intraepithelial neoplasia and anogenital squamous cell carcinoma. HPV type 16 is found in 50% to 60% of invasive carcinomas, and HPV type 18 is found in 10% to 20%.[3] Despite this association, only a subset of patients with type 16 or 18 HPV progress to invasive cancer.

Clinical Presentation

The clinical presentation of HPV infection may be latent, subclinical, or clinical. The incubation period is 3 weeks to 8 months. Patients are usually asymptomatic and present only after finding a lesion.

143

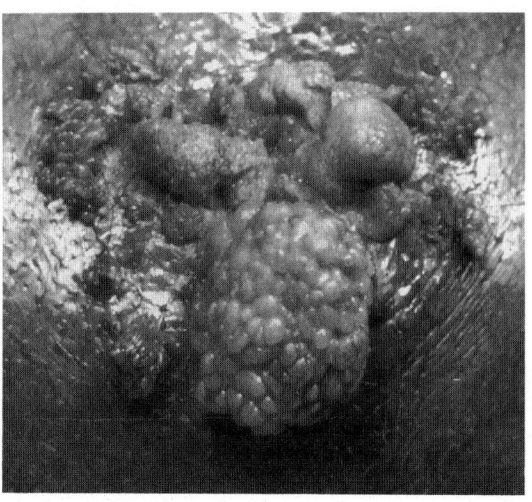

A

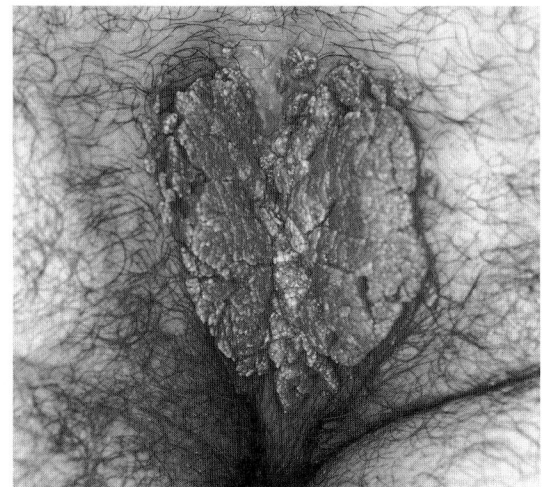

B

FIGURE 12.1. **A**, Condyloma acuminatum: cauliflower-like mass. **B**, Large sheet-like condyloma acuminatum surrounding the anus (photograph courtesy of Wayne Tuckson, M.D., Louisville, KY).

The gross appearance of condyloma acuminatum is raised, cauliflower-like masses (Figure 12.1**A**) that may form a sheet around the anus (Figure 12.1**B**). Occasionally they may appear as small sessile and keratotic papules or as flat lesions (Figure 12.2). If symptoms are present, pain, bleeding, discharge, perianal wetness, and itching are the usual complaints. Perianal lesions may be associated with intra-anal lesions, especially in patients who engage in receptive anal intercourse. The intra-anal lesions are usually at or below the dentate line, but warts may be found at the transition zone of the anal canal as well.

Clinical evaluation should include a detailed history, including a sexual history. Physical examination should include a thorough anogenital examination with anoscopy. Patients are at increased risk for other sexually transmitted diseases; therefore, an attempt should be made to screen for syphilis, gonorrhea, and chlamydia. Possible testing for human immunodeficiency virus infection should be discussed with the patient.

Diagnosis

The diagnosis of condyloma is usually made by inspection, and treatment is started based on the characteristic lesion. Although not routinely required, it is helpful, in some instances, to obtain a sample of tissue for pathological evaluation. Obtaining a sample should be strongly considered in cases where 1) a single lesion is greater than 10 mm in diameter, 2) the diagnosis is in doubt, 3) a lesion is unresponsive to standard treatment, 4) lesions are pigmented, 5) the condition worsens during therapy, 6) a patient is immunosuppressed, or 7) one or more lesions are indurated, ulcerated, or fixed to underlying structures.[4] Typing of HPV is of no

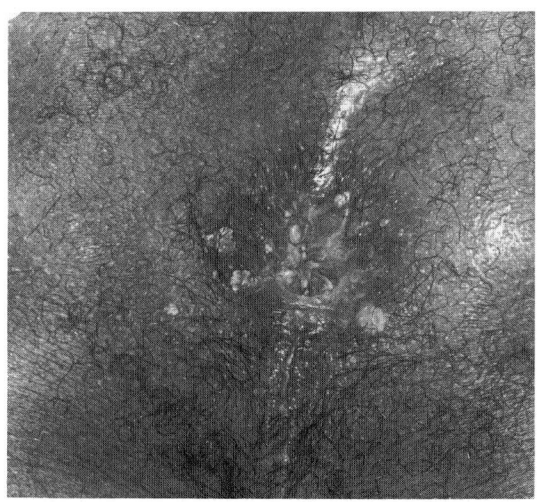

FIGURE 12.2. Small, scattered condylomata.

proven benefit in the diagnosis or management of patients with external anogenital condyloma.[4]

Subclinical disease may be made visible by enhancing techniques using the acetowhite test, which involves painting the areas in question with 3% to 5% acetic acid solution. This technique does have the limitation of a reported false-positive rate of 25%.[5] Flat warts may be difficult to visualize, and the acetowhite test may help locate these lesions, especially those located in the anal canal.[6] In latent disease, human papillomavirus DNA is present in areas with no clinical or histological evidence of HPV infection. These areas may account for the persistence of virus despite treatment.[7]

The differential diagnosis of condyloma acuminatum includes condyloma latum (syphilis), keratosis, lichen planus, skin tags, melanocytic nevi, and neoplasm. Bowenoid papulosis and Buschke-Lowenstein tumor represent variants of condyloma.

Buschke-Lowenstein tumor (Figure 12.3), a variant of a verrucous carcinoma, is a rare tumor with only 42 cases reported in the literature.[8] This tumor is slow-growing and locally aggressive and does not exhibit metastatic potential. The tumor is associated with HPV types 6 and 11 and occurs more commonly in men in the fifth decade of life. The recurrence rate has been reported as 66%, with an overall mortality of 20%. Wide local excision has been used, but patients may need abdominoperineal resection, especially in recurrent lesions. The effectiveness of chemotherapy and radiation are anecdotal.[8]

Treatment

Although spontaneous regression has been described, treatment for condyloma is usually necessary. The eradication of HPV is impossible with current therapeutic modalities. It appears reasonable, however, to treat visible lesions for aesthetic reasons and to reduce the viral burden and possibly the risk of transmission.[9] The association of certain HPV types with the subsequent development of carcinoma may also make the treatment of this disease important. There are numerous treatment options for the management of condylomata acuminata, but they are limited by high recurrence rates (25% to 90%). No single treatment is ideal for all patients. The basic treatment options, based on mechanism of action, include cytodestructive therapies, chemotherapeutic regimens, and immunomodulatory/antiviral therapies (Table 12.1).

Cytodestructive Therapy

The goal of cytodestructive therapy is to eradicate the population of HPV-infected cells. This category includes physical destruction of tissue or chemically induced cytotoxicity.

Surgical Excision

Excision alone may be used in the office to remove small lesions or in the operating room to remove

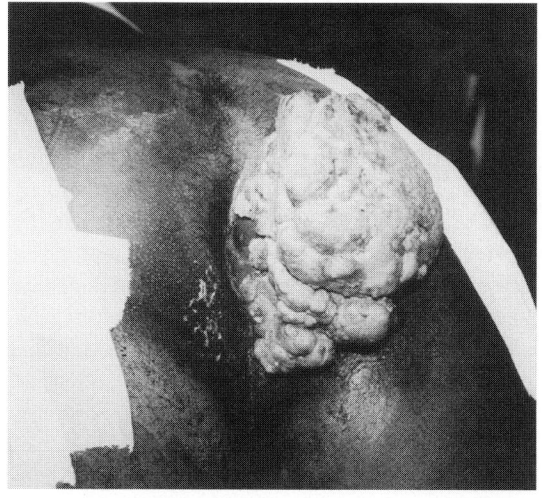

FIGURE 12.3. Buschke-Lowenstein tumor (photograph courtesy of Wayne Tuckson, M.D., Louisville, KY).

TABLE 12.1. Treatment for condyloma acuminatum.

Cytodestructive therapy
Surgery
Surgical excision
Electrocoagulation
Laser
Cryotherapy
Chemical
Bichloroacetic acid
Trichloroacetic acid
Chemotherapy
5-Fluorouracil
Podophyllin
Podophyllotoxin (podofilox)
Antiviral-immunomodulatory therapy
Interferon
Imiquimod
Autogenous vaccines

large ones. Local or general anesthesia is required. Care must be taken to avoid removing too much anoderm or mucosa. All visible condylomata are usually removed during the initial treatment. Pain, scarring, and anal stenosis may be complications of this technique. Response rates are good at 63% to 91%, with a recurrence rate of 25%.[6]

Electrocoagulation

Electrocoagulation requires the use of a local, regional, or general anesthetic. Cautery is very effective in the office to treat small lesions. The use of electrocoagulation requires some skill, and the user must control the depth and width of the wound. Large or numerous lesions are best handled in the operating room. Subcutaneous infiltration with 1% lidocaine with epinephrine is used to separate each condyloma to avoid damage to grossly normal perianal skin, anoderm, or mucosa. In most instances, it is prudent to excise a few condylomata for pathological evaluation. The condylomata are cauterized to a white coagulum. The wound created is usually a first- or second-degree burn and typically heals without significant scarring. Aggressive treatment, however, can lead to severe scarring, sphincter injury, and anal stenosis. A complete response rate of 94% and a recurrence rate at 1 year of about 25% are reported.[9] The combination of surgical excision and electrocoagulation is frequently used for extensive condylomata.

Laser Vaporization

Laser surgery destroys the HPV lesion by vaporization and thermocoagulation necrosis at the treatment site. Most series report the efficacy of laser therapy to be 60% to 90%, with recurrence rates between 5% and 10%.[10] Studies have not demonstrated laser therapy to be superior to other cytodestructive treatments,[10,11] and laser procedures require either local or general anesthesia. Disadvantages of laser therapy include high cost, scarring, potential infection, and transmission of viral particles in the laser plume.[4]

Cryosurgery

Cryotherapy destroys the condyloma by thermally induced cytolysis. The warts are frozen with liquid nitrogen or dry ice applied by spray, cryoprobe, or loosely bound cotton swab. Freezing, followed by thawing, destroys the condyloma but may cause significant discomfort. Local anesthesia may be useful in some instances. Improper application may result in undertreatment or overtreatment, poor outcome, and increased complications. Additional treatments may be necessary, as recurrence rates are reported at 24% to 37%.[12]

Chemical Agents

Other cytodestructive treatments include the caustic acids trichloroacetic acid and bichloracetic acid. These agents, which work by a chemical coagulation of proteins, can be used in the anal canal and can even be used during pregnancy. They must be applied only to the condyloma, and care must be taken to avoid normal skin or mucosa. Mild pain and burning or even severe pain may occur if too much acid is applied. If pain is a problem, sodium bicarbonate can be used to neutralize the acid. Multiple sessions are usually required to clear the condyloma. However, the acids should not be used to treat large areas of involvement. The method has approximately an 80% clearance rate with a recurrence rate of 36%.[10]

Chemotherapy

Podophyllin, podophyllotoxin, and 5-fluorouracil are the most frequently used chemotherapeutic agents in the management of condylomata acuminata. These agents work by the inhibition of cellular hyperproliferation.

Podophyllin and Podophyllotoxin (Podofilox)

Podophyllin, an antimitotic, is a resin extract from the roots of the May apple plant. This agent has been used for many years for external anogenital warts but varies widely in its therapeutic effect because of a large variation in the amount of podophyllotoxin (the active ingredient).[10] Podophyllin is applied to the condyloma and must be washed off in 6 to 8 hours. During application, pain and a burning sensation are common.

Multiple visits may be needed to clear the warts. Podophyllin has the disadvantage of causing a reversible dysplastic change in the condyloma that may cause confusion with malignancy in pathological diagnosis. Reported complications include scarring, fistula-in-ano, and necrosis. When used alone, cure rates of only 20% to 50% can be expected.[6] Podofilox solution, in contrast, contains purified podophyllotoxin and does not contain the known mutagens found in podophyllum. The 0.5% podofilox solution can be administered by the patient in 3-day treatment cycles. Currently, this drug is limited to treatment periods of 4 weeks and excludes patients with perianal warts. However, a recently published randomized, double-blind, multicenter study reported a 42% success rate in treatment of perianal condyloma and demonstrated that efficacy is improved if used up to 8 weeks. The most common adverse event was a burning sensation after application.[13]

5-Fluorouracil

The chemotherapeutic agent 5-fluorouracil (5-FU) has been used in the treatment of anogenital condyloma for many years but may produce significant discomfort and inflammation. An antimetabolite, 5-FU is a teratogen and should not be used during pregnancy. The greatest value of topical 5-FU may be in the prevention of recurrence after condyloma ablation, especially in immunocompromised patients.[6] An intralesional preparation of 5-FU with epinephrine and collagen matrix injected under the lesion has been shown to eradicate condyloma with few adverse effects. The treatments are given weekly for up to 6 weeks. Recurrence rates after 6 months ranged from 0% to 10%.[10] Disadvantages of the treatment are the required frequent visits and the route of administration. Further clinical trials are under way to assess the efficacy of intralesional 5-FU.

Immunomodulatory/Antiviral Therapy

The therapies discussed above are anticondyloma but not antiviral. The ideal treatment for papillomavirus infections would eliminate all lesions, eradicate the latent population of viral DNA, and permit the development of natural immunity to the virus. The agents currently available are interferon alfa and a new patient-applied treatment, imiquimod. Autogenous vaccines have good outcomes, and current investigations are attempting to develop recombinant vaccines based on more sophisticated molecular virology.[3]

Interferon

Interferons are naturally occurring proteins that boost local immunity and have antiviral effects. Topical, intralesional, and systemic interferon have been investigated in the treatment of anal condyloma. Results have been poor with topical and systemic interferon. Intralesional interferon alfa-2 has reported clearance rates of 47% to 62%.[10] Interferon treatment is not recommended for routine use because of the requirement for frequent office visits, the inconvenient route of administration, and the associated systemic side effects (i.e., flu-like symptoms). Interferon should be considered in recalcitrant condyloma. Intralesional interferon given after surgical ablation of lesions has met with some success.[14,15]

Imiquimod

Imiquimod (Aldara, 3M Pharmaceuticals, Saint Paul, MN) is a topical immunomodulator that stimulates monocytes, macrophages, and keratinocytes to produce interferon alfa and other cytokines. A newly approved treatment for external anogenital warts, imiquimod is not approved for use in the treatment of intra-anal condyloma. Imiquimod cream is administered three times a week for up to 16 weeks. It is patient applied and washed off in 6 to 10 hours. A randomized, double-blinded, placebo-controlled study has demonstrated a 56% clearance rate with use of 5% imiquimod cream. The recurrence rate was 13%.[16] Local inflammation and irritation were the most common adverse events. The disadvantage is that the treatment is quite prolonged, and systemic symptoms (i.e., flu-like symptoms) have been reported.[16]

Autogenous Vaccines

Immunotherapy is an effective method to treat anal condyloma. The use of autogenous vaccines has a reported success rate of 86% to 100%.[17,18] The technique has not met with widespread enthusiasm because of cost and the resources needed to prepare the vaccine.

Summary

There is no single effective treatment for anal condyloma. Therefore, surgeons must have expertise in the use of many therapies. In my practice, small lesions are treated with bichloracetic acid, and the patient is observed weekly until clearance is noted. Large lesions are treated with surgical excision and electrocoagulation with the patient under general or spinal anesthesia. Subcutaneous and submucosal infiltration of local anesthesia aid in the discrete removal of condylomata. Patient follow-up is scheduled on a weekly basis, and recurrent warts are treated with bichloracetic acid. Immunocompromised patients (those with human immunodeficiency virus disease and transplant recipients), who usually have large and numerous lesions, are treated aggressively with careful excision and electrocoagulation. Patients should be appropriately educated as to the natural history of the disease and that transmission is possible. The use of condoms should be emphasized, and sexual partners should be made aware of the problem and should seek medical attention.

Sacrococcygeal Pilonidal Disease

Pilonidal disease is a common condition familiar to the general and colorectal surgeon. Because of the uncertainty as to its etiology and the difficulty often encountered in its treatment, the literature bulges with references to this disease. In the past, the management of pilonidal disease has involved the use of extensive inpatient resources, but care in the ambulatory setting is now possible.

Anderson[19] first described this condition in 1847, and in 1880, Hodges[20] coined the term *pilonidal,* which is Latin for "nest of hairs." The name referred to the frequent occurrence of hair within the sinus tracts associated with this condition.

Symptoms of pilonidal disease rarely present before age 15 or after age 40. There is a 3:1 male predominance, and the incidence is highest among Caucasians.

Pathogenesis

There are two theories of pathogenesis: congenital and acquired. The congenital theory suggests that there is a preexisting epithelial lined tract in the midline of the natal cleft formed by squamous epithelium. The origin of this tract is believed to be a caudal remnant of the medullary canal or a faulty coalescence of caudal dorsal ectodermal segments.[21] The belief that pilonidal disease is congenital has provided justification that the surgical treatment should involve the complete removal of all malformed tissues. Surgeons soon found that extensive excisions resulted in prolonged wound healing and frequent recurrence of disease. Because of this experience, theories describing acquired etiology have become more plausible in pilonidal disease.

The mainstay of the acquired theory by Patey and Scarff[22] described the role hair plays in the cause of this condition. Bascom's histologic studies[23] outlined the stages in the development of pilonidal disease (Figure 12.4). The natal cleft hair follicle becomes distended with keratin. Anaerobic organisms are found in these follicles.[24] The distended follicle becomes inflamed and the resulting folliculitis produces edema that occludes the follicle opening. The obstructed follicle expands and eventually ruptures into the underlying subcutaneous fat to produce a pilonidal abscess. Bascom also explained the mechanics whereby the hair is drawn into the pilonidal abscess cavity by the suc-

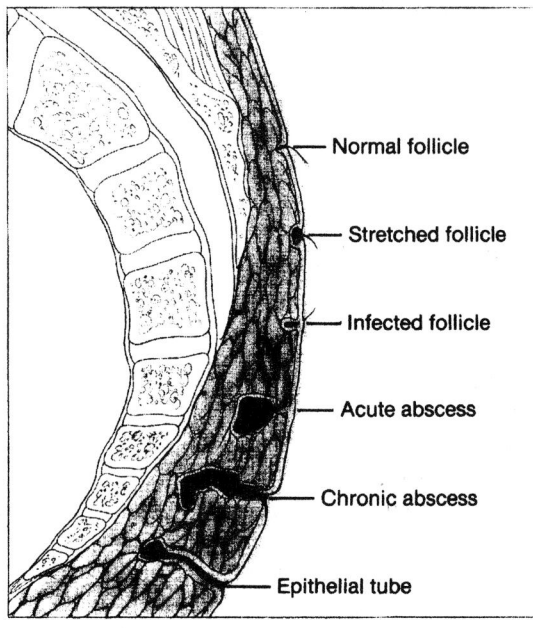

FIGURE 12.4. Pathogenesis of pilonidal abscess and sinus. Reproduced with permission from Nivatvongs.[21]

tion created by movement of the gluteal tissue. Bascom's theory explains the cause of pilonidal disease in the majority of patients. A significant number of men and women, however, have little if any natal cleft hair. In these patients, three gluteal cleft factors have been identified that foster pilonidal sinus formation: catch basin effect, gluteal cleft friction, and intergluteal cleft depth.[23]

Surgical Pathology

Pilonidal disease is a form of foreign body granuloma. Hair is found within the tract in about two-thirds of men and one-third of women.[25] The midline epithelial pit is lined with squamous epithelium. One percent of midline tracts may be lined by squamous epithelium, but the cavities typically do not have an epithelial lining. They are abscess cavities lined by granulation tissue. The tract extends cephalad for varying distances. Rarely, the tract may extend toward the anus and present like a fistula-in-ano.

Clinical Presentation

An accurate estimate of the prevalence of pilonidal disease is unknown. This condition peaks in the 16- to 20-year age range and declines after age 25.[21] Pilonidal disease is usually seen in obese, hirsute men, but many patients are female with only sparse truncal hair. Clinical presentations range from the finding of asymptomatic small midline pits in the presacral area (which may or may not contain hair) to an obvious painful and fluctuant mass situated approximately 5 cm above the anus, usually off the midline. A pilonidal abscess usually ruptures and leaves a chronically draining sinus (Figure 12.5).

The differential diagnosis should include actinomycosis, furuncle of the skin, hidradenitis suppurativa, fistula-in-ano, and other granulomatous conditions.

Treatment

With acceptance of the acquired theory as the probable etiology of most pilonidal disease, the treatment of this condition has shifted from extensive excisions to more conservative and less invasive management. The majority of patients with pi-

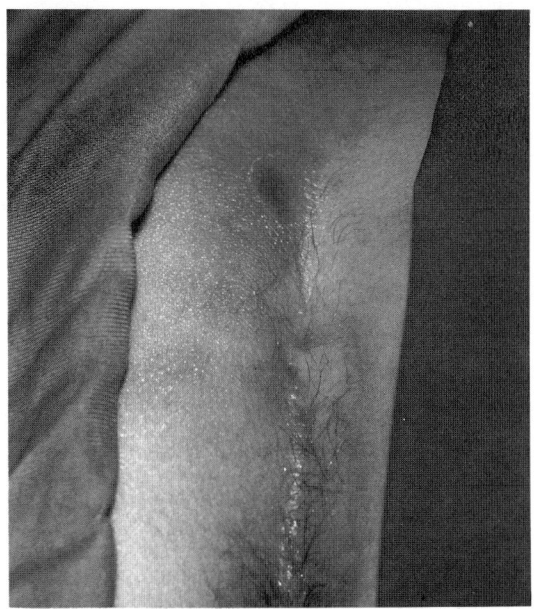

FIGURE 12.5. Pilonidal disease with midline pits and chronic sinus (photograph courtesy of Wayne Tuckson, M.D., Louisville, KY).

lonidal disease can receive their care in an ambulatory setting.

Pilonidal Abscess

A pilonidal abscess typically presents cephalad and lateral to the infected epithelial sinus. Immediate relief of symptoms will be achieved with incision and drainage under local anesthesia and removal of hair. The incision should be placed laterally to avoid the intergluteal cleft. Wounds in the cleft heal poorly. (*Editor's note:* It is our preference, John Bascom's teaching aside, to drain abscesses in the midline if the primary opening can be identified. A probe is inserted through the primary opening into the cavity and the abscess is unroofed with the cautery. Granulation tissue is removed and the wound is managed as described below. We have been able to achieve an unreported 80% "cure" rate with drainage and opening of the primary opening.) Large abscesses may require drainage under sedation or general anesthesia. Definitive treatment is not recommended at the time of drainage. The patient is instructed to take warm tub baths at least two times a day. Office visits are scheduled every other week for inspection of the wound and shaving of hair around the area. A cure rate of 60% has been reported after primary incision and drainage with appropriate postoperative care.[26] Definitive treatment is reserved for patients who do not heal after 3 months or in whom a chronic draining sinus develops. Bascom recommends excising the midline epithelial pits in conjunction with the laterally placed incision for drainage (Figure 12.6).[23]

Pilonidal Sinus

About 40% to 50% of patients with pilonidal disease will develop a chronic malodorous drainage.[25] The pilonidal cavity drains through a sinus. The large number of treatment options available for pilonidal sinus reflects the general controversy that exists concerning its management. The treatment options are as follows: nonoperative care, conservative excision, incision and marsupialization, and excision with or without primary closure. The majority of these procedures are carried out in the ambulatory setting.

Nonoperative Management

Conservative nonresectional therapy includes meticulous hair control by natal cleft shaving, perineal hygiene, and limited drainage of abscesses. Armstrong and Barcia reported success with this technique that significantly reduced the need for surgery.[27]

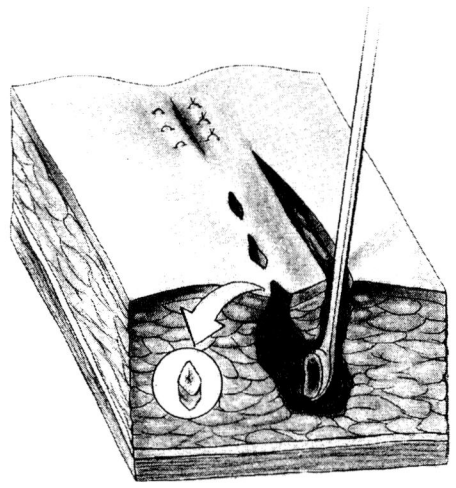

FIGURE 12.6. Treatment of pilonidal abscess: lateral incision into abscess with curetting of granulation tissues and excision of midline pits. Reproduced with permission from Nivatvongs.[21]

Conservative Excision

In 1965, Lord and Millar[28] described an outpatient treatment using local anesthesia. The midline pits are excised down to the underlying cavity through small elliptical incisions. The cavity is not removed, but all hair is removed. Hair in midline and lateral tracts is removed with a tiny nylon brush. Edwards[29] reported 102 patients treated in this fashion with postoperative shaving on a weekly basis. The recurrence rate was 11%. Patients who did not follow the postoperative routine had a much higher recurrence rate. Other methods of conservative excision include follicle excision with lateral sinus curettage, laying open all tracts with curettage, laying open all tracts followed by cryotherapy, and phenol treatment of sinus tracts.[21]

Excision

Excisional therapy is still commonly performed for pilonidal sinus disease. Wide excision of all affected pilonidal tissue down to the sacral fascia is unnecessary and should be abandoned. This technique has a high recurrence rate and is complicated by a high rate of unhealed wounds. (*Editor's note:* Since the pilonidal cyst is really not a cyst but a granulation tissue–lined cavity, there is no justification for the removal of the base of the cavity unless it has become epithelialized.)

Excision and Marsupialization

The excision and marsupialization procedure involves opening the tract, curetting the granulation tissue, and removing all hair (Figure 12.6). The skin edges are sutured to the edges of the cavity. The wound usually takes approximately 6 weeks to heal, and the recurrence rate has been reported to be between 6% and 10%.[25] (*Editor's note:* It has been our experience that when the skin edges are sutured to the base of the wound, primary healing rarely occurs. Patients in whom this is done also complain of more pain than do those without sutures. For these reasons, we have abandoned the idea of marsupialization of the edges and instead merely saucerize the wounds.)

Excision With or Without Primary Closure

All pilonidal tissue is removed to normal fat. The area is cleaned and packed open or closed primarily. The disadvantage of leaving the wound open is the long time required for healing. (*Editor's note:* Again, in our opinion there is no need or justification for excising the base of the cavity since it is fibrous tissue covered by granulation tissue.) Closing the wound is an attractive option, but wound infection and dehiscence may be a problem. There are many techniques for closure, and most require a small hospital stay. These techniques include Z-plasty, V-Y fasciocutaneous flap, rhomboid flap, gluteal myocutaneous flaps, and advancement flap operation (Karydakis operation).[21] (*Editor's note:* It is our experience that the vast majority of patients seen with recurrent pilonidal disease have undergone excision and closure techniques.)

Recurrent or Unhealed Pilonidal Disease

Recurrence increases with the length of follow-up after definitive treatment. Most recurrences occur within 3 years. Recurrence rates range from 3% to 40%. Unhealed wounds are a particularly distressing problem and usually require a wide excision and some type of flap closure. Bascom has described the cleft closure procedure for unhealed pilonidal wounds.[30] He stresses that the final suture line must lie off the midline on a ventilated, convex surface and not within the hazardous, anaerobic fold of the gluteal cleft (Figure 12.7). (*Editor's note:* Our experience with recurrent or unhealed pilonidal disease has not indicated a need for such radical procedures. Unhealed wounds frequently respond to curettage and saucerization [making the skin opening wider than the base of the wound] followed by meticulous wound care. In obese patients the concept of "reverse taping" is occasionally helpful. This involves taping the buttocks apart by passing tape from one buttock anteriorly around to the other buttock. This usually involves a lot of shaving and reapplication of the tape on a weekly basis, but it may result in healing of wounds that have not responded to less vigorous care. Patients who have had primary closure often present with a deep sinus extending the length of the primary excision wound. These often respond well to unroofing, curettage, and saucerization, performed in an ambulatory setting, followed by meticulous wound care.)

Pilonidal Disease and Carcinoma

Malignant degeneration is a rare occurrence in chronic pilonidal disease. As of 1994, 44 cases of car-

cinoma had been reported.[31] Most cases were squamous cell carcinoma and were preceded by pilonidal symptoms for a mean duration of 23 years. Eighty percent of the cases occurred in men with a mean age of 50 years. The tumor is locally invasive and may metastasize to inguinal lymph nodes. Treatment of choice is wide en-bloc resection to include the sacral fascia, but local recurrence is common. (*Editor's note:* The presence of carcinoma in a pilonidal wound *is* an indication for excision of the entire wound!) Chemotherapy and radiation therapy should be considered in the management of these patients.

Summary

Pilonidal disease is a very common problem whose origin appears to be acquired. A pilonidal abscess should be drained with the incision off of the midline. Careful shaving and follow-up are essential. If the wound heals, then no further treatment is needed. If a chronic sinus develops or the wound does not heal, then definitive treatment is appropriate. Consideration should be given to conservative excision methods and careful follow-up. Excision with marsupialization is still a good option. For recurrent disease or unhealed wounds, the cleft closure technique to flatten the gluteal cleft has met with success.

Fecal Impaction

Fecal impaction is a common health problem, but it is frequently ignored. This condition is usually the result of chronic constipation. However, there are many factors that can precipitate impaction. Fecal impaction is defined as the inability to evacuate a large mass of feces. It can occur in any age group but is especially common among elderly, incapacitated, and institutionalized patients. The problem is frequently overlooked and can lead to a number of medical and surgical complications. Impaction has been reported as the cause of intestinal obstruction in 1.3% of patients, but studies have shown an incidence up to 45% in the elderly and in spinal cord injury patients.[32]

Pathophysiology

Regardless of the cause of the impaction, the colon's normal absorption of salt and water contribute to the

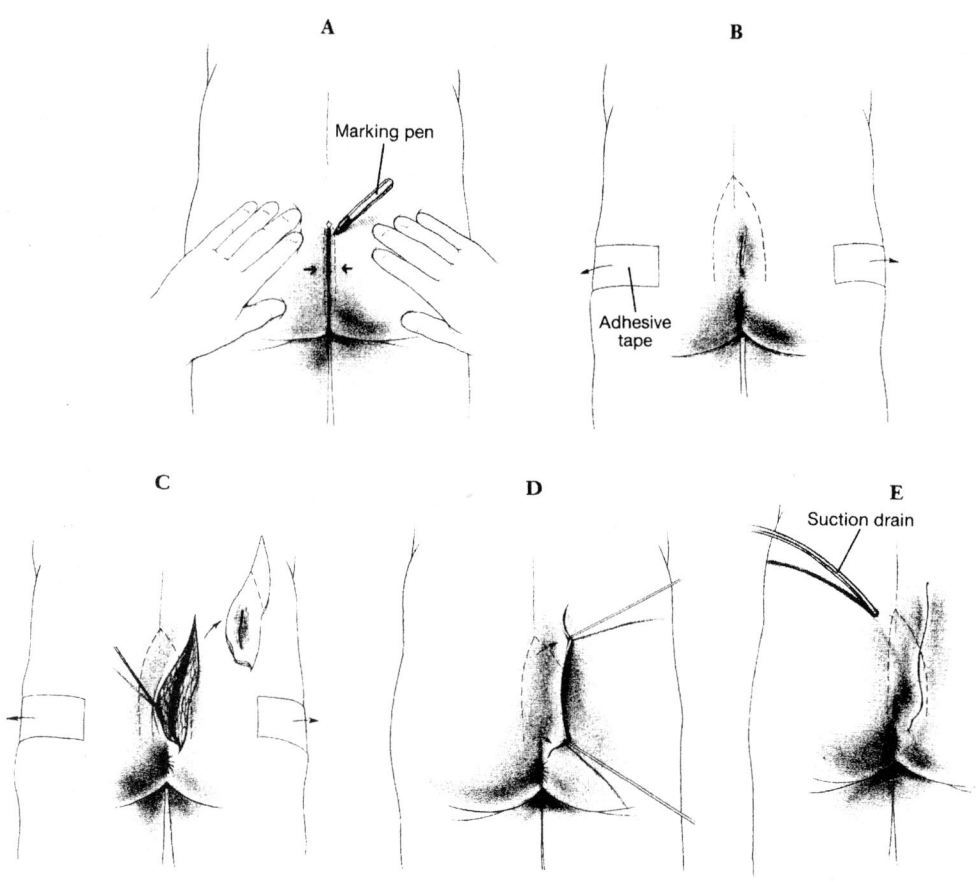

FIGURE 12.7. Cleft closure. Reproduced with permission from Nivatvongs.[21]

hardening of the stool, and its peristaltic activity causes packing of feces. The rectum has distention capability that allows the mass to reach a size that is too large to pass through the anal canal.[32]

Interestingly, once the impaction is present, fecal incontinence and paradoxical diarrhea may become the predominant problem. Fecal impaction is the most common cause of fecal incontinence in the elderly.[32] Fecal impaction is also a very common cause for encopresis in children. Physiologic studies suggest that this phenomenon is probably related to a combination of factors: an obtuse anorectal angle and low anal pressure, normally found in the elderly, and impaired anorectal sensation. These findings prevent conscious contraction of the external sphincter when the internal sphincter is relaxed.[33] The phenomenon of incontinence associ-

ated with fecal impaction may also be related to an exaggeration of the rectoanal inhibitory reflex.

The most common site of fecal impaction is in the rectum and sigmoid, although impactions have been reported higher in the colon. The fecal bolus can vary in size and may have a putty-like or hard consistency.

Etiology

By far the most common event preceding impaction is constipation. Fecal impaction may be caused by many factors: mechanical, neurologic, psychiatric, pharmacologic, dietary, environmental, systemic, and metabolic. Immobility of the patient may also contribute to the development of fecal impaction. Impactions may complicate anorectal surgery in 0.4% of cases.[34] In my experience, the figure is higher despite precautions.

Clinical Presentation

Symptoms vary, depending on the location and size of the impaction as well as the presence or absence of complications. Although evaluation of the patient with impaction may be in the hospital setting, many patients are referred for evaluation in the office.

The patient's complaints may be subtle and nonspecific. The patient may not be able to give an adequate history; therefore, information should be sought from a caregiver. A history of decreased frequency of bowel movements or sudden occurrence of diarrhea or incontinence should lead to a consideration of impaction. The patient usually complains of lower abdominal cramping pain, nausea, vomiting, anorexia, rectal pressure, and abdominal fullness. Symptoms may be related to other organ systems. In the elderly, acute states of confusion may complicate impaction. Urinary complaints, such as frequency, retention, and overflow incontinence may be caused by the mechanical effects of the fecal bolus.[32] A postoperative hemorrhoidectomy patient may present with increased pain, a sensation of perineal fullness, and inability to evacuate.

Low-grade fever and tachycardia may be present. The abdominal examination usually reveals distention, and feces may be palpated. The rectal examination is critical and will usually demonstrate a rectum full of clay-like feces. If the rectum is empty, impaction is not ruled out, because there may be a high impaction. In the case of high impaction, rigid proctosigmoidoscopy and/or a plain radiograph of the abdomen may be needed.

The characteristic finding of impaction on radiography is a mottled density of fecal matter in the rectum and/or colon (Figure 12.8).

If the patient presents with nausea and vomiting, admission to the hospital may be warranted to rule out intestinal obstruction. Appropriate laboratory studies are also obtained.

Complications

Intervention for fecal impaction is necessary not just to relieve pain and the inability to defecate but to prevent possible complications. The literature is

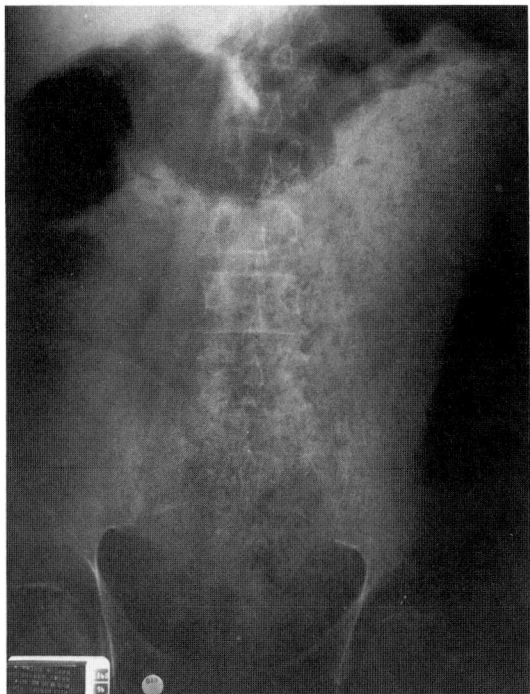

FIGURE 12.8. Abdominal radiograph showing fecal impaction with proximal colon dilated.

full of reports that describe unusual complications related to fecal impaction. However, the most common complication is fecal incontinence.[32] Intestinal obstruction may result from impaction in up to 50% of high-risk patients. With obstruction comes the risk of perforation. The many possible complications of fecal impaction include volvulus, megacolon, massive fecaloma, cerebrovascular accident, dystocia, urinary retention, incarcerated hernia, rectal prolapse, rectovaginal fistula, rectal fissure, hemorrhoids, pneumothorax (from straining), hepatic encephalopathy, and hypoxia.[35]

Stercoral ulceration is a very serious complication of fecal impaction that occurs in about 5% of impactions.[35] This condition is caused by pressure necrosis of the intestinal mucosa. The ulcerations may be multiple and are usually located on the antimesenteric border. The ulcers may perforate or bleed. A 55% mortality rate has been reported.

Treatment

The primary management of fecal impaction, in nonemergent situations, is to hydrate and soften the fecal bolus so that it can be removed or passed. Tap water, hypertonic phosphate, or oil-retention enemas will lubricate the bowel and soften the impaction. When giving enemas, care must be taken to avoid perforation of the rectal or colon wall.

Enemas and suppositories may eliminate some impactions, but manual fragmentation is usually required to fully relieve the impaction. Water-soluble contrast medium (meglumine diatrizoate) and whole-gut lavage have been used to treat nonobstructing impactions.[32] The use of stimulant laxatives to remove the impaction from above is usually not effective and only causes more abdominal pain and may lead to complications.

Fecal impactions are a frequent and recurring problem in neurologically impaired patients. Several reports have described successful treatment with the pulsed irrigation enhanced evacuation system (PIEE).[36,37] The PIEE system utilizes the mechanical action of pulsed water to disrupt dehydrated feces and stimulate colonic peristalsis. The freestanding unit is mobile. A recent report from Ohio evaluated 398 PIEE procedures performed in inpatient and outpatient settings. It was found to be a safe and effective method to treat impactions.[37]

A cooperative patient can undergo manual disimpaction in the office with careful dilation of the anus and digital fragmentation. A local anesthetic jelly should be used. After fragmentation and evacuation, enemas and suppositories are usually required to complete the process. Large impactions, on the other hand, are best managed in the operating room with the patient under some form of anesthesia. The patient is placed in the lithotomy position. A receptacle for the feces should be placed near the patient. Digital rectal examination with slow dilation will usually allow access to the fecal bolus. The bolus is then broken up by finger fragmentation. On occasion, careful instrumentation under direct vision may be needed to break up a hard impaction. If the bolus travels proximally beyond the reach of the finger, transvaginal or abdominal pressure may move the bolus distally.[32] The procedure is completed by irrigation of the colon with warm isotonic saline. In rare circumstances, an exploratory laparotomy may be needed to remove a hard concretion. Manual disimpaction is usually well tolerated. However, iatrogenic sphincter injury has been reported in situations that require repeated disimpactions.[38]

Prevention

Preventing recurrence of fecal impaction and correction of constipation should be addressed once the acute episode has been resolved, because recurrence is likely. Mechanical causes for impaction should be ruled out by total colorectal evaluation with air-contrast barium enema or colonoscopy.

Increased exercise, adequate hydration, treatment of underlying diseases, increased dietary fiber, and change in medications are a few measures that can be taken to control the problem. Bulk-forming laxatives are safe and effective but may not be effective in all patients. In some instances, the addition of a stool softener may be needed. Long-term use of stimulant laxatives is known to damage the myenteric plexus.[39] Bowel retraining and enema protocols should be used in the high-risk population.

Fecal impactions should be taken seriously. They should be treated as soon as the diagnosis is made, and every effort must be made to prevent subsequent episodes.

Examination Under Anesthesia

Anesthesia is rarely required for routine examination of the anorectum. Patients who present with a painful anal problem may be very hesitant and may refuse an examination. However, an attempt should be made to examine a fearful patient. Reassurance and the judicious use of lidocaine jelly may allow for inspection of the anus. Inspection may be enough to identify a perianal abscess, a thrombosed hemorrhoid, or the sentinel tag of a fissure. If these measures fail and the patient insists on being sedated, then examination under anesthesia (EUA) is the preferred method to identify the cause of the anal pain. The administration of anesthesia will allow a thorough examination to identify the reason for the anal pain. When obtaining informed consent, a discussion with the patient should include a list of possible findings. Also, the patient must understand that, if necessary, definitive treatment will be carried out.

It is usually clear when EUA is the best option to avoid a painful examination for evaluation of an anal complaint. In addition to the evaluation of an initial complaint of anorectal pain, EUA can be used to evaluate any number of anorectal problems. This discussion is by no means exhaustive but will suggest several indications for examination under anesthesia.

Evaluation of a Anorectal Abscess

The majority of perianal and ischiorectal abscesses can be drained in the office or the emergency department by using local anesthesia. Occasionally, the extent of an abscess cannot be accurately assessed, and therefore an EUA will help effect appropriate drainage. A patient who is suspected of having a horseshoe or intersphincteric abscess must be examined in the operating room. If such an abscess is found, it must be drained. A patient with a high intersphincteric abscess may show no external signs, but examination will demonstrate a palpable bulge into the rectum with an occasional opening in the anal canal with pus extruding.[40] Needle aspiration may assist in accurate localization of the abscess cavity.

Evaluation of Pain in a Neutropenic Patient

Neutropenia is usually the result of chemotherapy or leukemia. Perirectal pain may be a complaint in these patients. The cause is usually secondary to ulceration, fissure, or abscess.[41] The diagnosis of a perirectal abscess may be difficult, and an EUA may help to rule out a source of undrained sepsis.

Evaluation of Fistula-in-Ano

In suspected fistula-in-ano, office examination may identify a simple fistula. However, in many instances the internal opening cannot be identified except with adequate exposure under anesthesia. Meticulous examination will usually identify the type of fistula.

Evaluation of Perianal Crohn's Disease

Undrained abscess and multiple fistula tracts secondary to Crohn's disease are best assessed in the operating room and appropriate treatment given. Findings in this condition can be quite complex, and good visualization is important.

Evaluation of Posthemorrhoidectomy Bleeding

Early bleeding presenting after a hemorrhoidectomy is usually the result of technical error.

Control of hemorrhage is best managed by EUA with identification and ligation of the bleeding site. These patients are usually very uncomfortable because of recent surgery, and adequate exposure is crucial.

Evaluation of Postoperative Pain Following Anorectal Surgery

Since postoperative pain is expected, the patient should be prepared for it and appropriate analgesics should be prescribed. However, if unremitting pain, perineal pressure, and urinary retention occur, the patient should be evaluated to rule out fecal impaction, unresolved perianal sepsis, or new perianal or perirectal sepsis.[42] First, office examination should be attempted. If this is unsuccessful, then EUA is appropriate.

Minor Revisions of Intestinal Stomas

Restorative procedures for rectal cancer and inflammatory bowel disease have led to a reduction in the number of newly created permanent stomas. Despite this success, there are still many procedures that require the creation of a temporary or permanent stoma.

Intestinal stomas have a high complication rate ranging from 10% to 70%.[43] Stomal complications are characterized as early (within 30 days after surgery) or late (after 30 days). Appropriate measures should be taken to decrease the incidence of complications such as marking the stoma site preoperatively, placing the stoma through an appropriately sized aperture within the rectus abdominus muscle and providing education about stoma care. It has been shown that the practice of involving the enterostomal therapist in the care of any potential stoma patient decreases the incidence of adverse outcomes.[43] The surgeon needs to place significant importance on the creation of the stoma and not relegate its completion to a junior member of the surgical team.

The complications, which occur in association with ileostomy and colostomy, will be discussed together. Most of these adverse events are related to technical errors or the progression of the primary disease. The most frequent complications are related to skin problems. A well-trained enterostomal therapist can resolve many stomal problems. However, approximately one-third of stomas will require some form of revision. The revisions may be done locally at the site of the stoma or may require laparotomy. The majority of stomal complications requiring surgical correction are done in an inpatient setting. However, stenosis, retraction, prolapse, and small parastomal hernias may be revised using local procedures. Many of these corrective procedures may be performed in an ambulatory setting.

Stomal Retraction and Stenosis

Stomal retraction is frequently the result of a poorly placed stoma or one that is created under tension. Early stomal ischemia and mucosal sloughing may also lead to retraction. Thirty percent of ileostomies are complicated by retraction. The overall reported incidence of retraction in both ileostomy and colostomy is between 1% and 6%.[44] Patients usually present with leakage around the stomal pouch with skin irritation. Conservative treatment may be initiated with the use of a convex faceplate. Surgical correction may be needed.

Local measures may be attempted to gain length for an ileostomy. With the patient under intravenous sedation or general anesthesia, the retracted bowel wall is carefully grasped with clamps and the mucosa is everted above the level of the skin to the desired height. The stoma can be stabilized by multiple sutures, or a linear stapler without the blade may be fired three times (Figure 12.9). If these local measures to evert the stoma fail, the ileostomy will need to be completely separated from the skin and an attempt made to mobilize enough ileum to effect a new ileostomy. This procedure is more involved and may require a laparotomy and a hospital stay until the new stoma functions properly. Care should be taken not to injure the mesentery or the bowel. In revising a stoma, it is frequently advisable to make the incision on the mucosa adjacent to the skin edge rather than on the skin, so as not to increase the diameter of the skin opening and the base of the stoma.

Ileostomy stenosis is another problem that may be encountered. This may be at either the skin or fascia level. Ischemia or mucocutaneous separation usually causes scarring and subsequent stenosis. Skin level stenosis may be corrected on an ambulatory basis under local anesthesia by enlarging the skin opening and anastomosing the mucosa to the new skin edge. The correction of a fascial-level stenosis usually requires laparotomy with or without relocation of the stoma.

Colostomy retraction or stenosis (Figure 12.10) occurs in between 2% and 9% of patients in most series.[45] Retraction of a colostomy can be managed conservatively for the most part. If the patient has debilitating leakage with skin excoriation, revision should be undertaken. If the stoma has a significant stenotic component, an attempt at local correction can be performed using local anesthesia. After infiltration with a local anesthetic, a tangential incision is made from the mucocutaneous junction laterally down into the subcutaneous tissue. The bowel is mobilized and sutured to the skin edges of the incision.[44] Skin-level stenosis secondary to scar formation can be repaired by excising the scar and refashioning the stoma (Figure 12.11). Recurrence is a problem with simple scar excision. A Z-plasty can be done to treat skin-level stenosis. If local measures fail, laparotomy with relocation of the stoma is usually required.

Prolapse

Prolapse of an ileostomy is not common. Colostomy prolapse has been reported in 2% to 5% of cases.[45] There are two types of prolapse: fixed and sliding. The fixed type is usually the result of a stoma that was fashioned too long in the original procedure.[46] The sliding type moves in and out. Sliding prolapse may be associated with a parastomal hernia and is usually related to poor fixation, enlarged fascial opening, and/or redundant bowel.

A fixed prolapse can be repaired locally by a procedure that is similar to the rectosigmoidectomy. With the patient under general anesthesia, an incision is made on the mucosa of the stoma distal to the mucocutaneous junction, and the full length of the prolapsed bowel is mobilized. The excess colon or ileum is resected, and the stoma is refashioned with an anastomosis made to the cut edge of the original stoma (Figure 12.12). A sliding prolapse

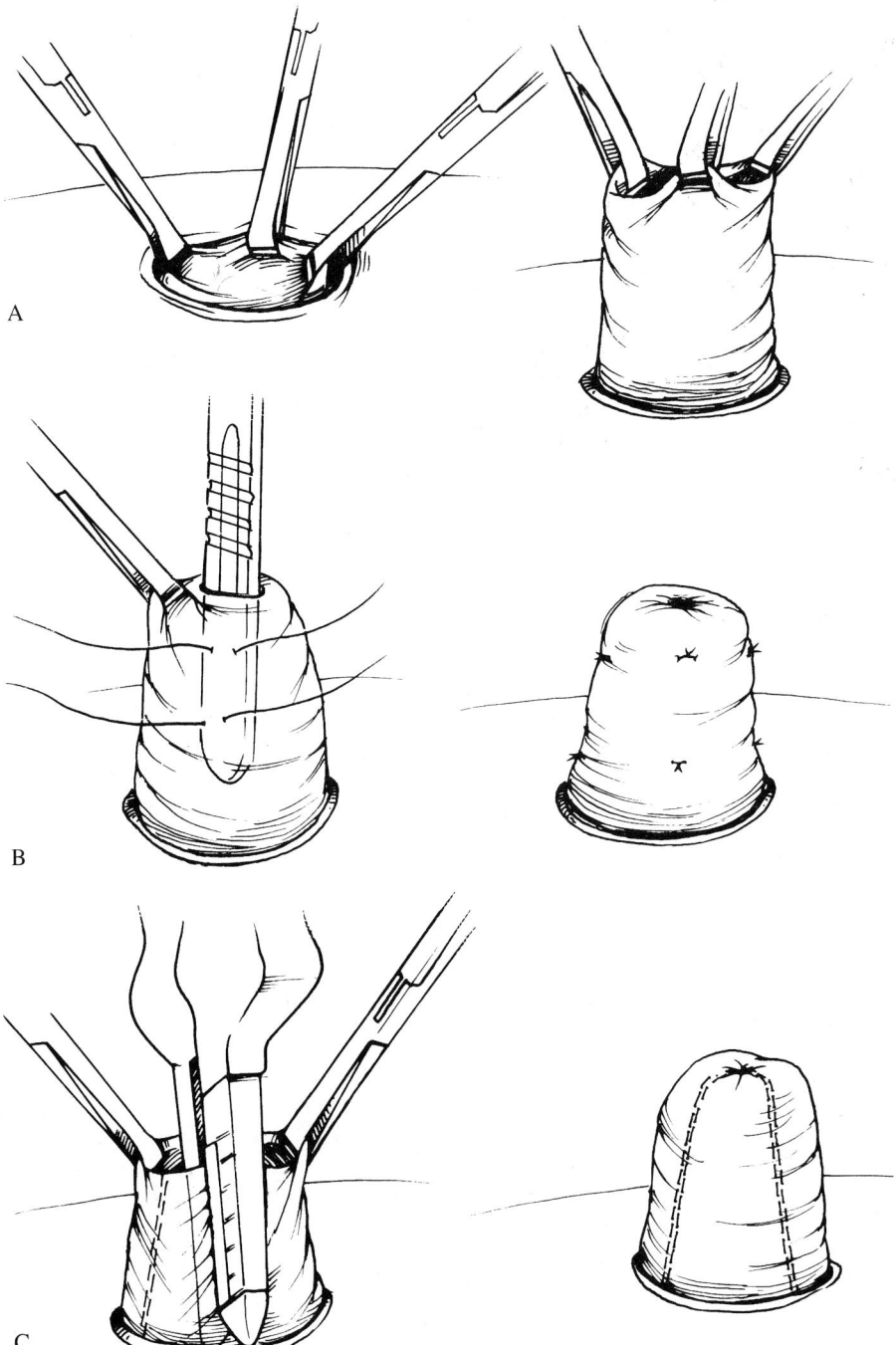

FIGURE 12.9. Revision of retracted ileostomy. **A**, The retracted bowel is drawn outward. **B**, The bowel is stabilized with sutures. **C**, The bowel is stabilized using a linear stapler. Redrawn from Keighley and Williams.[46]

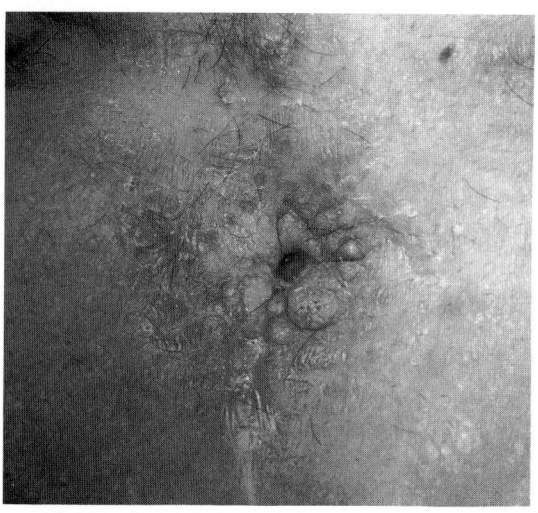

FIGURE 12.10. Colostomy stenosis (photograph courtesy of Wayne Tuckson, M.D., Louisville, KY).

mucosally to elevate all exposed mucosa. A circumferential mucosal incision is made 10 mm from the mucocutaneous junction. The mucosa is then dissected from the muscularis to the apex of the prolapse. Six to eight plicating absorbable sutures are placed in the muscular wall. The sutures are then tied, and the muscular cuff is reduced. The mucosal sleeve is then divided, and the cut ends of the mucosa are sutured together. If local procedures fail, laparotomy with relocation of stoma may be needed. The recurrence rate after surgery for prolapse has been reported to be as high as 65%.

Parastomal Hernia

Parastomal herniation is a frequent complication. The incidence is reported to be from 1% to 58%.[45] Clinically, the hernia may prevent proper placement of the stomal appliance, cause pain, and put the patient at risk for incarceration. The overall incidence of surgical repair is 10% to 20% for paracolostomy hernia and 50% to 70% for paraileostomy hernia.[48] The majority of hernia repairs will require relocation. A small symptomatic hernia may be repaired locally with approximation of the fascia with permanent sutures alone or with

usually requires a much more involved procedure that may require laparotomy and relocation of the stoma. A Delorme type procedure has been described to handle a symptomatic colostomy prolapse in a debilitated patient.[47] With the patient under local anesthesia, the prolapse is fully extended and 1:200,000 epinephrine is injected sub-

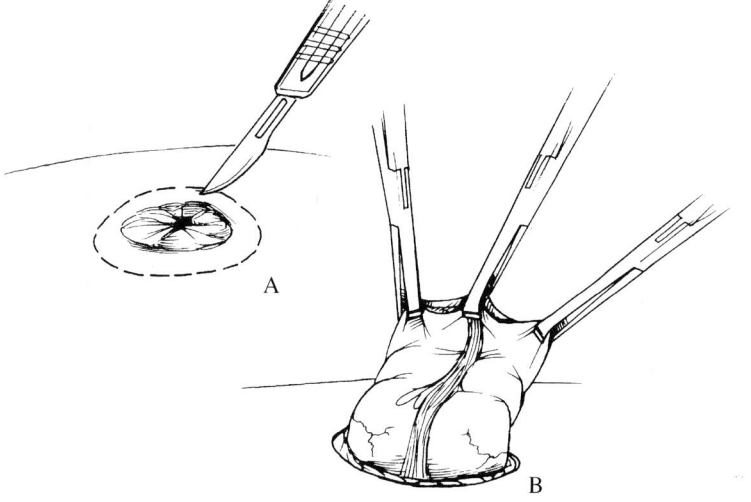

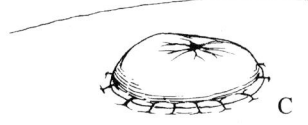

FIGURE 12.11. Revision of retracted or stenotic colostomy. **A**, The scar is excised. **B**, The colon is mobilized. **C**, The new stoma has matured. Redrawn from Corman ML (ed). Colon and Rectal Surgery, 4th edition. Philadelphia: Lippincott-Raven, 1998, p 1267.

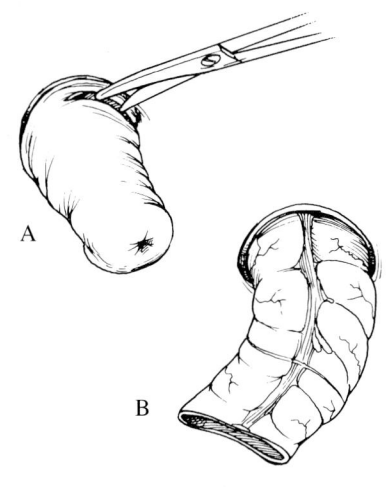

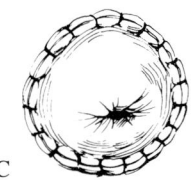

Figure 12.12. Revision of colostomy prolapse. **A**, An incision is made into the mucosa. **B**, Redundant bowel is removed. **C**, Maturation of new stoma. Redrawn from Corman ML (ed). Colon and Rectal Surgery, 4th edition. Philadelphia: Lippincott-Raven, 1998, p 1270.

mesh. This type of repair can be done in an ambulatory setting. A drain may be needed in the cavity created by the hernia.

Summary

There are many complications related to stomal creation. Minor revisions of an ileostomy or colostomy can be managed in an ambulatory setting with careful patient selection. Retraction, stenosis, prolapse, and parastomal hernias are amenable to local revision, and this should be done when possible.

References

1. Institute of Medicine (U.S.) Committee on Prevention and Control of Sexually Transmitted Diseases; Eng T, Butler WT (eds). The Hidden Epidemic: Confronting Sexually Transmitted Diseases. Washington, DC: National Academy Press, 1997, p 432.
2. Zurhausen H, Devilliers EM. Human papillomavirus. Annu Rev Microbiol 1994;48:427–447.
3. Phelps WC, Alexander KA. Antiviral therapy for human papillomavirus: rational and prospects. Ann Intern Med 1995;123:368–382.
4. Beutner K, Richwald GA, Wiley DJ, et al. External genital warts: report of the American Medical Association Consensus Conference, August 1997. Clin Infect Dis 1998;27:796–806.
5. Buntin DM. 1993 Sexually transmitted diseases treatment guidelines. Semin Dermatol 1994;13:269–274.
6. Congilosi SM, Madoff RD. Current therapy for recurrent and extensive anal warts. Dis Colon Rectum 1995;38:1101–1107.
7. Ferenczy A, Mitao M, Negai N, et al. Latent papillomavirus and recurring genital warts. N Engl J Med 1985;313:784–788.
8. Chu QC, Vezeridis MP, Libby NP, et al. Giant condyloma acuminatum (Buschke-Lowenstein tumor) of the anorectal and perianal region: analysis of 42 cases. Dis Colon Rectum 1994;37:950–957.
9. McDonald LL, Stites PC, Buntin DM. Sexually transmitted diseases update. Dermatol Clin 1997;15:221–232.
10. Baker GE, Tyring SK. Therapeutic approaches to papillomavirus infections. Dermatol Clin 1997;15:331–340.
11. Billingham RP, Lewis FG. Laser versus electrical cautery in the treatment of condylomata acuminata of the anus. Surg Gynecol Obstet 1982;155:865–867.
12. Gordon PH. Condyloma acuminatum. In Gordon PH, Nivatvongs S (eds). Principles and practice of surgery for the colon, rectum, and anus. St. Louis: Quality Medical Publishing, 1992, pp 301–316.
13. Tyring S, Edwards L, Cherry L, et al. Safety and efficacy of 0.5% podofilox gel in the treatment of anogenital warts. Arch Dermatol 1998;134:33–38.
14. Fleshner P, Freilich MI. Adjuvant interferon for anal condyloma: a prospective, randomized trial. Dis Colon Rectum 1994;37:1255–1259.
15. Armstrong DKB, Maw RD, Dinsmore WW, et al. Combined therapy trial with interferon alpha-2a and ablative therapy in the treatment of anogenital warts. Genitourin Med 1996;72:103–107.
16. Edwards L, Ferenczy A, Eron L, et al. Self-administered topical 5% imiquimod cream for external anogenital warts. Arch Dermatol 1998;134:25–30.
17. Wiltz OH, Torregrosa M, Wiltz O. Autogenous vaccine: the best therapy for perianal condyloma acuminata? Dis Colon Rectum 1995;38:838–841.

18. Abcarian H, Sharon N. Long term effectiveness of the immunotherapy of anal condyloma acuminata. Dis Colon Rectum 1982;25:648–651.

19. Anderson AW. Hair extracted from an ulcer. Boston Medical and Surgical Journal 1847;36:74.

20. Hodges RM. Pilonidal disease. Boston Medical and Surgical Journal 1880;103:485–486.

21. Nivatvongs S. Pilonidal disease. In Gordon PH, Nivatvongs S (eds). Principles and Practice of Surgery for the Colon, Rectum, and Anus. St. Louis: Quality Medical Publishing, 1992, pp 267–299.

22. Patey DH, Scarff RW. The hair of the pilonidal sinus. Lancet 1955;268:772–773.

23. Bascom J. Pilonidal disease: origin from follicles of hairs and results of follicle removal as treatment. Surgery 1980;87:567–572.

24. Marks J, Harding KG, Hughes LE, et al. Pilonidal sinus excision—healing by open granulation. Br J Surg 1985;72:647–650.

25. Allen-Mersh TG. Pilonidal sinus: finding the right track for treatment. Br J Surg 1990;77:123–132.

26. Jensen SL, Harling H. Prognosis after simple incision and drainage for a first-episode acute pilonidal abscess. Br J Surg 1988;75:60–61.

27. Armstrong JH, Barcia PJ. Pilonidal sinus disease: the conservative approach. Arch Surg 1994;129:914–918.

28. Lord P, Millar D. Pilonidal sinus: a simple treatment. Br J Surg 1965;52:298.

29. Edwards MH. Pilonidal sinus: a 5-year appraisal of the Millar-Lord treatment. Br J Surg 1977;64:867–868.

30. Bascom J. Pilonidal sinus. In Fazio V (ed). Current therapy in colon and rectal surgery. Toronto, Philadelphia: BC Decker, 1990, pp 32–39.

31. Davis KA, Mock CN, Versaci A, et al. Malignant degeneration of pilonidal cysts. Am Surg 1994;60:200–204.

32. Wrenn K. Fecal impaction. N Engl J Med 1989;321:658–662.

33. Read NW, Abouzekry L. Why do patients with faecal impaction have faecal incontinence. Gut 1986;27:283–287.

34. Buls JG, Goldberg SM. Modern management of hemorrhoids. Surg Clin North Am 1978;58:469–478.

35. Corman ML. Disorders of defecation. In Corman ML (ed). Colon and Rectal Surgery. Philadelphia: Lippincott-Raven, 1998, pp 368–400.

36. Kokoszka J, Nelson R, Falconio M, et al. Treatment of fecal impaction with pulsed irrigation evacuation. Dis Colon Rectum 1994;37:161–164.

37. Puet TA, Jackson H, Amy S. Use of pulsed irrigation evacuation in the management of the neuropathic bowel. Spinal Cord 1997;35:694–699.

38. Gattuso JM, Kamm MA, Halligan SM, et al. The anal sphincter in idiopathic megarectum: effects of manual disimpaction under general anesthesia. Dis Colon Rectum 1996;39:435–439.

39. Smith B. Effects of irritant purgatives on the myenteric plexus in man and the mouse. Gut 1968;9:139–143.

40. Kodner IJ. Anal procedures. In Wilmore DW, Cheung LY, Harken AH, et al. (eds). Scientific American Surgery CD-ROM. New York: Scientific American, 1998.

41. Nohr C. Non-AIDS immunosuppression. In Wilmore DW, Cheung LY, Harken AH, et al. (eds). Scientific American Surgery CD-ROM. New York: Scientific American, 1998.

42. Stamos MJ, Theuer CP, Headrick CN. General postoperative complications. In Hicks T, Beck D, Opelka F, Timmcke A (eds). Complications of Colon and Rectal Surgery. Baltimore: Williams & Wilkins, 1996, pp 118–139.

43. Bass EM, Del Pino A, Tan A, et al. Does preoperative stoma marking and education by the enterostomal therapist affect outcome? Dis Colon Rectum 1997;40:440–442.

44. Khubchandani IT. Stoma retraction. In Wexner SD, Vernava AM (eds). Clinical Decision Making in Colorectal Surgery. New York: Igaku-Shoin, 1995, pp 453–458.

45. Fleshman JW. Ostomies. In Hicks T, Beck D, Opelka F, Timmcke A (eds). Complications of Colon and Rectal Surgery. Baltimore: Williams & Wilkins, 1996, pp 357–381.

46. Keighley MRB, Williams NS. Ileostomy. In Keighley MRB, Williams NS (eds). Surgery of the Anus, Rectum and Colon. London: WB Saunders, 1993:139–199.

47. Abulafi AM, Sherman IW, Fiddian RV. Delorme operation for prolapsed colostomy. Br J Surg 1989;76:1321–1322.

48. Abcarian H. Peristomal hernias. In Wexner SD, Vernava AM (eds). Clinical Decision Making in Colorectal Surgery. New York: Igaku-Shoin, 1995, pp 449–452.

13

Rectal Prolapse and Rectocele

Richard P. Billingham, M.D., F.A.C.S.

Rectal Prolapse

Rectal prolapse is a surprisingly common disorder, most often seen in women in late middle age and beyond, which may begin with a number of minor symptoms of very gradual onset. Sufferers commonly ignore these symptoms or bring them to the attention of primary care physicians, who frequently fail to examine the patient and assume such symptoms are caused by hemorrhoids. If examination is carried out, the findings can be relatively subtle, and often the symptoms are attributed to "old age," "history of childbirth," or similar nonspecific and irreparable causes. Although this book is primarily aimed at the surgical specialist, it seems reasonable to review some of these issues, which may present initially to the primary care physician. Only through a better understanding of this problem will these providers consider this pathological entity at earlier stages of its development

Pathophysiology

True rectal prolapse is part of a continuum of events that may begin as prolapse of the internal hemorrhoids. With time, age, constipation, gravity, or other cause of loss of the normal support mechanisms of the rectum, sufficient mobility of the mid- and upper rectum can occur to the point where intussusception begins. Initially, this process can be thought of as occurring only with straining at stool, but with additional loss of support, intussusception may occur even without straining. Initially, the in-

tussusception may be confined to the mid-rectum and not be evident to the patient or physician ("internal rectal prolapse"), but, with time, the intussusception works its way through the anal sphincter, dilating the sphincter muscle. If unchecked, the intussusceptum can protrude chronically through the anal sphincter, even to the point of becoming incarcerated in that position.

There are three factors that keep the rectum in its normal anatomical position. The first is the normal fixation of the mid- and upper mesorectum to the presacral fascia. These attachments secure the rectum superiorly, up out of the pelvis, and posteriorly, allowing the normal rectum to follow the curve of the sacrum and coccyx. Thus, as the patient strains, the intraabdominal pressure on the anterior surface of the rectum forces it against the sacrum and coccyx, thus expelling its contents. Second, the so-called lateral ligaments account for the lateral support of the rectum, keeping it from descending into the pelvis during straining. Finally, the tone of the normal anal sphincter and its normal relaxation during defecation provide support and keep the distal rectum from descending during straining. Intussusception, which begins the process of rectal prolapse, is thought to begin in the mid-rectum, usually anteriorly, where there is little support. It is believed that continuation of this process first weakens the posterior attachments of the rectum to the sacrum and, later, the lateral ligaments as well. With intussusception poised just above the anal sphincter and with continued straining, the prolapse comes through the anal sphincter, dilating it repeatedly over the course of many months or years. It is not known whether the diminished sphincter tone seen in many patients with rectal prolapse is the result of the prolapse itself or antedates the prolapse and was one of the factors that allowed it to become clinically evident.

Mention should be made here of the causes of straining and increased abdominal pressure, which may be seen as precipitating factors in the development of prolapse. Idiopathic constipation and/or dysmotility may increase the requirement to strain in order to have a bowel movement. Pelvic floor abnormalities, such as nonrelaxing puborectalis muscle, may also increase the tendency of a person to strain, thus setting the stage for rectal prolapse as well as rectocele formation.

Clinical Presentation

In the earliest phases, patients are unaware of symptoms, although on close questioning, some will admit to intermittent slight seepage of mucus or stool, mild bleeding, or prolapse of tissue. The prolapsing tissue may be, or may appear to be, simply the internal hemorrhoids. In later stages, the patients may be aware of increasing amounts of tissue prolapsing through the anal canal. Typically, this symptom is first noticeable only at the time of bowel movements, with spontaneous reduction of the tissue. With progression of the condition, the prolapsing tissue becomes increasingly noticeable with slight straining at times not associated with bowel movements and may require manual reduction. In more advanced situations, the rectum may prolapse when the patient walks or stands and ultimately becomes irreducible or even strangulated.

Physical examination should include an abdominal examination to rule out masses, areas of tenderness, hernias, or other sources of straining. Although it is our usual practice to examine patients while they are in the left lateral position, the examination of the anorectum can also be carried out with the patient in either the prone jack-knife or the lithotomy position. Note should be made of the condition of the perianal skin and the presence of fissures or dermatitis. In addition, with the buttocks gently distracted, the patient should be asked to strain. This portion of the examination may enable the physician to determine whether there is any effacement of the anus itself, descent of the perineum, or evidence of protrusion of tissue from the vagina. Digital anorectal examination should as-

sess the sphincter tone, presence or absence of a rectocele, as well as the presence of masses. Anoscopy should be done, with particular attention to the presence of internal hemorrhoids and whether these alone may represent the source of the patient's symptoms, or if more proximal prolapse may be contributory. Asking the patient to strain during anoscopy is generally helpful here as well, to determine whether the prolapsing tissue is only the hemorrhoids or instead has its origin proximal to the hemorrhoid area. Rigid sigmoidoscopy is particularly useful in this situation to allow inspection of the mucosa for signs of erythema, solitary ulceration, or redundancy. The physician can also ask the patient to strain while the sigmoidoscope is in place, thus enabling confirmation of the presence of prolapse or intussusception.

One simple test that should be done, when the diagnosis is in doubt, is the toilet test. Although this test is primitive and slightly embarrassing to the patient, its potential for changing the diagnosis and therapy is too significant to ignore. During this examination, the patient is asked to sit on a conventional toilet seat and then slide and lean slightly forward while straining. From behind the patient, using a flashlight for better visualization, the physician can observe the presence and extent of prolapse. In attempting to refine this test a bit, some physicians have modified a commode chair to allow better visualization of the anorectal area with the patient in the sitting position. Others have suggested the use of a mirror attached to an extendable handle (such as those used by auto mechanics and available in auto supply stores) to get a better view of the perineum.

Because of the logistical difficulties and low technology of this examination, many physicians have abandoned the toilet test in favor of the video defecogram. The toilet test, however, is often diagnostic in situations where the video defecogram is not. Sometimes the patient is unable to reproduce the full extent of the prolapse during the scrutiny of the radiologic examination, whereas without as much fuss and expense, the prolapse can be more easily demonstrated in less threatening surroundings. Therefore, I believe that the toilet test is mandatory for the evaluation of the patient with suspected prolapse, whether or not video defecography is utilized.

Video defecography, introduced in 1968 by Broden and Snellman,[1] has been a great help to surgeons in the assessment and confirmation of rectal prolapse and other pelvic pathology, as well as providing a guide to therapy. In this test, the rectum and distal sigmoid are filled with a rather thickened mixture of barium, the consistency of which has been adjusted to mimic that of normal stool. (The consistency of this mixture is very different from that of the mixture used for a barium enema, which is quite thin and thus unsatisfactory for video defecography). After the instillation of barium, the patient is asked to sit on a specially designed (radiolucent) commode while video radiography is done. This is usually accomplished from the patient's left lateral position, so that a lateral view of the distal sigmoid, rectum, and anus is achieved with visualization of the relationship of this area to the sacrum and coccyx. The patient is then asked to tighten the sphincter, to cough, and to strain without evacuating to allow the physician to see the effects of these maneuvers on the position of the rectum and other structures. The patient is subsequently asked to defecate, so that during the straining and defecating process, the changing position of the rectum and the anal musculature can be noted. Findings that can be evaluated with such an examination include internal or complete rectal prolapse, separation of the rectum from the sacrum, nonrelaxing puborectalis muscle, the presence and extent of any rectocele, and whether the rectocele empties with defecation. In addition, when contrast medium is placed within the vagina and the small bowel, the presence of an enterocele, or vaginal or uterine prolapse, can also be confirmed.[2,3]

The examination has been criticized because the findings in the symptomatic patient may be indistinguishable from some of the findings in control subjects with no prolapse.[4] For this reason we believe that the results of such a study should be interpreted by the surgeon, who has the benefit of the history and office physical examination, and is thus able to put the radiographic findings into context.

Other tests that may be helpful in evaluating the anorectal area of patients with rectal prolapse include anorectal manometry, pudendal nerve terminal motor latency, and anal ultrasound imaging of the anal sphincter muscles. Anorectal manometry and pudendal nerve terminal motor latency are generally not as helpful diagnostically as video defecography, but they may be of value in incontinent patients in predicting the likelihood of return of nearly normal sphincter function and continence.[5] If there is prolonged conduction in the pudendal nerves, the likelihood of restoration of

tone and therefore continence is somewhat less than if the pudendal nerve conduction is normal.[6,7] Anal ultrasonography may be useful in identifying sphincter defects even when such defects may not be palpable.[8] These studies may be particularly valuable when obstetrical trauma is believed to be a potential source of diminished sphincter tone, even though the trauma may have occurred many decades before the clinical manifestation of the prolapse. If a sphincter defect is found, particularly anteriorly, this finding, in combination with the results of previously described studies, may help the surgeon decide whether to recommend sphincteroplasty, either at the time of the rectal prolapse surgery or in a staged manner, to improve continence.

Choice of Operative Procedure

"Medical" or "conservative" treatment generally has little or no place in the management of rectal prolapse. Since prolapse is a mechanical condition, it requires a mechanical solution. There are three categories of such mechanical solutions that are applicable for rectal prolapse. These are encirclement procedures of the anal sphincters, transanal approaches to resection, and abdominal approaches to fixation and/or resection.

Encirclement Procedures

Thiersch popularized the earliest of the encirclement procedures in the late 1800s.[9] In his procedure, a silver wire was placed beneath the perianal skin and outside the external sphincter muscle to limit the distensibility of the anal sphincter. The goal of the operation is to keep the intussuscepted rectum from prolapsing outside the anal verge, while still permitting stool to come through. The advantage of this procedure is its simplicity and the fact that it can be done under local anesthesia. Among the disadvantages, however, is the fact that the wire frequently either erodes into the sphincter or migrates through the perineum, thus necessitating removal of the wire. It is also very difficult to calibrate the tension on the wire satisfactorily. Ideally, it should be neither too tight, impeding bowel movements and causing increased chance of erosion or fecal impaction, nor too loose, allowing continued prolapse of the rectum.

Later modifications of this procedure have substituted other materials, such as sutures of various materials, a thin strip of Marlex mesh, or Dacron-impregnated silastic for the silver wire. Each of these materials had more or less the same advantages and disadvantages as the original silver wire, except that they provided a wider band of prosthetic material to diminish the chance of eroding into the muscle. The silastic was so nonreactive, however, that it discouraged tissue ingrowth and, therefore, fixation of the silastic. This caused an even higher migration and erosion rate than was seen with silver wire.[9] To counteract this tendency, Labow and associates suggested using silastic glue to attach Teflon felt to the outer surface of the silastic.[10] This change has allowed a lower incidence of erosion and migration, but the procedure itself is still unsatisfactory in approximately 30% of patients. It may still have some applicability in the inactive elderly person with multiple medical problems who is confined to a bed or chair.

Transanal Procedures

The two principal variants of the transanal approach, operating on the redundant rectum by going through the anal canal, are the Delorme procedure, and the Altemeier procedure. Delorme's procedure,

described in 1899, and thus prior to the development of antibiotics, has several principal advantages. First, in this procedure the peritoneal cavity is not entered, and therefore the risk of peritonitis and other morbidity is greatly reduced. In addition, since the procedure is done through the rectum in an area not supplied with pain fibers, there is generally very little postoperative discomfort. With the avoidance of laparotomy, the overall morbidity of this surgical procedure is considerably less. A further touted advantage is that imbrication of the rectal muscularis propria in an accordion fashion was thought to increase the length of the anal sphincter and thus improve continence for those in whom continence is impaired. A disadvantage of this procedure is that the recurrence rate in most series has been considerably higher than for other procedures.

In the Delorme procedure, the patient may be placed either in the lithotomy or the prone jackknife position. I find the latter much more satisfactory. An incision is made approximately 2 cm proximal to the dentate line, through the mucosa, but not through the muscularis propria (Figure 13.1). At this point, by means of needlepoint cautery or scissors, the mucosal dissection is begun and continues proximally. Some feel that it is helpful to inject the submucosa with a solution containing 1:100,000 or 1:200,000 epinephrine to aid hemostasis and facili-

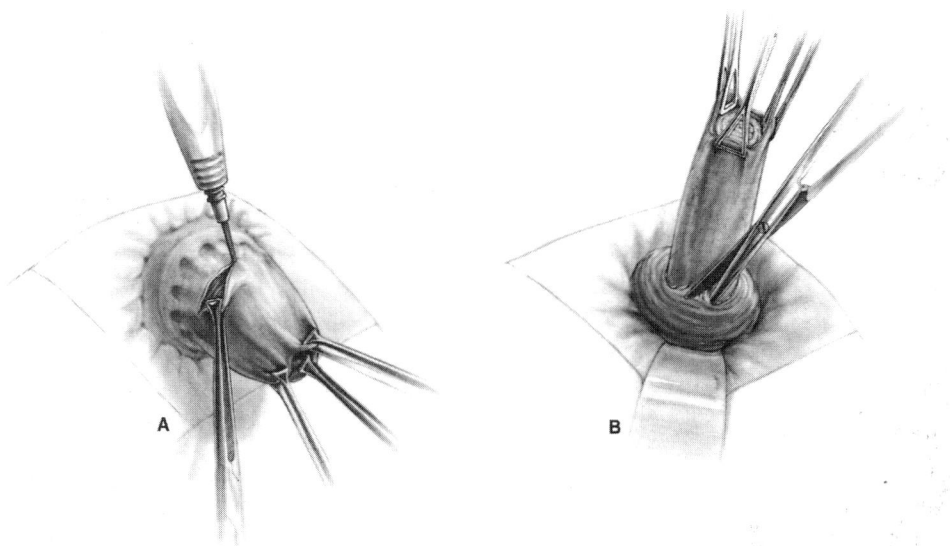

FIGURE 13.1. Delorme procedure. **A,** The mucosa is circumferentially incised above the dentate line. **B,** Submucosal stripping is carried out as far cephalad as possible. Reprinted with permission from Corman ML (ed). Colon & Rectal Surgery, 4th edition. Philadelphia: Lippincott-Raven, 1998, p 425.

tate the dissection. Bleeding is controlled with electrocautery. The dissection is continued proximally until the redundancy has been eliminated. The decision as to how high to dissect is one of judgment and is aided by a combination of visual inspection and traction on the dissected mucosal tube. The muscularis propria is then imbricated by using four to eight sutures of absorbable suture, such as 0 polyglycolic acid, to maintain it in an accordion-like position (Figure 13.2). Although the muscular imbrication was Delorme's original idea, Gundersen et al.[11] suggested incorporating less muscularis propria in the sutures. They described a stitch through the proximal muscularis propria, adjacent to the upper end of the mucosa to be transected, and a lower stitch through this muscle adjacent to the distal mucosal margin, to take tension off the ultimate anastomosis. The dissected redundant mucosa is then amputated, and an anastomosis is carried out between the proximal and distal edges of the rectum. This anastomosis may be done with sutures or staples in any of a number of satisfactory manners.

In the Altemeier procedure, the full thickness of the rectum is resected instead of only the mucosa. I believe that the anastomosis is generally more secure if a circular stapler is used. Although there are no data reporting a direct comparison of sutured versus stapled Altemeier anastomoses, several sources of data, collected in other anastomotic applications, lead to my conclusion that the stapled anastomosis is better. Foremost among these is the recent experience with ileal pouch–anal anastomosis (IPAA), performed with the circular stapler. In the early years (early 1980s) as this operation was evolving, anastomoses were generally done by hand. During that period, several authors attempted to perform the IPAA without covering ileostomies, and a high rate of anastomotic complications ensued. After the double-stapled technique for IPAA became more widespread, attempts were again made to avoid a diverting ileostomy, this time with multiple authors reporting success.[12–17] A similar trend has developed with colo-anal anastomoses, which were originally also believed to require a proximal stoma. Favorable experience has been recently gained with the combination of the stapled colo-anal anastomoses and the avoidance of such a temporary stoma.[18] Anastomotic leak rates of 1.5% and 0.5% have been reported in two recent series evaluating colo-anal anastomoses.[19,20] (*Editor's note:* We have a strong preference for the handsewn anastomosis with the Altemeier procedure. The anastomosis is technically very easy to perform with sutures. The bowel edges are in clear view and almost fall together. Obviously, the cost of sutures is also significantly less than that if the circular stapler is used. We use interrupted polyglycolic acid sutures for this anastomosis. Another

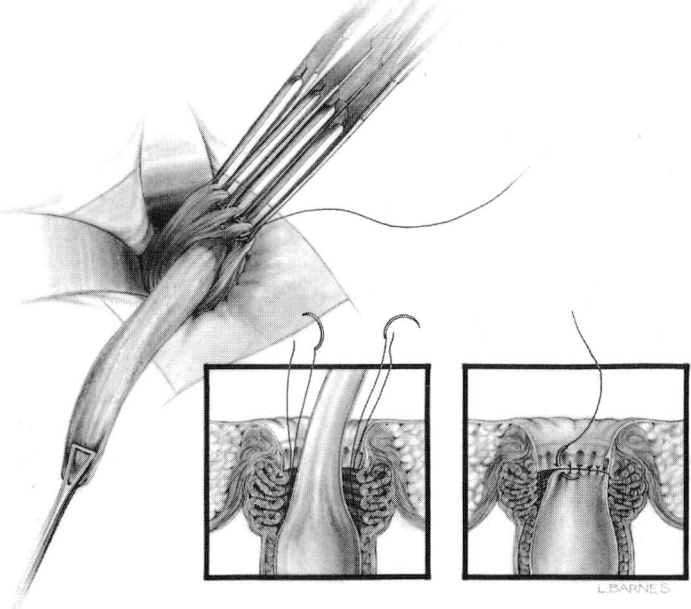

FIGURE 13.2. Delorme procedure. The circular muscle of the rectum is prepared for suturing by the placement of serial Allis clamps. Plication is carried out using 2–0 long-term absorbable sutures. The inset on the right illustrates the completed "anastomosis" after the redundant mucosa has been amputated. Reprinted with permission from Dis Colon Rectum 1990;33:573.

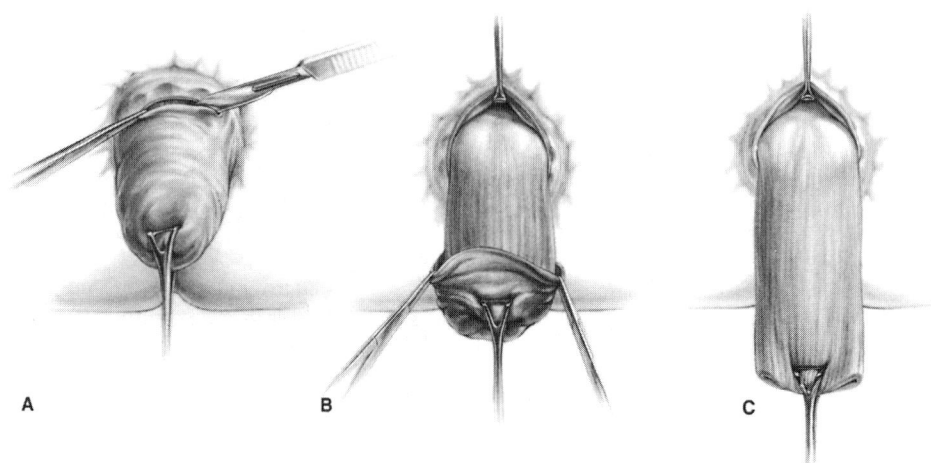

A   B   C

FIGURE 13.3. Altemeier procedure. **A**, Incision is made circumferentially in the anal canal above the dentate line. **B** and **C**, The rectum is mobilized and completely everted. Reprinted with permission from Corman ML (ed). Colon & Rectal Surgery, 4th edition. Philadelphia: Lippincott-Raven, 1998, p 421.

reason we do not favor the use of the stapler is that we find it difficult to perform the levatoroplasty in conjunction with the stapled anastomosis. After the anterior and posterior sutures are placed in the levator muscles, the opening at the pelvic floor is too small for me to fire or remove either the 29-mm or the 31-mm circular stapler.)

When planning to use a stapled anastomosis, it is my practice to make a circular incision through the entire thickness of the rectal wall approximately 3 cm proximal to the dentate line. Using Allis or Pennington clamps on the proximal bowel, dissection is carried upward in the plane just outside the muscularis propria (Figure 13.3), cauterizing bleeding points with the needlepoint electrode as they are encountered. Ultimately, when the degree of traction necessary to maintain the dissected segment outside the anal verge has been determined through visual inspection and tactile assessment, we decide that the redundant segment has been adequately mobilized. The dissection involves entering the peritoneal cavity through the deep cul-de-sac in almost all cases (Figure 13.4). In the presence of a complete bowel preparation and prophylactic systemic antibiotics, the intraabdominal dissection is certainly not cause for concern and is no less safe than an intraabdominal anastomosis.

When the dissection is complete (Figure 13.5**A**) and the redundant rectal segment has been amputated, a purse-string suture of 0 polypropylene is placed at the proximal end of the dissection, and through this open end of the upper rectum, the anvil and shaft of the appropriately sized circular stapling instrument is inserted and the purse-string suture secured. A similar purse-string suture is placed approximately 0.5 cm from the proximal edge of the remaining lower rectum (Figure 13.5**B** and **C**). (Thus, if the original incision was 3 cm from the dentate line, this purse-string suture would be placed at approximately 2.5 cm from the dentate line.) The anvil and shaft are attached to the remaining portion of the surgical stapler, which is closed just to the point of retaining the shaft, and the distal purse-string suture is tied around this shaft. The instrument is then closed, fired, and removed (Figure 13.5**D** and **E**). Both donuts are inspected to be sure they are intact. The anastomosis, which is located approximately 1.5 to 2 cm above the dentate line, can be carefully inspected and probed for defects, which can be repaired with sutures.

Debate continues on which of the transanal procedures give the best combination of low recurrence and minimal morbidity. Most authors report restoration of continence in approximately 90% or more of their patients, even with severe pudendal neuropathy. The recurrence rates for perineal operations range from 6% to 18%, with higher rates reported with longer duration of follow-up.[12-18] Both Delorme and Altemeier-type procedures can safely be repeated if recurrence of the prolapse should occur.[18,19]

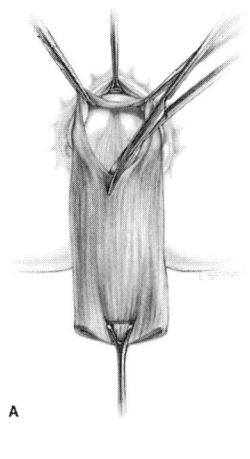

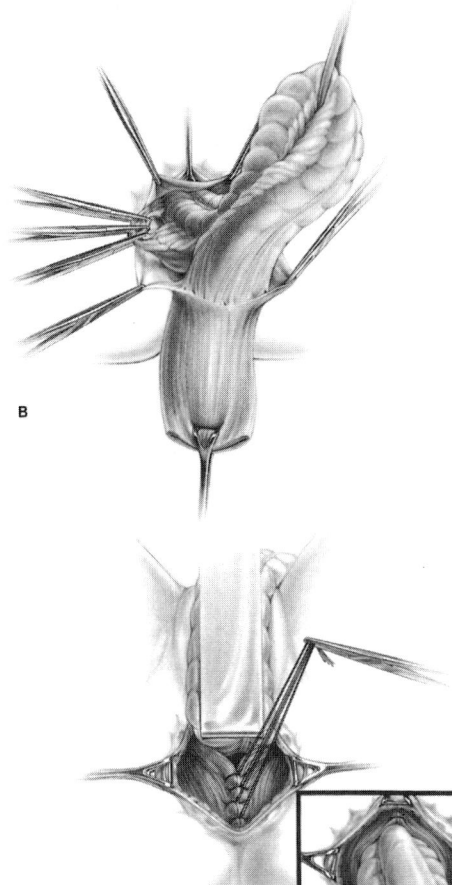

FIGURE 13.4. Altemeier procedure. **A**, The peritoneal reflection is identified and opened. **B**, Any redundant bowel is delivered through the peritoneal defect. **C**, The levator ani muscle is reefed anteriorly and posteriorly. Care should be taken to avoid narrowing the rectum. A finger should be able to pass easily through the defect (inset). Reprinted with permission from Corman ML (ed). Colon & Rectal Surgery, 4th edition. Philadelphia: Lippincott-Raven, 1998, p 422.

In conjunction with the Altemeier procedure, a levatoroplasty can be performed, anteriorly, posteriorly, or both, if the sphincter tone is diminished. Several reports attest to the improvement in continence when levatoroplasty is done.[12,17] Since it takes little time, does not increase morbidity, and improves continence in many cases, it is our practice to do a levatoroplasty (Figure 13.4**C**) whenever possible, using figure-of-eight sutures of 0 polyglycolic acid or a similar material. Generally, we perform the levatoroplasty after securing the anvil and shaft into the proximal bowel segment and before placing the distal purse-string suture.

Both the Thiersch-type procedures and the transrectal procedures lend themselves well to outpatient surgery. Even with the most extensive of these procedures, the Altemeier procedure, there is very little or no pain after surgery, very minimal surgical stress during and after the procedure, and no need for restriction of diet or activity in the postoperative period. Also, since these operative procedures involve a confined anatomic area, they lend themselves well to the use of regional anesthesia. The Thiersch-type procedures can be done under local anesthesia with sedation, but the limiting factor for the Delorme or Altemeier procedures seems to be the necessity for peritoneal traction, for which regional, but not local, anesthesia is helpful. (*Editor's note:* I have performed the Delorme procedure on multiple poor-risk patients with satisfactory results using only local anesthesia.)

In past years, patients undergoing the Delorme or Altemeier procedure were managed like other patients who had intestinal anastomoses. Their diets were held or restricted until bowel function was established. Extensive literature on laparoscopic colectomy with early feeding has shown dietary restriction to be largely unnecessary. With no

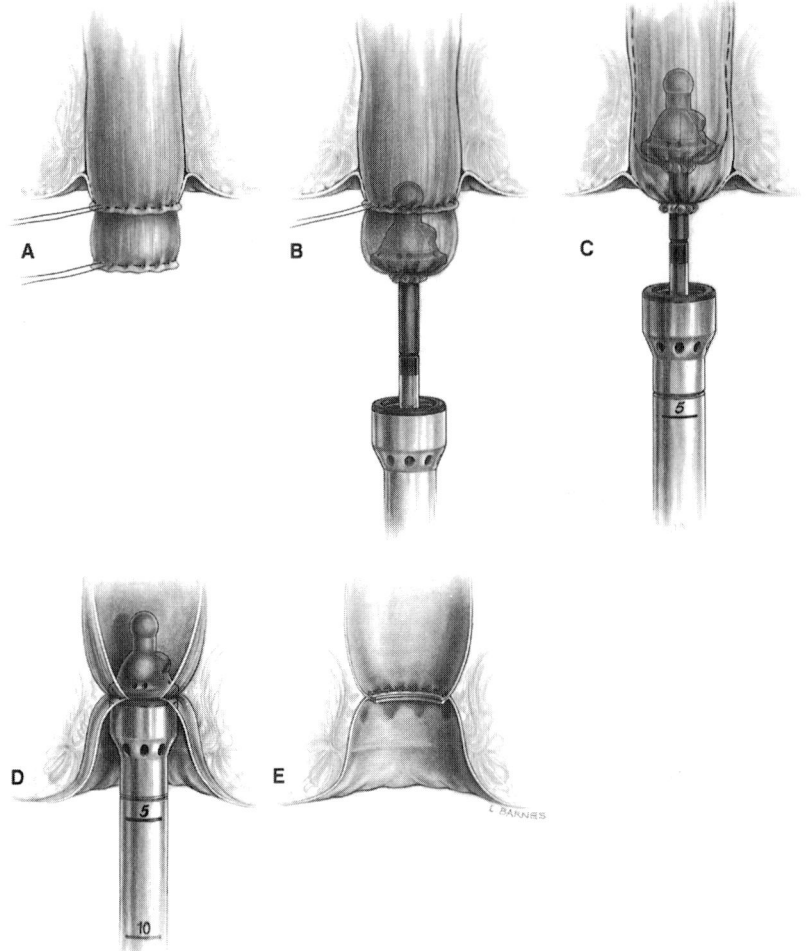

FIGURE 13.5. Altemeier procedure using the circular stapler. **A**, Purse-string sutures are attached to proximal and distal bowel after perineal resection. **B**, The proximal segment is secured over the anvil. **C**, The distal segment is secured. **D**, The instrument is closed and fired. **E**, The completed anastomosis. Reprinted with permission from Surg Gynecol Obstet 1983;156:85.

necessity for dietary limitation, and little or no pain after such procedures, there seems to be little advantage to the patient to remain in the hospital postoperatively unless other medical problems require such attention.

Abdominal Procedures

The third category of repair for rectal prolapse involves an intraabdominal approach. All such operations involve mobilization of the rectum, usually with rectopexy and possibly combined with sigmoid resection. These procedures generally involve a higher risk of perioperative complications in exchange for a somewhat lower risk of recurrence. Abdominal procedures allow correction of two of the three basic defects associated with the prolapse, permit fixation of the rectum superiorly and posteriorly against the sacrum, and provide the opportunity to remove redundant rectum and sigmoid. This operative approach compares with the transanal procedures, which remove only the redundant tissue (and possibly narrow the anal aperture). Criteria for the use of a transabdominal procedure include a patient under age 50 who is very active physically, the presence of another intraabdominal abnormality that would need simultaneous attention, and/or the presence of significant recto-sacral separation observed on video defecography. In the absence of these indications, we question the rationale for subjecting a patient to a procedure with significantly increased risks solely to diminish the recurrence rate. As mentioned above, if prolapse should recur after a transanal procedure, it can usually be managed with another transanal procedure with a much lower cumulative risk of surgery than there is after a single intraabdominal procedure.

Controversies such as whether to use prosthetic material in the performance of a rectopexy, whether to add a sigmoid resection, and whether to do either procedure laparoscopically continue to be debated, often with some passion. The part of the rectopexy procedure generally considered most important is the retrorectal dissection with freeing of the "lateral ligaments" to allow the rectum to be elevated from the pelvis. Methods of fixation include attachment of the rectum to the presacral fascia by using sutures through either the muscular wall of the rectum or the remaining lateral ligaments. Prosthetic materials such as polypropylene mesh (Marlex), Gore-Tex mesh, polyglycolic acid or polyglactin mesh (Dexon or Vicryl), and polyvinyl alcohol sponges (Ivalon) have been used[20] to secure the rectum to the sacral hollow. Duthie and Bartolo,[21] comparing the various techniques, found that continence was improved more with use of suture rectopexy than with prosthetic materials. Athanasiadis and colleagues,[22] who compared infection rates after rectopexy using Ivalon, Gore-Tex, and Marlex, found that after Ivalon was used, there was a slightly higher, but not statistically significant, infection rate. Novell et al.[23] compared suture rectopexy with the use of Ivalon and found a slightly higher complication rate with Ivalon and no difference in long-term results—data suggesting that the use of Ivalon is unnecessary. Overall, this is a moot point for many of us since the Ivalon sponge is not available in the United States. Sayfan and colleagues[24] also compared suture rectopexy with the use of Marlex and

came to a similar conclusion. Speakman and associates[25] have suggested that division of the lateral ligaments results in a lower incidence of recurrence but a higher incidence of postoperative constipation. We continue to use suture rectopexy, using 0 silk, and attaching the lateral ligaments to the sacrum as described above, and we do not see the additional advantage of prosthetic materials in open abdominal surgery. (*Editor's note:* We prefer to suture the muscular wall of the rectum directly to the sacrum, as we feel that using the lateral ligaments may result in narrowing or loss of distensibility of the rectum.)

The incorporation of sigmoid resection has also occasioned much discussion. The consensus seems to be that there is a lower rate of recurrent prolapse, a lower incidence of postoperative constipation, and no significant increase in morbidity when this is done at the same time as rectopexy.[13,20,21,24,26–28]

Some authors advocate the use of laparoscopic techniques for the intraabdominal approach to rectal prolapse. They suggest that when using this approach, morbidity is lower and hospital stay shorter, particularly if rectopexy is done without sigmoid resection. Most of the reported experience with laparoscopy involves rectopexy alone, using staple techniques for fixation of the prosthetic material to the tissues. Resecting a section of colon at the time of rectopexy currently requires an abdominal incision for removal of the specimen. Although laparoscopic resection and rectopexy are technically possible, these minimally invasive operations do not appear to be associated with any less morbidity, earlier return to work, earlier feeding, or shorter hospital stay than conventional laparotomy done for the same purpose.[29–34] Since limited experience has been reported to date using the laparoscopic approach, very few long-term data are available regarding recurrence rates and functional outcome. Therefore, I continue to believe that the intraabdominal approach to rectal prolapse is probably not feasible as a strictly outpatient procedure.

In summary, the repair of rectal prolapse lends itself well to an outpatient environment if an abdominal approach is not required. While the Thiersch procedure is the simplest of these approaches, its efficacy is limited by the tendency of the foreign material to migrate and require removal. It also does not really address the causative factors resulting in the rectal prolapse. The transanal procedures of Altemeier and Delorme do correct and resect the redundant segment of rectum and therefore have a lower recurrence rate and a very low morbidity rate and provide the ideal opportunity to perform this surgery on an outpatient basis. For the younger, more active patient, however, an intra-abdominal approach, combining sigmoid resection with suture rectopexy, may be the procedure of choice.

Rectocele

Many women with symptoms of rectal prolapse will be found during physical examination to also have a rectocele. A rectocele is a weakness of the rectovaginal septum that allows bulging of this septum anteriorly as the patient strains. When rectoceles become symptomatic, the patient must often put upward pressure on the perineum or posterior pressure on the back wall of the vagina to allow complete emptying of the rectum. It is widely speculated that the source of rectocele is related to weakness of the rectovaginal septum caused by birth trauma. Another theory that has gained increasing popularity is that the rectocele is really a large pulsion diverticulum. This develops because of increased intraabdominal pressure required by the failure of the levator and puborectalis muscles to relax appropriately at the time of defecation. This theory maintains that the rectovaginal septum is simply the path of least resistance in this anatomical region.[35] A parallel to this theory is seen in the situation of Zenker's diverticulum of the cervical esophagus.

Regardless of the etiology, when the rectocele is symptomatic it merits consideration of repair. Rectoceles may be repaired transrectally, transvaginally, or transperineally, and advantages and disadvantages have been advanced for each of these approaches. Advocates of the transvaginal approach argue that it diminishes contamination and does not result in entry of the bowel at any point. The vaginal approach is also logical if other transvaginal surgery such as cystocele repair, enterocele repair, or hysterectomy is required. The detractors of the vaginal approach point to a somewhat higher rate of recurrence of the rectocele than with repairs

done transrectally. They also make the theoretical point that it makes more sense to repair the defect from the rectal side since it is the "high-pressure" side of this septum. Nonetheless, transvaginally repaired rectoceles seem to be about as durable as those repaired by any other approach.

Advocates of the transperineal technique for repair of rectocele argue that this approach avoids entry into either the vagina or the rectum, thereby reducing infection and the possibility of a rectovaginal fistula. The implantation of prosthetic material such as polypropylene mesh into the septum has been described but has not gained widespread enthusiasm.[36] However, the transperineal repair is much more technically difficult and seems to be no more durable or safe than either the vaginal or rectal approaches.

When operations for rectal prolapse or other rectal abnormalities are being done, it makes excellent sense to simultaneously repair the rectocele by the transanal approach. When a rectocele repair is done as an isolated procedure, generally a segment of mucosa is removed from the anterior aspect of the rectum, from just above the dentate line to the top of the rectocele, possibly as high as the level of the pubic symphysis. The remaining mucosa is mobilized from approximately 120° of the anterior aspect of the rectum. One or two rows of imbricating sutures are placed in the circular muscle of the anterior rectum to increase the thickness of the rectovaginal septum and obliterate the rectocele. This imbrication may be done with interrupted, simple, or figure-of-eight sutures or with one or two continuous suture lines using a long-term absorbable suture such as 0 polyglycolic acid. This imbrication can be performed in either vertical or horizontal fashion or a combination of the two. Once the muscularis propria is approximated, any redundant mucosa is trimmed and the remaining mucosa is closed.

When rectocele repair is done in conjunction with the Delorme procedure, imbrication of the anterior muscularis propria is carried out before the accordion-style plication sutures are placed in this layer. When a rectocele repair is necessary, and an Altemeier procedure is planned, often no additional rectocele repair is required, since the segment of rectum containing the rectocele is removed. The only remaining area of weakness of the septum is that just distal to the line of resection, which is located 2 to 3 cm above the dentate line anteriorly. Sometimes the mucosa of this area can be partially everted prior to the anastomosis, allowing a few stitches to be placed in the muscularis propria. When an anterior levatoroplasty is performed along with the Altemeier procedure, no additional efforts are needed to repair the rectocele. When rectocele repair is required at the time of an intraabdominal approach to rectal prolapse, alternatives include performing the repair transvaginally or transrectally, or dissecting down between the rectum and vagina from the peritoneal approach and imbricating the front wall of the rectum, as described by Orkin (B.A. Orkin, personal communication, 1997).

Home Care After Outpatient Rectal Prolapse Repair

As mentioned earlier, patients who undergo either Delorme or Altemeier procedures are well suited to ambulatory surgical environments with either same-day or 23-hour hospital stays. Recently introduced antibiotics that provide both broad-spectrum coverage and high tissue levels when given orally are ideal for perioperative antibiotic coverage.

After perineal procedures for rectal prolapse, patients are essentially allowed unrestricted diet and physical activity. Discomfort from the anal dilatation required for these transrectal approaches may require mild to moderate-strength oral analgesics. We suggest that enemas and other instrumentation be avoided. Sitz baths may be of benefit in relieving pelvic muscle spasm, which often accompanies pelvic surgery.

Summary

Rectal prolapse and rectocele repairs lend themselves well to outpatient surgical management. Perineal procedures for rectal prolapse are associated with low morbidity and relatively low recurrence rates. Continence can be restored in a significant percentage of patients undergoing perineal repair of rectal prolapse. Since these operations can also be performed on an ambulatory basis, they can be associated with significant cost savings and patient satisfaction.

References

1. Broden B, Snellman B. Procidentia of the rectum studied with cineradiography: a contribution to the discussion of causative mechanism. Dis Colon Rectum 1968;11:330–347.
2. Archer BD, Somers S, Stevenson G. Contrast medium gel for marking vaginal position during defecography. Radiology 1992;182:278–279.
3. Sentovich SM, Rivela LJ, Thorson AG, et al. Simultaneous dynamic proctography and peritoneography for pelvic floor disorders. Dis Colon Rectum 1995;38(9):912–915.
4. Pfeifer J, Oliveira L, Park UC, et al. Are interpretations of video defecographies reliable and reproducible? Int J Colorectal Dis 1997;12(2):67–72.
5. Rao SS, Sun WM. Current techniques of assessing defecation dynamics. Dig Dis 1997;15(suppl 1):64–77.
6. Birnbaum EH, Stamm L, Rafferty JF, et al. Pudendal nerve terminal motor latency influences surgical outcome in treatment of rectal prolapse [see comments]. Dis Colon Rectum 1996;39(11):1215–1221.
7. Pfeifer J, Salanga VD, Agachan F, et al. Variation in pudendal nerve terminal motor latency according to disease. Dis Colon Rectum 1997;40(1):79–83.
8. Rieger N, Sweeney J, Hoffmann D, et al. Investigation of fecal incontinence with endoanal ultrasound. Dis. Colon Rectum 1996; 39:860–864.
9. Horn H, Schoetz D, Coller J, Veidenheimer M. Sphincter repair with a silastic sling for anal incontinence and rectal prolapse. Dis Colon Rectum 1985; 28:868–872.
10. Labow S, Hoexter B, Moseson M, et al. Modification of silastic sling repair for rectal procidentia and anal incontinence. Dis Colon Rectum 1985;28:684–685.
11. Gundersen A, Cogbill T, Landercasper J. Reappraisal of Delorme's procedure for rectal prolapse. Dis Colon Rectum 1985;28:721–724.
12. Agachan F, Reissman P, Pfeifer J, et al. Comparison of three perineal procedures for the treatment of rectal prolapse. South Med J 1997;90(9):925–932.
13. Jacobs LK, Lin YJ, Orkin BA. The best operation for rectal prolapse. Surg Clin North Am 1997;77(1):49–70.
14. Johansen OB, Wexner SD, Daniel N, et al. Perineal rectosigmoidectomy in the elderly. Dis Colon Rectum 1993;36(8):767–772.

15. Muller-Lobeck H. [Therapy: perineal operation]. Langenbecks Arch Chir Suppl Kongressbd 1997; 114:914–917.

16. Thorne MC, Polglase AL. Perineal proctectomy for rectal prolapse in elderly and debilitated patients. Aust N Z J Surg 1992;62(10):791–794.

17. Williams JG, Rothenberger DA, Madoff RD, Goldberg SM. Treatment of rectal prolapse in the elderly by perineal rectosigmoidectomy. Dis Colon Rectum 1992;35(9):830–834.

18. White S, Stitz RW. Rectal prolapse: Delorme or Ripstein repair. Aust N Z J Surg 1992;62(3):193–195.

19. Fengler SA, Pearl RK, Prasad ML, et al. Management of recurrent rectal prolapse. Dis Colon Rectum 1997;40(7):832–834.

20. Winde G, Reers B, Nottberg H, et al. Clinical and functional results of abdominal rectopexy with absorbable mesh-graft for treatment of complete rectal prolapse. Eur J Surg 1993;159(5):301–305.

21. Duthie GS, Bartolo DC. Abdominal rectopexy for rectal prolapse: a comparison of techniques. Br J Surg 1992;79(2):107–113.

22. Athanasiadis S, Weyand G, Heiligers J, et al. The risk of infection of three synthetic materials used in rectopexy with or without colonic resection for rectal prolapse. Int J Colorectal Dis 1996;11(1):42–44.

23. Novell JR, Osborne MJ, Winslet MC, Lewis AA. Prospective randomized trial of Ivalon sponge versus sutured rectopexy for full-thickness rectal prolapse. Br J Surg 1994;81(6):904–906.

24. Sayfan J, Pinho M, Alexander-Williams J, Keighley MR. Sutured posterior abdominal rectopexy with sigmoidectomy compared with Marlex rectopexy for rectal prolapse. Br J Surg 1990;77(2):143–145.

25. Speakman CT, Madden MV, Nicholls RJ, Kamm MA. Lateral ligament division during rectopexy causes constipation but prevents recurrence: results of a prospective randomized study. Br J Surg 1991;78(12):1431–1433.

26. Huber FT, Stein H, Siewert JR. Functional results after treatment of rectal prolapse with rectopexy and sigmoid resection. World J Surg 1995;19(1):138–143; discussion, 143.

27. Luukkonen P, Mikkonen U, Jarvinen H. Abdominal rectopexy with sigmoidectomy vs. rectopexy alone for rectal prolapse: a prospective, randomized study. Int J Colorectal Dis 1992;7(4):219–222.

28. McKee RF, Lauder JC, Poon FW, et al. A prospective randomized study of abdominal rectopexy with and without sigmoidectomy in rectal prolapse. Surg Gynecol Obstet 1992;174(2):145–148.

29. Wexner SD, Reissman P, Pfeifer J, et al. Laparoscopic colorectal surgery: analysis of 140 cases. Surg Endosc 1996;10(2):133–136.

30. Reissman P, Weiss E, Teoh TA, et al. Laparoscopic-assisted perineal rectosigmoidectomy for rectal prolapse. Surg Laparosc Endosc 1995;5(3):217–218.

31. Herold A, Bruch HP. [Laparoscopic therapy of functional disorders of the rectum and pelvic floor]. Langenbecks Arch Chir Suppl Kongressbd 1997;114:905–908.

32. Graf W, Stefansson T, Arvidsson D, Pahlman L. Laparoscopic suture rectopexy. Dis Colon Rectum 1995;38(2):211–222.

33. Boccasanta P, Rosati R, Micheletto G, et al. [Video laparoscopic surgery and rectal prolapse. Our experience in rectopexy]. Minerva Chir 1997;52(12):1417–1423.

34. Darzi A, Henry MM, Guillou PJ, et al. Stapled laparoscopic rectopexy for rectal prolapse. Surg Endosc 1995;9(3):301–303.

35. Mellgren A, Lopez A, Schultz I, Anzen B. Rectocele is associated with paradoxical anal sphincter reaction. Int J Colorectal Dis 1998;13:13–16.

36. Watson S, Loder P, Halligan S, et al. Transperineal repair of symptomatic rectocele with marlex mesh: a clinical, physiological and radiologic assessment of treatment. J Am Coll Surg 1996;183:257–261.

14

Colonoscopy

J. Byron Gathright Jr., M.D.

History

Although certain advances in medicine, such as Fleming's discovery of penicillin, have a clear-cut beginning, colonoscopy has many parents. Turell, in 1963, using a modified gastroscope, was able to get a limited view of the colon.[1] Two years later, again using a gastroscope, Provenzale and Revignas used a swallowed plastic tube to pull the instrument through the colon.[2] In 1965 the first instruments designed specifically as colonoscopes appeared in Japan. Oshiba and Watanabe[3] have been credited with the initial report of the use of the colonoscope. In the same journal, two other reports were printed that described the use of colonoscopes.[4,5] Soon thereafter, colonoscopes were being manufactured in Japan and in the United States. These early models were crude and difficult to use, but users made suggestions and the manufacturers listened and made important improvements.

Some early models would flex only up and down, requiring rotation of the entire instrument to turn left or right. These were soon replaced with instruments having handles permitting movement in four directions. Though an improvement, these were quite stiff and did not flex beyond 90°. Improved design led to the familiar two-wheel control seen on modern instruments. Increased flexibility at the tip and variable flexibility through the length of the instrument have been additional design improvements.

All of the early instruments had fiberoptic viewing so that only the operator was able to see the colon. The introduction of teaching heads with their dual viewing systems permitted the assistant to also see what was happening. The use of the teaching head was achieved at the cost of light reduction and some problems with focus of the image. The current instruments have replaced the optical viewing system with a microchip, which relays the image to a large-screen television monitor, thus permitting the entire team to view the procedure.

Wolff and Shinya's groundbreaking work showed that it was possible to remove colonic polyps with a wire snare cautery.[6] This development changed the colonoscope from a purely diagnostic instrument, only capable of small biopsies, to a therapeutic instrument as well.

Recently, the radiological literature has described the technique "virtual colonoscopy." With this technique a computer-generated image of the colonic wall is made from a contrast spiral computed tomographic scan.[7,8] The obvious problem with this technology is that it cannot identify lesions beyond those seen on the radiograph, and thus it may be no better than a well-done barium enema. As currently described, virtual colonoscopy is also unable to provide details of color and texture of the colonic wall seen so well with the colonoscope. Virtual colonoscopy may represent a great technical advance, but does it actually have merit? It suffers from the same drawbacks as other colonic imaging studies, namely, that if a lesion is found, colonoscopy is then necessary to perform biopsy, remove, or do any other indicated thing to the lesion. As with traditional imaging studies, many virtual colonoscopic reports may carry the disclaimer "clinical correlation recommended."

Indications for Colonoscopy

The indications for colonoscopic examination have been widely debated, resulting in a large number of guidelines. Organizations publishing guidelines for colonoscopy include the American Cancer Society, the American College of Gastroenterology, the American Gastroenterological Association, the American Society for Gastrointestinal Endoscopy, the Crohn's and Colitis Foundation of America, the Oncology Nursing Society, and the Society for American Gastrointestinal Endoscopic Surgeons, as well as Medicare and the American Society of Colon and Rectal Surgeons.[9] The wonder is not that so many groups have produced guidelines and indications for colonoscopy, but that in spite of such diverse parentage, these guidelines are remarkably similar. Table 14.1 represents a synthesis of many of the guidelines referenced above.

At this point, we must explore the differences between screening and surveillance and their application as indications for colonoscopy. Screening is the examination of a whole population or an average risk segment thereof, whereas surveillance involves the monitoring of persons who are considered to be in a high-risk group, such as those who have had a colonic malignancy.[10,11] Naturally, the indications for screening and surveillance are different.

Surveillance

Most authorities agree that surveillance of high-risk patients is a valid indication for colonoscopy. The controversy regarding the high-risk group centers primarily on the frequency of examination.[12–15] This is largely tempered by the physician's experience with surveillance and the patient's willingness to undergo examination versus his or her fear of another lesion. There is nearly universal agreement on the need for surveillance of patients who have had colon cancer, patients with long-standing inflammatory bowel disease[16] (especially chronic ulcerative colitis [CUC]), patients with a strong family history of colon cancer (one or more first-degree relatives with that disease), patients with a family history of inherited colonic malignancy syndromes such as familial adenomatous polyposis and hereditary non-polyposis colon cancer. Less agreement is found regarding patients with a history of adenomatous polyps. If a patient has more than two polyps, or has a polyp that is large or dysplastic or has a villous component, I prefer to place that patient under surveillance after treatment of the initial lesions.[12,17]

Screening of the General Population

Screening of the general population for colonic disease with the colonoscope is much more controversial than surveillance of persons at high risk. Even the most enthusiastic endoscopists will admit that colonoscopy is costly. These costs include tangibles such as the initial equipment investment, hospital and physician fees, as well as patient, physician, and hospital personnel time. The rate of discovery of significant disease in a population with age as the only risk factor is simply too low to justify the cost.

Occult Bleeding

Chief among the other indications is the detection of the source of lower gastrointestinal bleeding. Episodic small episodes of blood per anus and iron deficiency anemia are both indications for colonoscopy.[18] Vascular ectasias of the colon are easily identified with the colonoscope and can be treated with the heater probe, the bi-cap electrode, or the laser. Right-sided colon cancer and polyps are frequent sources of iron deficiency anemia.

Ogilvie's Syndrome

Patients with nonobstructive megacolon (Ogilvie's syndrome) have been successfully treated by colonoscopic decompression. Removal of all possible air and liquid while severely limiting air insufflation may allow the distention to be relieved. The decompression can be repeated as often as is necessary.[19]

Volvulus

Treatment of volvulus by colonoscopy has been successfully accomplished. When the site of volvulus is in the sigmoid colon, detorsion may of course be accomplished with the rigid or flexible sigmoidoscope, but volvulus involving the transverse

TABLE 14.1. Early detection of colorectal polyps and cancer.

Risk category	Recommendation	Age to begin	Interval
Average risk			
All people 50 yr or older who are not in the categories below	One of the following: FOBT plus flexible sigmoidoscopy or TCE	Age 50	FOBT every year and flexible sigmoidoscopy every 5 yr, colonoscopy every 10 yr or DCBE every 5–10 yr
Moderate risk			
People with single small (<1 cm) adenomatous polyp	Colonoscopy	At time of initial polyp discovery	TCE within 3 yr after initial polyp removal; if normal, as per average risk recommendations (above)
People with large (>1cm) or multiple adenomatous polyps of any size	Colonoscopy	At time of initial polyp discovery	TCE within 3 yr after initial polyp removal; if normal, TCE every 5 yr
Personal history of curative-intent resection of CRC	TCE	Within 1 yr after resection	If normal, TCE in 3 yr; if still normal, TCE every 5 yr
CRC or adenomatous polyps in 1st degree relative younger than 60 yr or in two or more 1st degree relatives of any age	TCE	Age 40 or 10 yr before the youngest case in the family, whichever is earlier	Every 5 yr
CRC in other relatives (not included above)	As per risk recommendations (above); may consider beginning screening before age 50		
High risk			
Family history of familial adenomatous polyposis	Early surveillance w/endoscopy, counseling to consider genetic testing, and referral to a specialty center	Puberty	If genetic test positive or polyposis confirmed, consider colectomy; otherwise endoscopy every 12 years
Family history of hereditary non-polyposis colon cancer	Colonoscopy and counseling to consider genetic testing	Age 21	If genetic test positive or if patient has not had genetic test, colonoscopy every 2 yr until age 40 yr, after every year
Inflammatory bowel disease	Colonoscopies w/biopsies for dysplasia	8 yr after start of pancolitis; 12–15 yr after the start of left-sided colitis	Every 1–2 yr

Abbreviations: FOBT, fecal occult blood test; TCE, total colon examination (either DCBE or colonoscopy); DCBE, double-contrast barium enema; CRC, colorectal cancer.

colon, cecum, and splenic flexure may require colonoscopy.[20] In fact I have often used the colonoscope for sigmoid volvulus because of its superior picture quality. After decompression of sigmoid volvulus, the instrument can be used to carry a large tube beyond the point of twisting to allow splinting of the bowel to prevent recurrent volvulus (while the tube is in place). The splint should be left in place only long enough to prepare the patient for definitive surgery. Splinting of more proximal segments after detorsion of the colon has not been attempted.

When attempting to treat volvulus endoscopically, the operator must remain cognizant of the possibility of ischemic changes, even full-thickness gangrene of the colonic wall. Perforation under these circumstances increases the mortality rate several fold. It is safest to discontinue the procedure and prepare for immediate surgery upon encountering evidence of ischemic necrosis.

Surveillance in Inflammatory Bowel Disease

Monitoring the course of inflammatory bowel disease by colonoscopic surveillance has become standard practice.[21] There is debate regarding the timing of initiating the monitoring after the diagnosis of CUC or Crohn's colitis, but almost all agree as to the desirability of such monitoring. Random sampling of the mucosa searching for dysplasia has become standard practice in CUC. In patients with Crohn's disease, the goals of colonoscopic evaluation include biopsy for dysplasia as well as identification of the extent of disease, disease activity, and stricturing. A biopsy should be performed for any unusual feature and every stricture.

Annual or even more frequent examination should be planned in patients with CUC, depending on the level and extent of dysplastic changes. The interval between examinations in patients with Crohn's colitis is less clear, but it can certainly be longer than in CUC. The incidence of cancer in Crohn's colitis is believed to be higher than that occurring in the general population, but it does not reach the frequency seen in CUC.[22]

Diverticular Disease

The role of colonoscopy in diverticular disease is quite limited. It can be used to clarify between diverticular disease and cancer and is occasionally useful in differentiating between bleeding from vascular ectasias and diverticular bleeding. Colonoscopy is clearly contraindicated in the face of acute diverticulitis.

Preparation

Preparation for the colonoscopic examination is crucial to the success of the procedure. With inadequate preparation and decreased visibility, significant lesions may be overlooked, there is an increased possibility of perforation, and finally the rare but real possibility of the presence of explosive mixtures of gas exists.[23]

There is no "standard" preparation favored by all endoscopists. The majority, however, use a polyethylene glycol (PEG) base with added electrolytes to offset losses that may occur with the whole-gut lavage produced by the PEG. The usual protocol consists of 48 hours of clear liquids followed by rapid (8 oz every 10 to 15 minutes) ingestion of 2 to 4 L of PEG solution. This is adequate to fully cleanse the colon in most patients; however, those with a history of chronic constipation may require stimulant laxatives at the start of the preparation to attain satisfactory cleansing of the bowel. There are several variants of the PEG preparation solution with different flavorings and slight variations on the electrolytes used, but all produce approximately the same result.[24]

Another preparation using sodium phosphate is reported to be as effective as the PEG-based solutions. Reports of renal failure following use of sodium phosphate have made most physicians cautious in prescribing it for the elderly, even for patients with apparently normal renal function.[25] The reduced volume of fluid that must be ingested may, on the other hand, make sodium phosphate more acceptable to younger patients.

When is the quality of the preparation acceptable to the endoscopist? If liquid feces with solid particles are encountered in the left colon, the view of the cecum is likely to be compromised. If attempts to wash and suction the bowel clean are not easily accomplished, the procedure may be postponed and further preparation attempted. If the patient can drink more PEG, he or she may be allowed to do so in a private place with access to a toilet. If the patient is unable to drink more, the preparation solution may be administered via a small feeding tube. Elderly and unwell patients may need to be examined on a subsequent day after continuing with clear liquids and taking additional laxatives to achieve a clean bowel. Decisions must be made in the face of inadequate preparation as to what is best for the individual patient. Few colonoscopic examinations are true emergencies, but in the face of an urgent situation, a preparation that would otherwise be considered inadequate may have to be accepted.

Sedation

Colonoscopic examinations performed without sedation have been reported from some centers. The vast majority of endoscopists and patients, however, favor some form of sedation.[26,27] General anesthesia has been used in the past, but the current practice in most areas is to utilize "conscious sedation." The patient receives a combination of meperidine and midazolam, which are titrated to the point of drowsiness or light sleep. Some physicians now utilize fentanyl to replace meperidine. I have no experience with fentanyl. Our preference is to have intravenous access with fluids running at a slow rate. This makes access to the bloodstream instantly available and lessens the chemical phlebitis commonly seen at the site of direct intravenous injection. Fluids can also be administered if the patient develops transient hypotension.

It is best to achieve an adequate level of sedation before beginning the procedure, as pain and apprehension caused by too little sedation may require "catch-up" doses of medication that can result in oversedation. Monitoring of the level of sedation as well as other vital signs (blood pressure, pulse rate, respiratory rate, oxygen saturation, and electrocardiogram) is performed by the registered nurse. His or her only other duty is to give intravenous sedation at the direction of the endoscopist. Although blood pressure and oxygen saturation monitoring are routinely used, electrocardiographic monitoring is utilized only in selected cases.[28] The physician and endoscopy suite personnel should be trained in resuscitative procedures in the event of marked oversedation or idiosyncratic reaction to the medication. Oxygen, endotracheal tubes, and the associated equipment and drugs for resuscitation must be readily accessible in the endoscopy suite.

The average-sized healthy patient can usually be safely started with 25 to 50 mg of meperidine and 1 to 2 mg of midazolam. Obviously, evaluation of the size and status of the individual should guide the physician in the choice of initial dose. During the course of the procedure, additional sedation may be required. This is usually administered in increments of 20 to 25 mg of meperidine and 1 mg of midazolam. Total drug doses given depend obviously on the patient's size and level of fitness. Doses of 150 mg of meperidine and 5 mg of midazolam are near the maximum doses that I am comfortable giving. These are maximum doses for a large, fit patient given over the course of the entire examination. The drugs are administered incrementally, as needed, throughout the procedure. Once the cecum is intubated, it is not usually necessary to give additional medication. Withholding additional sedation during the withdrawal phase

of the examination allows the patient to begin recovery a bit sooner.

(*Editor's note:* We have used fentanyl in place of meperidine for the past 15 years with very satisfactory results. Fentanyl has a shorter half-life and produces much less histamine release than does meperidine. The patients seem to awaken more quickly and have less hypotension and bradycardia than we experienced when we used meperidine. Doses of 50 to 100 μg of fentanyl are administered and are well tolerated.)

In the past, diazepam was widely used to sedate patients for endoscopic procedures. The much shorter half-life of midazolam and the availability of drugs to reverse its action have made it the drug of choice in most instances. Midazolam has the additional advantage of rarely causing the chemical phlebitis that so commonly occurs with diazepam injections.

As noted, general anesthesia has been used by some rather than conscious sedation. We have avoided general anesthesia, believing that it is important to know the patient's level of discomfort to be sure not to exert undue pressure on the bowel that can lead to possible perforation. In certain cases in which the patient is known to have a particularly difficult colon to intubate, very heavy sedation monitored by an anesthesiologist, or even light general anesthesia may prove to be the best choice.

Technique

There are probably as many variations on colonoscopy techniques as there are endoscopists. I will therefore describe the method most often used in the Ochsner Clinic Department of Colon and Rectal Surgery.

Before beginning the colonoscopy, a brief history is taken to reveal any significant medical problems. Physical examination is carried out with special attention to the heart and cardiopulmonary systems. A consent form is then read by the patient and questions are answered by the physician before it is signed. Ideally, the consent is obtained during the patient's clinic visit when discussion and questions can be covered in a less threatening environment. If consent was not previously obtained, it must be completed prior to beginning sedation. No sedation is given until the baseline vital signs are obtained.

The patient is placed in the left lateral (Sims') position, and conscious sedation is initiated. A gentle digital examination is performed to lubricate the anal canal, to dilate the sphincters slightly, to locate any low-lying anal or rectal lesions that might escape detection otherwise, and to permit easier insertion of the colonoscope. If not previously done in the clinic, anoscopic examination may be performed to visualize the anal canal and lower rectum. Villous tumors located in this area are notoriously difficult to palpate.

The colonoscope is "rotated" into the anus from anterior to posterior by the index finger pressing the side of the scope and turning the end into the anal canal at the same time. This method is preferable to straight-ahead insertion because it produces less pain.

It is our practice to have the operator control both the wheeled control knobs and the forward motion of the scope. (*Editor's note:* It is our usual practice for the operating endoscopist to operate the controls while an assistant advances and withdraws the endoscope under the verbal control of the endoscopist. We find that with modern endoscopes, it is rarely necessary to torque the scope during insertion. Twisting the scope may result in broken fibers and stretching of the control cables and may lead to more frequent repairs than if torque is infrequently used.) The assistant, often a resident in our clinic, may be needed for abdominal compression or to operate the snare or biopsy forceps at the appropriate time

Once the instrument is in place, insertion is gently begun, with the lumen in sight whenever possible. Insertion is usually accomplished by a series of in and out motions described as "dithering" but always attempting to move forward. If the patient becomes uncomfortable, a loop has probably been created in the instrument. This may be confirmed by palpation of the abdomen, or better, by withdrawing the scope and observing that there is little outward movement of the tip until the loop has been removed. The presence of paradoxical motion is also indicative of looping. With paradoxical motion, forward motion of the instrument results in backward motion of the tip and vice versa. When the loop has been removed, forward insertion may begin again. Removal of the loop is confirmed by

resumption of appropriate motion of the instrument.

Because of the anatomical configuration of the colon, the mobile sigmoid colon is the most frequent site of looping, followed by the transverse colon. The remedy remains the same regardless of the location. Persistent sigmoid looping may be dealt with by first removing the loop, turning the patient to the supine position, and having an assistant apply pressure over the sigmoid colon as the instrument is advanced.[29] When the descending colon has been reached, the pressure may no longer be required.

Two additional techniques, which are occasionally used to facilitate difficult examinations, need to be mentioned. Fluoroscopy has been employed by some endoscopists as a means of detecting loops and facilitating straightening of the scope, as well as to confirm intubation of the cecum. An external splinting device or overtube is occasionally slipped over the scope to straighten the sigmoid colon and prevent looping. With increasing experience by the endoscopist, neither of these adjuncts is commonly needed.

After the sigmoid colon has been intubated, the patient is rotated to the supine position and the location of the light from the instrument may be used to gauge progress. During the course of the procedure when there is difficulty in advancing the instrument, other positions such as right lateral or prone may be tried, but for most patients left lateral (Sims') and supine are the only positions needed.

Both flexures may be sites of difficulty with intubation, especially a high and acutely angulated splenic flexure, and numerous cases of splenic injury have been reported in association with colonoscopy.[30] Continued gentle searching for the lumen and utilization of the marked flexion possible in modern instruments will reward the patient endoscopist. It is tempting to use "slide by" at the flexures and other difficult areas. Slide-by is a technique of pushing ahead without visualizing the lumen. Brief and gentle use of this method is acceptable, but the endoscopist must realize that it carries a substantial risk of perforation if pursued aggressively. When using slide-by, excess pressure is indicated when the visible surface of the bowel blanches, turning from red or pink to white. At this juncture, slide-by should be abandoned and a search made for the lumen. After the splenic flexure is passed, progress across the transverse colon is generally not difficult, as the lumen tends to stay open with little additional air insufflation.

Regarding the amount of air insufflated into the bowel, the dictum less is better applies without exception. Visualize a long slender balloon such as those used by clowns to make toy Dachshunds. The more air that is blown into the balloon, the longer it gets, and the more the wall is stretched. The colon is surely elongated by the presence of excessive air and the wall is certainly stretched. Distention of the bowel also stretches the peritoneal surface and causes pain. If one is in doubt, it is always a good practice to remove air from the colon.

The hepatic flexure is usually less difficult to pass than the splenic flexure because it is less acutely angled and the lumen is larger. There may be difficulty, however, because of the length of colonoscope already inserted and the distention of the right colon by air. Continued gentle forward motion in the dithering fashion accompanied by removal of air until the lumen begins to collapse will usually be rewarded by progression to the cecal cap. In order to be certain that complete colonoscopy has been accomplished it is mandatory that the ileocecal valve be identified. Lesions can be hidden just below the valve and escape detection unless the endoscopist has an unobstructed view of the cecal cap. The identification of the appendiceal orifice may provide further confirmatory evidence that a complete examination of the colon has been accomplished.

Although it is not always necessary, I believe that it is sound practice to attempt intubation of the ileocecal valve in every case. Routine ileocecal intubation allows the endoscopist to attain the skill of doing so for the cases in which it is critical, such as in inflammatory bowel disease. Viewing the ileal mucosa also provides positive confirmation of total colonoscopy. The tip of the endoscope should be placed deep in the cecal cap and angled toward the valve. Then the instrument is slowly withdrawn. The tip will then slip through the ileocecal valve into the terminal ileum.[31] The rate of ileal intubation will increase as the endoscopist practices this maneuver.

Although the colonic wall is inspected as the colonoscope is inserted, the best examination is possible as the scope is withdrawn. For this reason, withdrawal should be slow and deliberate, and any areas that slip by too rapidly should be re-intubated for a thorough inspection. It is important, usually at the completion of the procedure, to obtain a careful look at the lower rectum. (*Editor's note:* Although retroflexion of the colonoscope to allow examination of the distal rectum is commonly practiced by gastroenterologists, we prefer, like Dr. Gathright, to examine this area with the anoscope or rigid sigmoidoscope. Retroflexion is uncomfortable for the patient and may lead to a higher rate of endoscope repair.)

Remember that no endoscopist (not even I) can examine every colon to the cecum. One should use good judgment and carry on resolutely as long as undue pressure is not required and as long as the patient is not experiencing undue discomfort. If the endoscopist does not recognize his or her limitations and ventures beyond them, complications may be lurking.

At the completion of the procedure, the patient is taken to a recovery area for observation while the effects of the conscious sedation gradually resolve. While in recovery, the patient is encouraged to pass the insufflated air, thereby reducing both postprocedure discomfort and the possibility of social embarrassment. A certain number of patients may complain of bloating and intermittent cramping for up to 72 hours after an otherwise uneventful examination without biopsy or polypectomy. Whether this discomfort is due to overinflation with air, unrecognized trauma during the examination, or unusual sensitivity on the part of the patient is unclear, but in the absence of other symptoms or findings, reassurance is all that is needed. In case of a change in symptoms (increasing abdominal pain, bleeding, or fever) the patients are instructed to immediately report the change to their physician (during office hours) or to the physician on call.

All patients are required to bring with them a responsible adult who can drive them home and observe them for problems that might arise after they leave the outpatient area. Our nurses then follow up the next day with a telephone call to ensure that the patient is experiencing no ill effects from the examination. If there are problems, a call is then made to the patient by the attending physician. In the case of an extremely difficult examination, or where polypectomy has resulted in a worrisome depth or breadth of burn, it may be prudent to admit the patient overnight for observation. If a complication arises, it can then be quickly recognized and treated.

Although it is uncommon, delayed perforation, which results in signs of peritoneal irritation, can certainly occur. One reason for the rarity of peritonitis following colonoscopy is that small perforations may be sealed off by omentum, mesentery, or small bowel. In addition, large areas of the colon are at least partially retroperitoneal, thereby covering small perforations and rendering them asymptomatic or minimally symptomatic. Perforations between the leaves of a fat mesentery may also be concealed.

Therapeutic Colonoscopy

Thus far, we have concentrated on colonoscopy indications, preparation, sedation, and technique. Now we will discuss biopsy and polypectomy techniques, the "dos and don'ts" for avoiding complications of these operative procedures.

Sampling for histology and destruction of small (less than 5 mm) polyps can be accomplished with the "hot biopsy" forceps. Its cup-shaped jaws are used to obtain a specimen and then an electric current is applied to completely destroy any remaining polypoid tissue.[32] During the electrocoagulation, the polyp should be lifted slightly from the bowel wall but should not be pulled hard enough to create a thin neck of tissue. Excessive traction may concentrate the electrical energy in a small area. This may produce a deeper burn, creating the possibility of serosal injury or even full-thickness perforation. Slightly larger sessile polyps may be dealt with by two or three applications of the hot biopsy forceps followed by surface cauterization of any suspected residual neoplastic tissue.

Cold biopsy—biopsy without utilizing the electrocautery—is often used when taking multiple samples of tissue when monitoring patients with inflammatory bowel disease for dysplasia. Cold biopsy can also be employed in sampling tissue from a suspected carcinoma.

Pedunculated polyps are best removed utilizing the wire snare and electrocautery.[6] With the polyp under direct vision, the operator and the assistant maneuver the snare over the head of the polyp in a coordinated effort. The loop should be brought down near the base of the pedicle, slightly above the bowel wall. (*Editor's note:* It is our practice to attempt to place the snare closer to the head of the polyp and slightly farther from its base. Although this technique may leave some of the stalk behind, we feel that the risk of significant hemorrhage following removal of large polyps may be diminished. The stalk, which is composed of normal mucosa and submucosa, will resolve spontaneously over a few months and will not be visible at the time of follow-up colonoscopic examination.) As the snare is slowly tightened, the electrical current is applied, dividing the pedicle and coagulating vessels feeding the polyp. If the pedicle is short, or especially if it is broad-based, great care should be taken to avoid using sufficient current to produce damage to the bowel wall. The addition of a small amount of cutting current to the coagulating current may help in dividing the pedicle while avoiding injury to the wall. Polyps whose heads are 3 to 4 cm in diameter can easily be dealt with in this fashion. Larger polyps require more skill, experience, and luck, but if the snare can be passed over the head, most pedunculated lesions can be safely removed. Recent advances in polypectomy technique to make the procedures safer have included the injection of the polyp base with a saline-epinephrine mixture prior to polypectomy, the use of smaller snares to prevent inadvertent damage to the tissues beyond the polyp, and the application of the argon laser for noncontact hemostasis.[33–35]

After division of its pedicle, the polyp will occasionally "disappear." Generally, it will be found in the nearest colonic fold, either proximally or distally. Occasionally, the polyp will have been pulled into the suction channel of the colonoscope. Backwashing this channel will usually yield the polyp. Every effort should be made to locate the polyp, as failure to retrieve the polyp for histologic evaluation can have future consequences for the patient and possible legal consequences for the physician.[36]

Sessile polypoid lesions may present a different challenge. Small sessile polyps can be managed in the manner previously described. Larger ones can be removed by multiple biopsy and coagulation treatment. As the size of the polyp increases, so does the possibility of its harboring malignancy. This is especially true if the lesion has a villous component, as is frequently found in larger sessile polyps. Since the malignant portion of the polyp in these cases is often found deep within the lesion, surface biopsies may be misleading. The ideal management of sessile lesions greater than 2.5 cm in diameter is surgical resection of the segment of bowel containing the tumor. The segmental resection should be carried out as if there was known malignancy present, resecting not only the bowel but also the appropriate node-bearing mesentery. For sessile polyps that seem to be amenable to snare cautery excision, pre-polypectomy injection of saline and epinephrine can reduce the likelihood of a perforation.

In patients deemed unable to withstand resective therapy, multiple biopsies and fulgurations may destroy the lesion. Because the risk of complications, including perforation, is significant with this technique, dismissal of the surgical option should not be made without careful consideration. Introduction of the laser to fiberoptic technology has added a newer, and possibly safer, method of dealing with sessile lesions.[37] Only large series will determine if use of laser is both safe and efficacious.

Polypectomy technique using multiple "scoops" of the snare to remove such sessile lesions has been advocated, and illustrations of this technique make it appear quite simple.[38,39] I suggest that the next time you have an opportunity to assess the thickness of the cecal wall, you consider what the scooping technique could do to this thin membrane with or without saline and epinephrine injection. Even when the submucosal injection technique is used, it is possible to create a false pedicle containing bowel wall or even serosa with the snare. Heroics with large polyps may be best left to the well-insured experts. Multiple polyps present yet another problem in management. Despite the many advances in the design of colonoscopes, it remains necessary to withdraw and reinsert the instrument each time a polyp larger than 5 to 8 mm in diameter is removed. If insertion of the colonoscope is difficult, or the number of polyps is great, two other options are available. If the polyps are restricted to one segment of the bowel, resection may be considered. Alternatively, as many polyps as is feasible (preferably the largest ones) can be removed initially, then another session can be scheduled in a few weeks. (*Editor's note:* Some larger polyps may be removed through the suction channel of the endoscope. This technique may, however, result in fragmentation of the polyp.

Other techniques for retrieving multiple polyps include the use of the splinting device mentioned earlier or cutting off multiple polyps and then irrigating the right colon with a hyperosmolar solution such as sodium phosphate to flush out the polyps. With the latter technique, polyps may be lost and never retrieved.)

In dealing with pedunculated polyps, which are found to contain invasive carcinoma, we have used Haggitt's classifications in determining therapy[40,41] (Figure 14.1). Most polyps restricted to levels 1 and 2 and many that reach level 3 do not require further therapy unless there is high-grade malignancy or evidence of lymphatic or vascular invasion. Many level 3 polyps can also be treated by polypectomy alone. Again, the presence of high-grade malignancy or vascular or lymphatic invasion mandates resective treatment. Polypectomy can be considered adequate therapy as long as there is an adequate tumor-free (more than 2 mm) margin in the pedicle, and both the patient and physician understand the fact that tumor cells in the submucosa have access to the lymphatics and can, in a small percentage of cases, recur or metastasize. Multiple studies have indicated that polypectomy alone is a safe option.[42,43] The management of these lesions must always be carefully individualized. Discussion of the histologic findings with a pathologist may be wise.

All level 4 polyps have access to the lymphatics of the submucosa and muscularis propria of bowel wall and thus should be treated by a cancer operation with removal of an appropriate length of bowel and its accompanying mesentery.[44]

There is a well-recognized entity called post-polypectomy syndrome that occurs after polypectomy. The low-grade signs of peritoneal irritation may be due to injury of the serosa by the electrocautery. This condition requires no specific treatment, but it should be recognized for what it is and vigilant follow-up should be instituted.[45] Late perforation should be suspected anytime symptoms worsen.

Complications

Complications of colonoscopy are fortunately uncommon, and are, for the most part, easily remedied. They can be classified as major or minor,

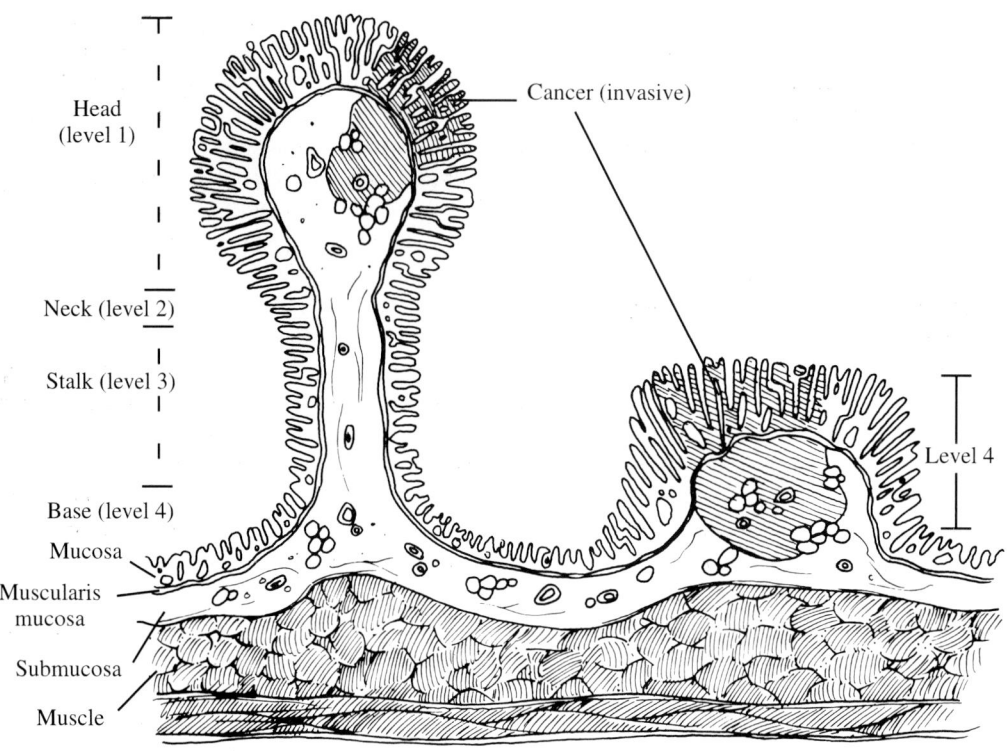

FIGURE 14.1. Pedunculated and sessile polyps illustrating Haggitt's classification of levels of invasion.

depending primarily on the possible need for surgical intervention.

Heart failure, coronary thrombosis, and stroke have been reported in association with colonoscopy, but these are more of a reflection of the age group of patients most often requiring colonoscopy. Bacteremia may occur during or immediately after colonoscopy and can result in the development of bacterial endocarditis. Patients with valvular heart disease should receive antibiotic prophylaxis following the guidelines of the American Heart Association and other organizations whose task forces have studied the problem [46-48]

Minor complications after colonoscopy may include the following: 1) minor bleeding after biopsy or polypectomy; 2) electrolyte imbalance from the preparation (rare with the use of balanced electrolyte solutions); 3) abdominal distention and cramping secondary to excessive air insufflation; 4) aggravation of hemorrhoids, fissures, or other anorectal problems; 5) colitis and diarrhea secondary to mucosal injury from incomplete removal of cleaning solution from the endoscope's sheath[49];

and 6) oversedation, resulting in hypoxia and/or prolonged recovery time. The reader will likely have several other minor complications to add to this list. As can be seen, most of these complications can be avoided if their existence is known.

Bleeding after biopsy or polypectomy is, however, not one of those complications that can always be easily avoided. Grasping the bleeding site with hot-biopsy forceps and coagulating the area will suffice in controlling the hemorrhage in many cases. Utilization of this ball-tipped electrode produces satisfactory coagulation with very little depth of penetration, and it may often be the safest tool available. Many gastroenterologists favor the heater probe to control bleeding, but we have little experience with this device. The theoretical advantages of the heater probe are the minimal penetration of its burn and, thereby, very little tissue destruction.

Pulsatile arterial bleeding encountered following division of the stalk of a polyp can be a thrilling experience, but fortunately, this bleeding is easily controlled in most instances. Prompt reapplication of the snare to the stalk with enough pressure to stop the bleeding begins the solution. Steady pressure, insufficient to cut through the tissue, is applied while waiting for three to five minutes. The snare is then loosened, and if no bleeding occurs the end of the stalk is coagulated for good measure. If bleeding recurs, reapplication of the snare and pressure for another 5 minutes is usually successful. Should persistent bleeding continue, the stalk or base may be injected with a 1:10,000 adrenaline solution via a sclerotherapy needle. Failure to stop bleeding after three tries should send the operator back to the chart looking for some previously undetected coagulopathy. As a last resort, a pitressin drip via a radiologically placed intraarterial catheter may be used. If this measure fails, surgical intervention will be necessary. At the Ochsner Clinic, no postpolypectomy bleeding in recent years has required laparotomy for its control. (*Editor's note:* Although it is occasionally possible to resnare the bleeding pedicle, the amount of bleeding is often such as to rapidly obscure vision through the scope and prevent such a maneuver. If the bleeding does cease following "squeezing" of the stalk, I am reluctant to apply electrocautery for fear of causing the bleeding to begin anew. When we are unable to resnare the stalk, we remove the colonoscope and wait. Frequently, in a few minutes, the bleeding will cease spontaneously due to swelling of the stalk from the cautery effect.) Another bleeding problem that may be occasionally encountered is late bleeding, which occurs 7 to 14 days after polypectomy. This type of bleeding may require transfusion but rarely operative intervention. The incidence of late bleeding in our practice has diminished significantly since we began to instruct patients to avoid aspirin and nonsteroidal anti-inflammatory drugs for 2 weeks after polypectomy.

The most serious complications of colonoscopy involve injury to the bowel or another intraabdominal organ. Bowel injury is generally of three types: mucosal injury with or without hematoma, serosal injury from either splitting or full-thickness cautery burn, and frank perforation from either mechanical trauma or cautery injury. While they do not always require surgical intervention, these complications do require that the physician contemplate the need for surgery. Only the first of these injuries may occur without peritoneal signs. Early bleeding may occur as a result of a mucosal stripping injury, whereas late postcolonoscopy bleeding may occur when a submucosal hematoma evacuates spontaneously. Observation is usually the only treatment required in these injuries. I have never even seen transfusion required in such cases.

Serosal injury without true perforation is the most common of these major injuries. This condition requires careful monitoring of the patient's abdominal symptoms and physical signs but does not typically require surgical intervention. There is sometimes a very fine line between a small complete perforation and serosal injury without perforation. The surgeon with experience caring for patients with peritonitis is the best person to monitor and decide on treatment of such a patient. Even complete perforation can, under certain circumstances, be treated nonsurgically.[49-53]

Anatomically the right colon, both flexures, and most of the descending colon are at least partially retroperitoneal structures. Injuries to the retroperitoneal portion of the bowel or between the leaves of a fat mesentery will often resolve with bowel rest, administration of fluids and appropriate antibiotics, and careful observation. Small areas of perforation or serosal injury may be walled off by adjacent bowel or omentum, as is seen in diverticular disease. An extreme example of the occasionally benign course of retroperitoneal perforation was seen in a patient who came to our emergency room 8 hours after flexible sigmoidoscopy by the gastroenterology department. His chief complaint was swelling of the neck. Upon examination, he was found to have crepitus from the base of his skull to the mid-thorax. X-ray examination confirmed retroperitoneal and subcutaneous air. He was admitted to the hospital for observation, but, because he had no fever or elevation in his white blood cell count, was treated with only bowel rest. Despite the uneventful course of this patient, all perforations must be regarded as potentially lethal situations.

Suspected perforation with peritoneal signs that are localized to a small area of the abdomen may be treated expectantly with bowel rest, fluids, and antibiotics. Repeated examinations of the patient's abdomen at intervals of 4 hours or less by an experienced physician are required. If the area with peritoneal signs is found to be expanding, immediate plans for surgical exploration of the abdomen should proceed. Since the bowel is already cleansed mechanically, the ideal time for surgical intervention may be early rather than late in the course of the injury.

The findings at the time of laparotomy, as always, will dictate the procedure that needs to be performed. In our experience, resection is almost never needed unless dictated by the primary disease process (e.g., Crohn's disease, ulcerative colitis, or ischemic colitis). If a perforation occurs near a cancer or a lesion such as a villous tumor that would require resection in any case, then segmental resection is obviously advisable. Perforations that occur distant to these lesions can be closed in conjunction with resection of the primary lesion.

Cautery burns can be débrided until healthy bleeding tissue is encountered, and the wound can then be closed with sutures. Tears likewise can be oversewn. Closure along the long axis of the bowel is usually possible and does not constrict the lumen to a significant degree. (*Editor's note:* Long, linear tears, particularly in patients with significant diverticular disease, may be better managed by resection.)

The list of major complications seen after colonoscopy includes injury to other organs. The spleen is the organ most often injured and the only one I have seen reported.[54,55] It is certainly possible that injuries could also occur to the liver from tears of the capsule by traction on the hepatocolic ligaments and to the small bowel from full-thickness cautery burns.

A disastrous complication, which appears now to be of only historic importance, is explosion of gases within the bowel. With poor or inadequate bowel preparation, explosive gas mixtures were occasionally present in the bowel, especially with poor evacuation of the colon or with mannitol-based preparations.[56] A cautery spark could ignite these gases. Avoidance of the use of cautery should be the inviolate rule in the occasional patient having an unprepared colonoscopy or exhibiting a heavy fecal load despite attempts to prepare the bowel.

Prevention of complications should always be our goal. The complications discussed above can be avoided by gentleness by the examiner, constant visualization of the lumen when advancing the scope, awareness of looping of the instrument, and, finally, by fearful application of the electrocautery. Unfortunately, the latter technique is the product of experience, but one should always assume that the cautery could be burning more deeply than is expected.

Special note should be made of the risks of lower gastrointestinal endoscopy in patients with suspected ischemic colitis or inflammatory bowel disease. The colon in these patients may be more easily perforated, a situation that is particularly true in patients in whom nearly full-thickness ischemia has occurred. Examination in the face of ischemia should be done by only the most experienced endoscopists and should be terminated immediately if full-thickness ischemic changes are encountered or strongly suspected.

The colon wall of patients with ulcerative colitis may be quite thin or may even have undergone spontaneous perforation in the situation of toxic dilatation. Even in Crohn's disease, toxic dilatation can occur and thus increase the risk of perforation during colonoscopic evaluation. Crohn's disease produces thickening of the bowel wall and may thereby lessen the possibility of perforation. On the other hand, such thickening may diminish the natural elasticity of the bowel, making perforation more likely to occur, especially in deeply ulcerated areas of the bowel.

Conclusion

Fiberoptic colonoscopy has clearly revolutionized the diagnosis and management of many colorectal diseases. Few other medical modalities so adroitly meld diagnostic and therapeutic capabilities. In addition, refinements in the instrumentation and optics should continue to improve visualization and permit safer biopsies and polypectomies. It is important, however, to fully consider the limitations of the colonoscope to avoid unnecessary complications.

References

1. Turell R. Fiber optic colonoscope and sigmoidoscope. Am J Surg 1963;105:133–136.
2. Provenzale L, Revignas A. An original method for guided intubation of the colon and rectum. Gastrointest Endosc 1969;16:11.
3. Oshiba S, Watanabe A. Endoscopy of the colon. Gastroenterol Endosc Tokyo 1965;7:400–402.
4. Niwa H. Endoscopy of the colon. Gastroenterol Endosc Tokyo 1965;7:402–408.
5. Kanazawa T, Tanaka M. Endoscopy of the colon. Gastroenterol Endosc Tokyo 1965;7:398–400.
6. Wolff WI, Shinya H. Polypectomy via the fiberoptic colonoscope: removal of neoplasms beyond reach of the sigmoidoscope. N Engl J Med 1973;288:329.

7. Alquist DA. Computed tomographic colography and virtual colonoscopy. Gastrointest Endosc Clin N Am 1997;7(3):439–452.

8. Johnson CD. Computed tomographic colonography (virtual colonoscopy): a new method for detecting colorectal neoplasms. Endoscopy 1997;29(6):454–461.

9. The Standards Task Force American Society of Colon and Rectal Surgeons. Practice parameters for the detection of colorectal neoplasms—supporting documentation. Dis Colon Rectum 1992;35(4):389–394.

10. Lieberman D. How to screen for colon cancer. Annu Rev Med 1998;49:163–172.

11. Markowitz AJ, Winawer SJ. Screening and surveillance for colorectal carcinoma. Hematol Oncol Clin North Am 1997;11(4):580–608.

12. Beck DE, Opelka FG, Hicks TC, et al. Colonoscopic follow-up of adenomas and colorectal cancer. South Med J 1995;88(5):567–570.

13. Patchett SE, Mulcahy HE, O'Donoghue DP. Colonoscopic surveillance after curative resection for colorectal cancer. Br J Surg 1993;80:1330–1332.

14. Atkin WS, Morson BC, Cuzick J. Long-term risk of colorectal cancer after excision of rectosigmoid adenomas. N Engl J Med 1992;326(10):658–661.

15. Winawer SJ, Zauber AG, O'Brien MJ, et al. Randomized comparison of surveillance intervals after colonoscopic removal of newly diagnosed adenomatous polyps. N Engl J Med 1993;328(13):901–960.

16. Solomon MJ. Cancer and inflammatory bowel disease: bias, epidemiology, surveillance and treatment. World J Surg 1998;22(4):352–358.

17. Beck DE, Opelka FG, Hicks TC, et al. Colonoscopic follow-up of adenomas and colorectal cancer. South Med J 1995;88(5):567–570.

18. Church JM. Analysis of the colonoscopic findings in patients with rectal bleeding according to the pattern of their presenting symptoms. Dis Colon Rectum 1991;34:391.

19. Jetmore AB, Timmcke AE, Gathright JB Jr, et al. Ogilvie's syndrome: colonoscopic decompression and analysis of predisposing factors. Dis Colon Rectum 1992;5:1135–1142.

20. Ghazi A, Shinya H, Wolff WI. Treatment of volvulus of the colon by colonoscopy. Ann Surg 1976;183:263.

21. Waye JD. Endoscopy in inflammatory bowel disease: indications and differential diagnosis. Med Clin North Am 1990;74:51–65.

22. Ekbom A, Helmick C, Zack M, et al. Increased risk of large-bowel cancer in Crohn's disease with colonic involvement. Lancet 1990;336:357–359.

23. Bigard MA, Gaucher P, Lassalle C. Fatal colonic explosion during colonoscopic polypectomy. Gastroenterology 1979;77:1307–1310.

24. DiPalma JA, Brady CE, Stewart DL, et al. Comparison of colon cleansing methods in preparation for colonoscopy. Gastroenterology 1984;86:856.

25. Keeffe EB. Colonoscopy preps: what's best? Gastrointest Endosc 1996;43(5):524–528.

26. Phillips MS. Drugs and sedation for colonoscopy. Prim Care 1995;2(3):433–443.

27. Herman FN. Avoidance of sedation during total colonoscopy. Dis Colon Rectum 1990;33:70–72.

28. Council on Scientific Affairs, American Medical Association. The use of pulse oximetry during conscious sedation. JAMA 1993;270(12):1463–1468.

29. Waye JD, Yessayan BA, Lewis BS, et al. The technique of abdominal pressure in total colonoscopy. Gastrointest Endosc 1991;37:147–151.

30. Ahmed A, Eller PM, Schiffman FJ. Splenic rupture: an unusual complication of colonoscopy. Am J Gastroenterol 1997;92(7):1201–1203.

31. Marshall JB, Barthel JS. The frequency of total colonoscopy and terminal ileal intubation in the 1990's. Gastrointest Endosc 1993;39:518–520.

32. Williams CB. Small polyps: the virtues and dangers of hot biopsy. Gastrointest Endosc 1991;37:394–395.

33. Shirai M, Nakamura T, Matsuura A, et al. Safer colonoscopic polypectomy with local submucosal injection of hypertonic saline-epinephrine solution. Am J Gastroenterol 1994;89(3):334–338.

34. Waye JD. New methods of polypectomy. Gastrointest Endosc Clin N Am 1997;7(3):413–422.

35. Greene FL. Colonoscopic polypectomy: indication, technique and therapeutic implications. Semin Surg Oncol 1995;11(6):416–422.

36. Waye JD, Lewis BS, Atchison MA, et al. The lost polyp: a guide to retrieval during colonoscopy. Int J Colorectal Dis 1988;3:229–231.

37. Mathus-Vliegen EMH, Tytgat GNJ. The potential and limitations of laser photoablation of colorectal adenomas. Gastrointest Endosc 1991;37:9–17.

38. Nivatvongs S, Snover DC, Fang DT. Piecemeal snare excision of large sessile colon and rectal polyps: is it adequate? Gastrointest Endosc 1984;30:18–20.

39. Walsh RM, Ackroyd FW, Shellito PC. Endoscopic resection of large sessile colorectal polyps. Gastrointest Endosc 1992;38:303–309.

40. Haggitt RC. Management of the patient with carcinoma in an adenoma. Prog Clin Biol Res 1988;279:89–99.

41. Haggitt RC, Glotzbach RE, Soffer EE, Wruble LD. Prognostic factors in colorectal carcinomas arising in adenomas: implications for lesions removed by endoscopic polypectomy. Gastroenterology 1985;89(2):328–336.

42. Nivatvongs S, Rojanasakul A, Reiman HM, et al: The risk of lymph node metastasis in colorectal

polyps with invasive adenocarcinoma. Dis Colon Rectum 1991;34(4):323–328.

43. Pollard CW, Nivatvongs S, Rojanasakul A, et al. The fate of patients following polypectomy alone for polyps containing invasive carcinoma. Dis Colon Rectum 1992;35(10):933–937.

44. Kafka NJ. Endoscopic management of malignant colorectal polyps. Surg Oncol Clin N Am 1996;5(3): 633–661.

45. Waye JD. The postpolypectomy coagulation syndrome. Gastrointest Endosc 1981;27:184.

46. Dajani AS, Bisno AL, Chung KJ. Prevention of bacterial endocarditis: recommendations, by the American Heart Association. JAMA 1990;264: 2919–2922.

47. Standards of Training and Practice Committee, American Society for Gastrointestinal Endoscopy. Infection control during gastrointestinal endoscopy: guidelines for clinical application. Gastrointest Endosc 1988;34(suppl):37S.

48. Standards Task Force, American Society of Colon and Rectal Surgeons. Practice parameters for antibiotic prophylaxis-supporting documentation. Dis Colon Rectum 35:278–285, 1992.

49. Dolce P, Gourdeau M, April N, et al. Outbreak of glutaraldehyde-induced proctocolitis. Am J Infect Control 1995;23(1):34–39.

50. Lo AY, Beaton HL. Selective management of colonoscopic perforations. J Am Coll Surg 1994;179: 333–337.

51. Damore LJ. Colonoscopic perforations. Etiology, diagnosis and management. Dis Colon Rectum 1996;39(11):1308–1314.

52. Vernava AM. Complications of endoscopic polypectomy. Surg Oncol Clin N Am 1996;5(3):663–673.

53. Hall C, Dorricott NJ, Donovan IA, et al. A perforation during colonoscopy: surgical versus conservative management. Br J Surg 1991;78:542.

54. Heath B, Rogers A, Taylor A, et al. Splenic rupture: an unusual complication of colonoscopy. Am J Gastroenterol 1994;89(3):449–450.

55. Doctor NM, Monteleone F, Zarmakoupis C, et al. Splenic injury as a complication of colonoscopy and polypectomy: report of a case and review of the literature. Dis Colon Rectum 1987;30:967.

56. Avgerinos A, Kalantzis N, Rekoumis G, et al. Bowel preparation and the risk of explosion during colonoscopic polypectomy. Gut 1984;25:361.

15

Local Treatment
of Rectal Cancer

Julio Garcia-Aguilar, M.D., Ph.D.
Charles O. Finne III, M.D., F.A.C.S.

The surgical treatment of rectal cancer assumes that the cancer starts as local disease that disseminates in an orderly fashion from the site of origin to the regional lymph nodes, and from there to the bloodstream to establish distant metastases.[1] Until recently the lymph node status could not be determined preoperatively. Consequently, in the absence of distant metastasis, rectal cancers have been treated by radical en bloc resection of the rectum and its lymphatic drainage. For tumors located in the upper and mid rectum, a radical resection and adequate oncologic distal margin can usually be accomplished with a sphincter-preserving operation.[2] However, in distal rectal tumors the requirement for an oncologically acceptable distal margin often mandates an abdominoperineal resection.[3]

Although these radical procedures are still considered the gold standard in the surgical treatment of rectal cancer, they are often associated with significant morbidity, mortality, and poor functional results. The operative mortality for anterior resection is approximately 2%, and the operative mortality ranges from 1% to 6% for abdominoperineal resection.[3] The overall complication rate after radical proctectomy ranges between 50% and 75%.[3] Up to 40% of these patients develop urinary complications, and 5% to 69% complain of sexual dysfunction.[4-7] Of patients undergoing an abdominoperineal resection, 16% develop an infection, dehiscence, or herniation of their perineal wound and 11% have complications related to the colostomy. Even patients who are able to undergo anterior resection frequently complain of urgency, tenesmus, and incontinence to stool.[8,9]

In addition, a significant number of rectal cancer patients do not benefit from the potential advantages of these radical procedures.[10] Some individuals are diagnosed when their cancer is still localized to the bowel wall and can be cured by less radical operations. Other patients with seemingly localized tumors will die of disseminated distant metastases despite extensive resection. Both of these groups of patients undergo an unnecessarily radical procedure. Therefore, it is not surprising that many surgeons are increasingly interested in developing alternatives to radical resection in patients with rectal cancer.[11]

Local excision has always been an acceptable alternative in the surgical treatment of rectal cancer in patients unfit for a major radical operation because of advanced age or comorbid conditions. The experience accumulated in the last decades with the treatment of breast cancer has demonstrated that for patients with early-stage disease, local therapy consisting of lumpectomy and breast irradiation can provide similar tumor control and long-term survival compared with radical excisions.[12] However, local therapy for rectal cancer has never gained widespread acceptance for the treatment of the average-risk patient, largely because of the inability to preoperatively identify patients with early tumors who may benefit from less radical operations. The development of new diagnostic tools, especially endorectal ultrasound, that facilitate the preoperative staging of these patients, has increased the interest in local treatment of early rectal cancers.

Many retrospective studies have revealed that in properly selected patients, local treatment of rectal cancers results in similar tumor control compared with radical surgery but without the need for a major operation or permanent colostomy. Recurrence and survival are similar with different forms of local therapy in patients with identical tumor stage. Excisional procedures are preferred because they provide a specimen for confirmation of the diagnosis, assessment of the completeness of the excision, and staging of the depth of tumor penetration of the rectal wall. This information from the excised specimen can be readily used to change the plan of therapy, compare results between similar groups of patients, and obtain prognostic information. The ablative techniques, endocavitary radiation and electrocoagulation, are useful when the tumor cannot be excised transanally or when the patient is too fragile to tolerate radical surgery.

Local Excisional Techniques

Selection Criteria

The optimal treatment of rectal cancer requires consideration of tumor characteristics such as size, location, depth of invasion, nodal status, and histology. Patient-related factors include operative risks, functional status, and patient desires. Only anatomically accessible tumors that are localized to the rectal wall are potential candidates for curative local excision. Once the tumor has spread outside the rectal wall, either by direct extension into the perirectal fat or by invasion of the regional lymph nodes, it cannot be reliably cured by local excision alone. Thus, in the absence of distant metastasis, decisions regarding local excision are based on the depth of tumor penetration and the involvement of the regional lymph nodes.

The depth of mural invasion is of particular importance because the incidence of lymph node metastasis increases with tumor penetration into the deeper layers of the rectal wall. This incidence of nodal metastasis ranges between 6% and 12% for tumors infiltrating the submucosa, between 20% and 26% for tumors limited to the muscularis propria, and between 51% and 66% for tumors infiltrating the perirectal fat.[13-15] The depth of mural invasion and the presence of lymph node metastasis can be assessed either clinically or with the help of special diagnostic tests.

TABLE 15.1. Clinical staging system for rectal cancer.

Stage	Definition	Pathological correlation
CS I	Freely mobile	Submucosa
CS II	Mobile	Muscularis propria
CS III	Tethered mobility	Perirectal fat
CS IV	Fixed/tethered fixation	Adjacent structures

Clinical Examination

Clinical assessment of a rectal cancer by digital rectal examination provides valuable information about size, distance from the anal verge, accessibility, and fixation, but digital examination permits only a gross estimation of the depth of tumor invasion. Mason introduced a clinical staging system for rectal cancer based on tumor mobility on digital examination (Table 15.1).[16] Nicholls et al. compared this clinical staging system with pathologic examination in 70 patients with rectal cancer and found that digital assessment was poor at predicting tumor spread to the individual layers of the rectal wall.[17] Digital examination was, however, able to differentiate between tumors confined to the rectum or slightly invading the mesorectum from those with moderate or extensive perirectal invasion in greater than 80% of the patients.[17] Unfortunately, the accuracy of digital examination at detecting lymph node invasion was significantly lower. Two-thirds of the nodes thought to be involved by digital examination were confirmed to be involved by the pathologist, but only 50% of the nodes containing metastases were correctly assessed by digital examination. Therefore, clinical examination is more accurate in staging locally advanced cancers than it is in staging early tumors that may be amenable to local therapy. Not surprisingly, the accuracy of digital assessment varies significantly with the experience of the examiner.[17] While the accuracy of digital examination in predicting the depth of invasion has been surpassed by newer diagnostic modalities, palpation of the tumor remains a critical component of the clinical assessment of rectal cancer patients because it provides direct, although subjective, information to the surgeon performing the procedure.

Macroscopic Features

For many years, only tumors smaller than 3 cm in diameter were considered for local excision. Although larger tumors tend to be more advanced, several studies have demonstrated that, when corrected for histologic grade and depth of invasion, tumor size is not an independent risk factor for lymph node metastasis and overall prognosis.[14,18] Other macroscopic tumor characteristics, such as the morphologic configuration, do not appear to be independent predictors of lymph node metastasis.[13-15] Tumor size and morphology are not considered contraindications to local excision when the lesion is localized to the rectal wall, located in an accessible area, has a favorable histology, and technically can be completely removed.

Tumor Histology

Histopathologic features provide information concerning the biological aggressiveness of the tumor and the incidence of lymph node metastasis. The risk of lymph node metastasis increases with tumor grade, as does the reported rate of local recurrence after local excision of poorly differentiated tumors.[11,13-15,19,20] Lymphatic and blood vessel invasion is also associated with a higher incidence of lymph node metastasis, local recurrence, and decreased survival.[13-15,19] Although there is no agreement regarding the mucin content required for the diagnosis of mucinous carcinoma,[21] a rectal cancer with a mucinous component has a higher risk of local recurrence and a poorer prognosis.[21-23] Local excision as the sole form of treatment is contraindicated in patients with these unfavorable histopathologic criteria. Unfortunately, discrepancies in the assessment of tumor grade are very common between the initial biopsy and the resected specimen.[24]

Endorectal Ultrasonography

Endorectal ultrasonography (ERUS) can discriminate between the different layers of the rectal wall and can be used to reliably assess tumors up to about 12 cm from the anal verge (Figure 15.1). In recent years ERUS has become the diagnostic modality of choice for the preoperative staging of rectal cancers.[25] The ability to image tumor invasion through the different layers of the rectal wall led to the development of an ultrasonographic staging system that corresponds to the TNM classification[26] (Figure 15.2). When compared with histopathologic staging, the accuracy of ERUS in predicting the

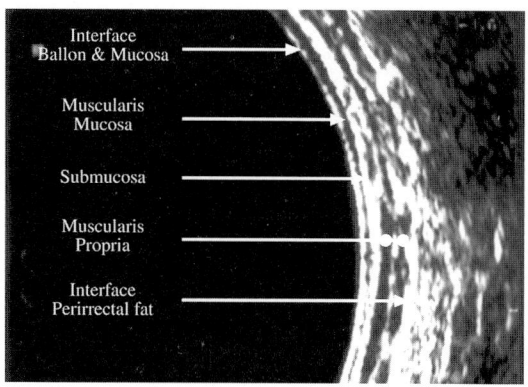

Figure 15.1. Partial view of an endorectal ultrasound image of the rectal wall represented as a seven-layer model. The white line separating the outer dark line represents the interface between the circular and longitudinal layers of the muscularis propria.

depth of mural invasion ranges between 85% and 91%[27-33] (Table 15.2). We have recently reviewed the University of Minnesota experience with the preoperative staging of 278 rectal neoplasms, in which the ERUS could be correlated with the pathologic stage. None of these lesions were treated by preoperative chemoradiation therapy. We found an overall accuracy of 79% for depth of wall invasion, with 13% of the tumors overstaged and 8% understaged. This accuracy varied with the stage of the tumor, being 94% for uT0, 65% for uT1, 76% for uT2, and 75% for uT3 lesions (unpublished data).

The accuracy of ERUS in identifying metastasis to the perirectal lymph nodes is lower than that for assessment of depth of mural invasion. Normal perirectal lymph nodes are isoechoic with the perirectal fat and are therefore not visualized on ERUS. The diagnosis of lymph node metastasis is based on visualization of a well-defined hypoechoic image[34] (Figure 15.3). Neither the size of the node nor the ultrasonic characteristics are reliable predictors of lymph node metastasis. The accuracy of ERUS on the diagnosis of perirectal lymph node metastasis ranges between 61% and 83%[28-33] (Table 15.2). In our own series of 102 patients who underwent radical surgery without preoperative radiotherapy, the overall accuracy was 65%, with 45% of the patients overstaged and 31% understaged. These relatively poor results, however, are based on a selected group of patients that excluded

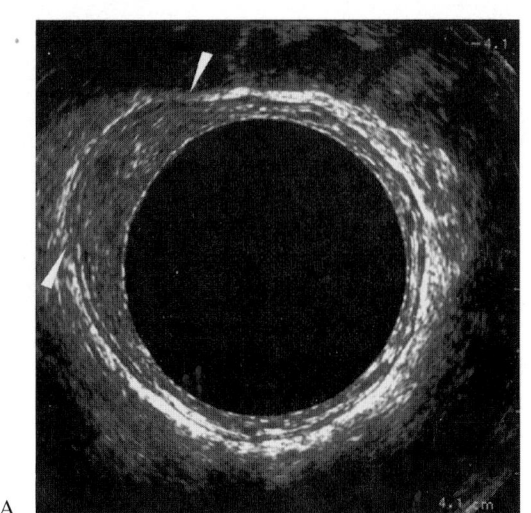
A

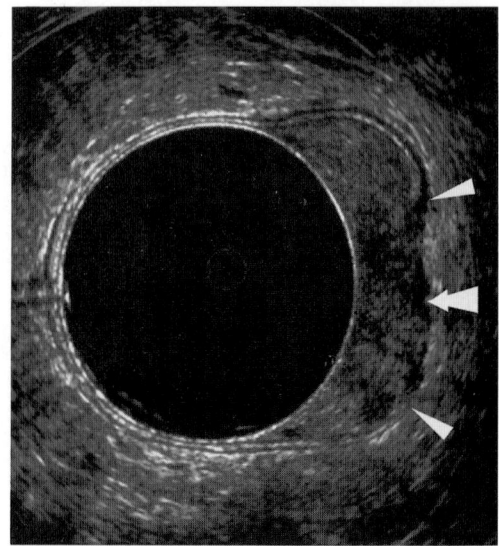
B

FIGURE 15.2. **A**, Ultrasound image of a T1 lesion. The arrows indicate the breach in the submucosa (middle white line). **B**, Ultrasound image of a T2 lesion. The thickening of the muscularis propria is evident in the central portion of the lesion (large arrow). The breach of the submucosa is seen laterally (small arrows).

TABLE 15.2. Accuracy of endorectal ultrasound on the preoperative staging of rectal cancer.

Author	Year	Tumor invasion		Nodal metastasis	
		No.	Accuracy (%)	No.	Accuracy (%)
Beynon[26,28]	1986/1989	42	91	95	83
Holdsworth[29]	1988	36	86	36	61
Milsom[30]	1990	52	83	17	70
Hinder[31]	1990	25	80	20	80
Lok Tio[32]	1991	61	80	37	72
Herzog[33]	1993	118	89	111	80
Authors' series[a]	1998	278	79	102	65

[a]Unpublished data.

uT3 or uN1 tumors that received chemoradiation therapy before radical surgery, and uT1 uN0 and uT2 uN0 tumors that were treated by local excision. Our overall accuracy in assessing lymph node metastases would probably be higher if these groups were included in the analysis. Biopsy of suspicious lymph nodes is not routinely performed due to both the difficulty in accessing the node without traversing the tumor and the risk of tumor seeding the needle tract.

Sources of error in tumor staging with ERUS include technical limitations, characteristics of the tumors, peritumoral inflammatory reaction, location of the tumor within the rectum, operator experience, and interpretation biases.[35] Overstaging of a

rectal carcinoma may result in denying a patient the potential benefits of local excision, whereas understaging is more likely to affect the chance of cure. Local excision of a tumor with penetration of the perirectal fat or lymph node invasion not detected by ERUS may require a second procedure or may result in early recurrence and compromised survival. Because of the fear of undertreating patients, overstaging is more common than understaging in most reported series.

Tridimensional ultrasonography may facilitate imaging of stenotic tumors and allow biopsy localization of suspicious perirectal lesions, but it does not provide significantly improved accuracy over

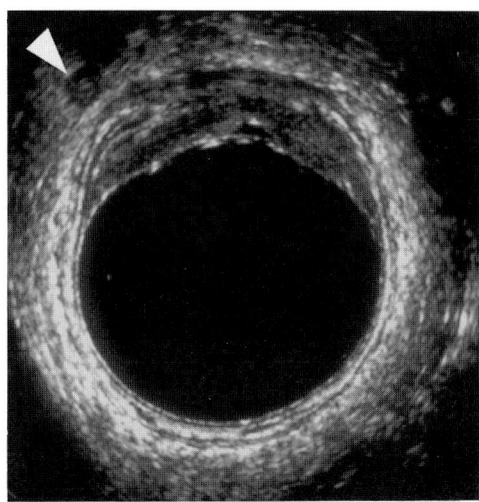

FIGURE 15.3. Endorectal ultrasound image of a perirectal. lymph node (arrow).

conventional ERUS.[36,37] The addition of color-flow and pulsed Doppler imaging may enhance the accuracy and specificity of the conventional gray scale ERUS in the evaluation of perirectal lymph nodes.[38]

(*Editor's note:* Several comments regarding ERUS seem warranted. First, the ideal instrument for rectal evaluation is one that provides a 360° view of the wall. Second, evaluation of mid to upper rectal lesions frequently requires that the probe be placed above the lesion by means of a special proctoscope 15 cm in length and with a diameter sufficient to allow passage of the probe. Finally, I would make a plea for surgeons to perform their own ERUS. Although the radiologist may have sophisticated equipment and experience in interpreting ultrasound, he or she frequently lacks either the interest or the skill needed to properly position the probe and interpret the study in light of the clinical situation.)

Computed Tomography

Computed tomography (CT) scanning, even when using intrarectal contrast, cannot distinguish the individual layers of the rectal wall. CT assesses rectal wall invasion and lymph node metastasis based on size criteria.[39] Wall thickness greater than 6 mm and lymph node diameter above 1.0 cm are considered pathologic. However, many early cancers can measure less than 6 mm in thickness. Nodal size is not a reliable indicator of metastasis, as approximately 18% of lymph nodes smaller than 5 mm harbor metastasis. The reported accuracy of CT scanning in the assessment of tumor invasion ranges between 53% and 77% and is even lower (40% to 45%) in detecting lymph node metastasis.[40-44] Nichols et al. have reported that CT scanning is no more reliable than a digital examination in the assessment of rectal cancers,[17] and most comparative studies have found that CT scanning is less accurate than ERUS.[45,46] The diagnostic accuracy of CT scanning increases with the stage of the tumor, and CT scanning is more reliable for assessing extrarectal invasion than for selecting patients for local therapy. Extrarectal invasion is suggested by small strands of tissue extending into the perirectal fat and by loss of normal tissue fat planes surrounding structures such as the vagina. Some of these changes should be interpreted with caution, however, because they may represent normal anatomical variants, inflammation, or scarring. CT is useful in the selection of patients with advanced tumors for preoperative adjuvant therapy and to exclude liver metastasis.

Magnetic Resonance Imaging

Conventional surface coil magnetic resonance imaging (MRI), like CT, has difficulty defining the layers of the rectal wall. The overall accuracy of MRI in the staging of rectal cancer ranges between 66% and 82% for mural invasion and between 60% and 72% for lymph nodal metastasis.[47-49] Comparative studies have reported slightly increased accuracy over CT scanning but less accuracy than ERUS.[47-49] New MRI technology (such as rapid scanning technique, paramagnetic contrast agents, and endorectal surface coils) provides higher spatial resolution of the different layers of the rectal wall. Initial results suggest that endorectal coil MRI provides comparable images and more accurate staging than ERUS[50-53] (Table 15.3). However, prospective studies comparing both techniques have not confirmed a significant advantage of endorectal coil MRI over ERUS.[54-57] Early results with high-resolution MRI suggest that, at best, it is as accurate as ERUS in the preoperative staging of rectal cancers (Table 15.3). Potential advantages of endorectal coil MRI over ERUS include its deeper penetration with improved definition of

TABLE 15.3. Accuracy of magnetic resonance imaging (MRI) and endorectal ultrasound (ERUS) on preoperative staging of rectal cancer.

		Accuracy (%)			
		Mural invasion		Nodal Metastasis	
Author	No. patients	MRI	ERUS	MRI	ERUS
Conventional MRI					
Waizer[47]	13	77	84[a]	—	—
Thaler[48]	37	82	88	60	80
Starck[49]	34	66	88	72	71
High-resolution MRI					
Joosten[54]	9	77	67[b]	—	—
Meyenberger[55]	6	40	83[c]	66	66
Zagoria[56]	10	80	70[d]	—	—
Kulling[57]	13	77[e]	85[e]	62	62

[a]Different ultrasound grading system.

[b]5-MHz biplanar probe.

[c]7.5-MHz echo colonoscope.

[d]Differences not statistically significant.

[e]Endoscopic magnetic resonance and endoscopic ultrasound.

perirectal extension, simultaneous body imaging for the assessment of distant metastasis, and less operator-related variability in technique and interpretation. MRI, however, is much more expensive and uncomfortable for the patient, lacks portability, and does not allow the optimal positioning of the probe in relation to the tumor that can be achieved with ERUS.

Patient Criteria

Every patient with a rectal tumor that conforms to the selection criteria is a candidate for local excision with curative intent. However, a patient who is already incontinent may not benefit from the hypothetical benefits of local therapy. Local excision, with or without adjuvant chemoradiation therapy, may be the procedure of choice in patients who have more advanced disease but who are physically unfit to undergo major surgery, and in patients who may not benefit from more radical procedures because of the presence of distant metastasis.

Patient Evaluation

The preoperative evaluation of patients with rectal cancer should include a medical history and general physical examination. A digital rectal examination

is essential to assess the location, size, and fixation of a distal tumor. The examination may also provide useful information about anal sphincter function. The diagnosis is confirmed by endoscopy and biopsy. Whereas a complete colonoscopy is performed to exclude synchronous colon cancer or polyps, rigid proctoscopy is preferred to record the characteristics of the tumor, such as distance from the anal verge, size, and macroscopic appearance. If necessary, a larger biopsy can also be obtained through the rigid proctoscope. A chest radiograph and abdominal and pelvic CT scans are obtained to exclude pulmonary and liver metastases and to check for the presence of pelvic extrarectal invasion. Except in clinically advanced tumors, an ERUS examination should be performed.

Technical Considerations

There are four technical approaches to local excision: transanal, transcoccygeal, transsphincteric, and transanal endoscopic. Patient selection for local excision is usually based on the results of ERUS, and therefore only tumors that are within the reach of the ERUS probe are candidates for local excision with curative intent. Most of these tumors can be excised through the anus. The transsacral and transsphincteric approaches do not

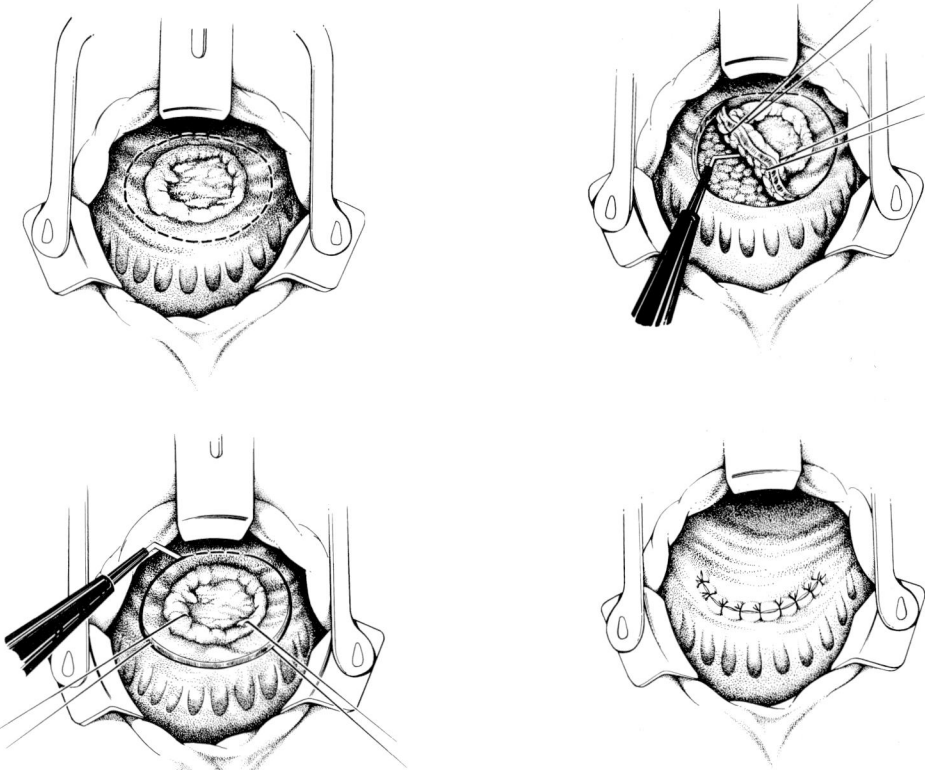

FIGURE 15.4. Technique of transanal full-thickness excision of early rectal cancer. Reprinted with permission from Bailey et al.[80]

provide a significant technical advantage over the transanal approach and carry the risk of the patient's developing a fecal fistula and/or anal incontinence. Transanal endoscopic microsurgery (TEM) may be a useful alternative in selected tumors of the upper rectum that cannot be removed by standard transanal techniques. Although some have advocated using TEM for all local excisions, we have not found that approach to be necessary.

Transanal Excision

Full-thickness excision of rectal tumors requires mechanical bowel preparation including oral antibiotics, and perioperative prophylactic intravenous antibiotics. A bladder catheter is routinely inserted. The procedure is usually performed under general or regional anesthesia, but in certain circumstances it can be done under local anesthesia with intravenous sedation. A pudendal nerve block is frequently used to relax the sphincter and help control postoperative pain. Most local excisions are performed in the prone jack-knife position. However, some posterior lesions may be better approached using the modified lithotomy position. An operating headlight is essential in providing good illumination. Taping the buttocks apart exposes the perianal area, and the Lone Star Retractor™ (Lone Star Medical Products, Houston, TX) is used to efface the anus and facilitate exposure of the distal rectum. A Pratt bivalve anoscope is commonly used to dilate the anus and localize the lesion, but we prefer the Sawyer, Hill-Ferguson or Ferguson Moon retractors to expose the rectum and excise the lesion. This type of retractor exposes approximately 50% of the circumference of the rectum and can be easily rotated within the rectum. More proximal lesions may require longer retractors such as narrow malleables, Wylie renal vein retractors, or narrow Deavers.

The line of resection is marked with the electrocautery unit, preserving a 1.0-cm margin of normal mucosa around the tumor (Figure 15.4A). Proximal lesions are brought closer to the anus with traction sutures placed in the rectal wall lateral and distal to the tumor. Using electrocautery, a full-thickness incision, which extends into the perirectal fat, is begun at the distal line of resection (Figure 15.4**B** and **C**). As the incision is extended proximally, traction sutures are sequentially placed around the area of excision to maintain control of the rectal wall. In anteriorly located lesions, care must be taken to avoid injury of adjacent structures, such as the vagina, prostate, or urethra. An opening into the peritoneal cavity can be safely closed. The excised specimen should be oriented and pinned out for fixation and then evaluated by formal histologic study. Resection margins should be inked. The rectal wall defect is usually closed in a transverse fashion with a single layer of full-thickness absorbable sutures (Figure 15.4**D**). A proctoscopic examination at the end of the procedure is essential to ascertain that the rectal lumen was not inadvertently closed or narrowed.

(*Editor's note:* The editors use the Parks' retractor for full-thickness transanal excision and find that it provides excellent exposure of the lesion and operative field. The illustrations show the Parks' retractor in place.)

Postoperative pain is usually minimal, requiring only mild analgesics. Clear liquids are started on the same evening after surgery, and the diet is advanced as tolerated. Most patients are discharged within 48 hours of the operation. (*Editor's note:* Our practice has evolved toward earlier discharge following local excision of rectal tumors. Our patients are given a regular diet after surgery and discharged either the same day [with 24 hours of broad-spectrum oral antibiotics] or the following morning. We have had no regrets about this policy of early discharge.) Complications of local excision include urinary retention, hemorrhage, and infection of the perirectal tissue.

Transcoccygeal Excision

Before the abdominoperineal resection became the standard therapy for rectal cancers, Kraske introduced the transsacral posterior proctotomy in 1885.[58] After the introduction of the Miles procedure, the Kraske operation lost popularity but remained in the surgical armamentarium for the local treatment of selected rectal cancers. The transcoccygeal excision is always performed with the patient in the prone jack-knife position. The buttocks are taped apart and the sacrococcygeal and perineal regions are prepared with antiseptic solution. An incision is made adjacent to the distal sacrum and coccyx down to the upper margin of the external anal sphincter. The skin and subcutaneous tissue are incised to expose the coccyx and the anococcygeal ligament. The anococcygeal ligament is opened in the midline, and the coccyx is excised by cutting though the sacrococcygeal joint. Lateral retraction of the levator muscles exposes the mesorectal fat covering the posterior wall of the rectum. Anteriorly located lesions are exposed and excised through a posterior proctotomy. Lesions on the posterior wall of the rectum are localized by simultaneous palpation and digital rectal examination and are excised with a 1.0-cm margin of normal rectum. The excision site and the proctotomy are closed with one layer of full-thickness interrupted absorbable sutures. The integrity of the suture lines is tested by insufflating the rectum with air while the operative field is filled with sterile saline. The levators and the anococcygeal ligaments are then approximated in the midline, and the subcutaneous tissue and the skin are closed with interrupted absorbable sutures. Postoperative care is similar to that of patients undergoing transanal excision. Fecal fistulae develop in 5% to 29% of patients,[52,59,60] but in the absence of tumor recurrence, most of these fistulae heal with temporary fecal diversion.

Transsphincteric Approach

The transsphincteric approach, introduced by Bevan in 1917,[61] was reintroduced and popularized by York Mason in 1970[62] to treat tumors located on the anterior wall of the rectum. The patient is positioned and prepared as described for the transanal and transcoccygeal approaches. A paracoccygeal incision is made from the lower end of the sacrum down to the anal verge. The components of the sphincter complex are sequentially divided, with each being tagged to facilitate tissue re-approximation. The incision in the posterior wall of the rectum is extended cephalad to expose the tumor, and the operative field may be further extended by removal of the coccyx. The tumor is removed by full-thickness excision of the anterior rectal wall including a 1.0-cm margin of normal tissue. The excision site is closed in transverse fashion with interrupted absorbable sutures, and the rectum and the sphincter musculature are carefully re-approximated in a stepwise fashion. Wound abscesses and anal incontinence are common complications of this approach,[63] and therefore it is rarely used today.

Transanal Endoscopic Microsurgery

With TEM, the rectum is approached through a large operating proctoscope that permits the introduction of a stereoscopic telescope and specially designed instruments.[64] Exposure is provided by a constant carbon dioxide insufflation system. The equipment is attached to the operating table, and therefore precise location of the tumor within the circumference of the rectum is extremely important for the positioning of the patient. In theory, tumors located as high as 20 cm from the anal verge can be removed by TEM. In practice, only carcinomas located below the peritoneal reflection are removed with this technique, because of inability to maintain insufflation with the peritoneum open. There is also the theoretical potential for tumor spread into the peritoneal cavity. Furthermore, tumors beyond the reach of the ERUS probe cannot be preoperatively staged and accurately selected for curative local excision.

TEM is technically challenging and requires significant training in the use of the instruments and equipment. Smith et al. recently reported the combined TEM experience of several institutions within the United States.[65] Forty-five of their initial 153 patients were treated for rectal cancer. These authors list a wide variety of technical problems and complications in the entire group, but they reported no operative mortality and a mean hospital stay of 2.2 days. The recurrence rate was 10% for T1 tumors, 40% for T2 tumors, and 66% for T3 tumors. All patients with local recurrence, except two considered unfit for laparotomy, underwent radical resection. (*Editor's note:* Although the TEM data may reflect the learning curve associated with the technique, the results are worse regarding local recurrence than most series using conventional means. I feel that this underlines the idea that this technique has relatively limited applicability and does not need to be available in all centers where rectal cancer is treated.) The applicability of this technique to the local treatment of early rectal cancer has also been demonstrated by Mentges et al. They have recently reported a 4% recurrence rate after 29 months of follow-up in 52 patients with well-differentiated or moderately well-differentiated pT1 tumors excised by TEM.[66] Although the results of TEM in a few centers is promising, the indication for this technique is probably limited to only a few posteriorly located rectal cancers that can be staged by endorectal ultrasound but are not removable by standard transanal approach.

Results

The results of local treatment of rectal cancer are difficult to interpret, because the literature is dominated by retrospective studies of heterogeneous groups of patients who underwent local excision for diverse reasons. Most of the reports include patients unfit for major surgery who underwent local excision with curative intent and patients with metastatic disease requiring local palliation.[10,18,20,67,68] Few reports contain information regarding preoperative staging, and most of them include patients who underwent surgery before the introduction of ERUS. Many of these series also include patients with tumors extending outside the rectal wall and poorly differentiated tumors.[10,18,20,67,69–71] References to lymphatic and vascular invasion are frequently missing. There are also significant variations in the surgical approach. Although most tumors have been excised transanally, others were excised by posterior proctotomy,[67] by transsphincteric approach,[18,20] or endoscopically.[72] Some series include patients with positive or compromised resection margins,[18,69,73] clearly an oncologically unacceptable procedure. The role of rescue surgery after local excision is often not clearly stated, particularly in series with patients who underwent local excision because they were unfit for radical resection. Despite all these limitations, the combined experience of these individual reports has helped to define the role of local excision.

Local recurrence after transanal excision ranges from 0% to 11% for T1 lesions and from 11% to 23% for T2 lesions (Table 15.3). Local recurrence is higher for poorly differentiated tumors and for tumors with compromised resection margins. Salvage radical resection is possible in 25% to 100%

of patients with recurrence after local excision. The cancer-specific survival is related to stage, differentiation, and histologic grade and ranges between 77% and 91%.

Between 1987 and 1996, a total of 180 patients with rectal cancer underwent local treatment at the University of Minnesota.[74] Of those, 85 patients met the criteria for local excision (i.e., moderately and well-differentiated tumors, without vascular invasion, and localized to the rectal wall), and their tumors were excised transanally with curative intent. All the tumors were contained within the muscularis propria (uT1, uT2) and were node negative (uN0) by ERUS. The tumor and a margin of normal tissue were excised full thickness. All tumors were confirmed to be T1 or T2 and had negative margins on pathologic examination. None of the patients received any form of adjuvant therapy. The patients have been followed up for a mean of 52 months under a protocol of proctoscopic examination and ERUS every 4 months for the first 3 years, then every 6 months for an additional 2 years. The overall recurrence rate was 23%. Not surprisingly, it was lower for the T1 (15%) than for the T2 tumors (39%). Most recurrences occurred within 2 years of the operation (average 20 months). The overall and cancer-specific survival rates were 82% and 97% for T1 tumors and 61% and 84% for T2 tumors, at 55 and 48 months, respectively.[74]

Adjuvant chemoradiation therapy, given before or after radical surgery, decreases the incidence of local recurrence and improves the survival rate in patients with rectal cancers having perirectal fat or lymph node invasion.[75,76] Given the significant rate of local failure after local excision of rectal cancers, several authors have tried to extrapolate the beneficial effects of chemoradiation therapy to patients with rectal cancer treated by local excision. In the last decade several institutions have reported their experience with the treatment of early rectal cancer by local excision and adjuvant chemoradiation therapy.[19,59,77–87] As with the reports of patients treated by local excision alone, most of these series are also retrospective and heterogeneous regarding the selection of patients, tumor stage and histology, type of treatment, adjuvant therapy, and length of follow-up. Recurrence rates vary from 0% to 24%, and the overall survival rates vary between 77% and 100%. The two series that have followed their patients prospectively[59,81] also have problems with

patient selection and uniformity of treatment. Bleday et al.[59] report an 8% local recurrence rate and 4% tumor-specific mortality rate with a mean follow-up of 40 months. All tumors that eventually recurred infiltrated the perirectal fat, had lymphatic invasion, or were incompletely resected. These authors had no recurrences among the 21 T2 patients treated by local excision with adjuvant chemoradiation therapy. However, among this subgroup of patients, the percentages of poorly differentiated tumors and tumors with lymphatic invasion or with positive resection margins are not stated.

The difficulty in interpreting the data on the effect of adjuvant therapy in locally excised rectal cancers is complicated by the lack of uniformity in the indications, dosage, and sequence of both the chemotherapy and radiation therapy. For example, in the series by Bleday et al.,[59] T2 patients received postoperative chemoradiation, whereas in the series by Otta et al.,[81] patients with T2 rectal cancers received postoperative radiotherapy alone; chemoradiation was used on T3 lesions and in T2 tumors with vascular invasion. The total dose of radiation even in the same series has varied from 4500 cGy to 7380 cGy.[78] These reports individually suggest a beneficial effect of chemoradiation therapy on local control of locally excised T2 rectal cancers, but they do not allow the establishment of definitive indications for the use of adjuvant chemoradiation therapy in the different subsets of locally excised rectal cancer (Table 15.4).

A prospective multi-institutional trial to evaluate the efficacy of local excision and postoperative chemoradiation was initiated by the Cancer and Leukemia B study group in 1989. The enrolled patients had mobile uT1-uT2 N0 M0 cancers, less than 4 cm in diameter, involving less than 40% of the circumference of the rectum, and located within 10 cm of the anal verge. The trial closed in 1995 having accrued 180 patients. Of the 164 patients who underwent full-thickness local excision, 48 were ineligible because of involved margins, size greater than 4 cm, or stage higher than T2 or lower than T1. Sixty T1 patients were treated solely with local excision, and 52 T2 patients were treated by full-thickness local excision followed by chemoradiation therapy. After 24 months of follow-up, 4 patients had died of their malignant disease. Two additional patients who developed isolated local recurrence and underwent rescue radical surgery were alive at the time of the

TABLE 15.4. Results from selected series of patients with rectal cancer treated by local excision alone with curative intent.

Author	No. patients	Margins	Stage	Local recurrence (%)	Salvage surgery[a] (%)	Cancer-specific survival (%)	Follow-up (months)
Morson[69]	91	Negative	T1, T2	3	66	100	
Hager[72]	36	Negative	T1	8	NS	90	33
	18	Negative	T2	17	NS	78	40
Heimann[67]	14	Negative	T1, T2	21	100	93	48
Obrand[73]	19	Negative	T1, T2 (one T3)	26	60	82	58
Garcia-Aguilar[74]	57	Negative	T1	15	70	97	48
	28	Negative	T2	39	87	84	55

[a]Percentage of patients with local recurrence undergoing radical operation.

NS, not specified.

study report, bringing the local recurrence rate up to 5.3%. Although the follow-up is still short, the preliminary results of this study are better than average, particularly considering that patients with unfavorable histology were not excluded.[88]

Two institutions have reported their experience with the use of preoperative radiation therapy followed by local excision, with or without brachytherapy of the tumor bed, for early rectal cancers.[89–91] Their incidence of local failure was comparable to series of local excision alone or local excision followed by radiation therapy. However, this technique overtreats many patients with early cancers, and it destroys histologic information that may have therapeutic and prognostic significance.

Follow-Up

Early diagnosis of local recurrence is important, since radical surgery may effectively control such recurrences. Therefore, every patient undergoing curative local excision for rectal cancer should be closely monitored postoperatively for local recurrence. We perform digital rectal, proctoscopic, and endorectal ultrasonographic examinations as a baseline, then every 4 months for 3 years and every 6 months for 2 additional years. Any area suspicious for recurrence should have a biopsy performed.

Indications for Local Excision With Curative Intent

The review of the surgical literature and our own experience indicate that only patients with well-differentiated or moderately well-differentiated tumors limited to the submucosa (uT1, uN0) and without distant metastasis are candidates for curative local excision (Figure 15.5). If the formal histologic examination after local excision reveals a more advanced tumor (i.e., T2, T3, or N1, an undifferentiated tumor, a mucinous component, or vascular or lymphatic invasion), a radical resection should be performed. If the margins after local excision are not clear of cancer, either re-excision or more aggressive treatment by radical resection should be undertaken.

Tumors infiltrating the muscularis propria (T2) should not be treated by local excision alone (Figure 15.5). The results of several retrospective studies, and the preliminary reports of a prospective randomized trial, suggest that T2 rectal cancers can be effectively treated with local excision followed by chemoradiation therapy (Table 15.5). The question of whether this form of therapy will provide equivalent local tumor control and long-term survival compared with radical surgery still needs to be answered in a prospective randomized trial.

Nonexcisional Techniques

Endocavitary Radiation

Endocavitary contact radiation therapy as the sole form of treatment in early rectal cancer was introduced by Papillon in France over 30 years ago and has been popularized in the United States by Sischy et al.[92,93] This technique is suitable only for the same small superficial cancers that are candidates for local excision and therefore requires careful patient selection. The advantages of endocavitary

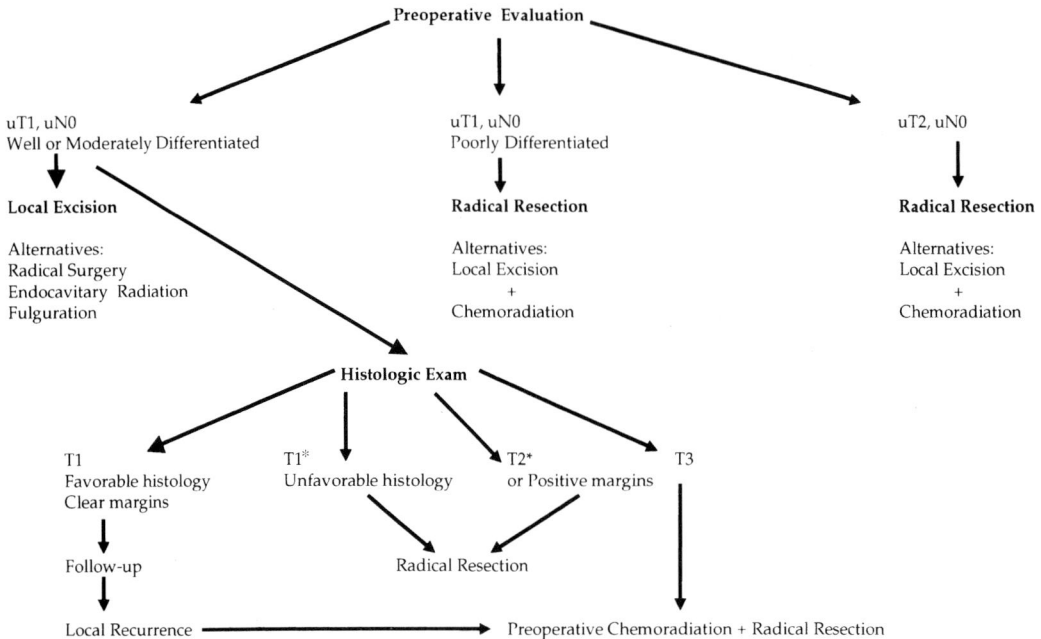

FIGURE 15.5. Algorithm for local treatment of rectal cancer.

TABLE 15.5. Results of selected series of patients with rectal cancer undergoing local excision and postoperative radiation.

Author	No. patients	Negative margins (%)	Stage	Radiation (cGy)	Chemo-therapy	Local recurrence (%)	Salvage surgery[a] (%)	Survival (%)	Follow-up (months)
Rosenthal[79]	16	100	2 T1 9 T2 5 T3	2700–5700	No	12.50	100	94 (3 years)	33
Bailey[80]	53	100	35 T1 18 T2	4500–5000[b]	No	8	50	90	44
Minsky[78]	22	95	4 T1 12 T2 6 T3	4500–7380	Variable	18	75	79 (4 years)	37
Fortunato[87]	21	66	2 T1 15 T2 4 T3	2700–6300	10%	19	75	58	56
Ota[81]	46	100	16 T1 15 T2 15 T3	5300	Variable	8	NS	NS	35
Bleday[59]	21	100	21 T2	5400	Yes	0	—	100	43

[a]Percentage of patients with isolated local recurrence undergoing radical operation.

[b]Only 54% of the patients received radiotherapy.

NS, not specified.

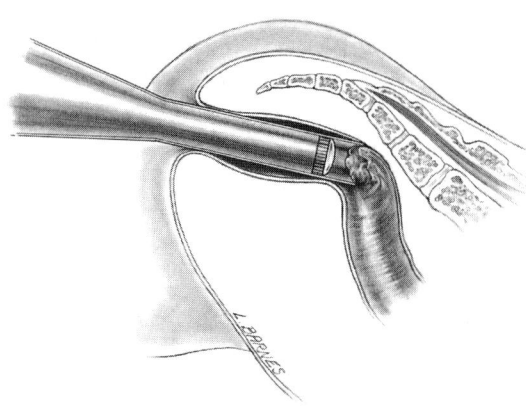

FIGURE 15.6. Endocavitary radiation: Technique of application via special proctoscope. Reprinted with permission from Corman ML (ed). Colon & Rectal Surgery, 4th edition. Philadelphia: Lippincott-Raven, 1998, p 843.

radiation include minimal enema preparation of the rectum, ability to perform the procedure using conscious sedation on an outpatient basis, essentially no recovery period, and suitability for almost all patients.

The radiation is delivered directly to the tumor with a hand-held 50-kv x-ray source that has an aperture 3.0 cm in diameter and is inserted through a special proctoscope (Figure 15.6). With an intrarectal focal distance of 4.0 cm, the output is approximately 20 Gy per minute. These 50-kv x-rays have low penetration: the percentage depth dose is 100% at surface, 44% at 5 mm, 23% at 10 mm, and 9% at 20 mm. They are therefore ineffective for the treatment of bulky or deep tumors. The low penetrance and negligible scatter maximize tumor exposure and minimize irradiation of the surrounding normal tissues.

Patients are treated as outpatients under conscious sedation in the knee-chest position. Typically, the treatment is given in three or four fractions of 30 Gy, spaced 2 to 4 weeks apart. Each application lasts no more than 2 minutes and produces rapid shrinkage of the tumor. The operator can adjust the dose and the focus at every session. A boost dose of 20 to 30 Gy to the tumor bed using iridium-192 wire implants is frequently used in France. Treatment is usually well tolerated, with rare symptoms related to radiation therapy in a few patients. Radiation ulcers spontaneously heal in

most patients, and there is no risk of hemorrhage, sexual or bladder dysfunction, and anal incontinence.

Local control with endocavitary radiation, supplemented with iridium-192 boost in selected patients, ranges from 76% to 95% for T1 and T2 rectal cancers. These results improve to 82% to 99% after surgical salvage of local recurrences. Five-year overall survival rates ranging from 60% to 90% and 5-year tumor-specific survival rates between 74% and 94% have been reported.[94] Most of these patients maintain a functionally competent rectum.

The University of Minnesota experience with endocavitary radiation includes 64 patients treated with curative intent. The overall recurrence rate was 23% and was higher for uT2 tumors (37%) than for uT1 tumors (4%). With two exceptions, all recurrences have manifested within 14 months of the initial diagnosis. Half of the patients who developed a recurrence were successfully salvaged by radical surgery. The overall disease-free survival rate was 84% at 3.4 years after the initial diagnosis. Recurrence rates were higher for lesions larger than 3.0 cm in diameter and for distal lesions extending within 3.0 cm of the anal verge.

Our current policy is to offer endocavitary radiation as an alternative to patients who are candidates for transanal local excision. This technique is useful for patients medically unfit for anesthesia, for those who refuse an operation, and for patients with a lesion located such that local excision is technically impossible. Because of the limited field of radiation, endocavitary radiation should not be used to treat tumors greater than 3.0 cm in diameter. The main disadvantage of endocavitary radiation therapy is that it does not provide a specimen to confirm the level of invasion.

Electrocoagulation

Byrne introduced the use of electrocoagulation to treat rectal cancer more than a century ago. Although this technique has never gained widespread acceptance, it has been used with good results at some institutions.[95] Advocates claim that electrocoagulation is less likely to seed viable tumor cells than is local excision. The disadvantages of electrocoagulation include the lack of pathology specimen for staging, the reliance on visual and tactile information to confirm tumor eradication, the morbidity of postoperative fever and hemorrhage, and the frequent need for additional operations.

Electrocoagulation can be used for cure or palliation. When intended for cure, patient selection is critical. The preoperative workup, the indications for the procedure, and the selection criteria are very similar to those described for local excision. Only tumors localized to the bowel wall should be treated by electrocoagulation for cure. Tumors should be mobile, exophytic, less than 4.0 cm in diameter, and located below the peritoneal reflection. Tumors located anteriorly are less suited for electrocoagulation because of the proximity to the peritoneal reflection and the potential for damage to the prostatic capsule or rectovaginal septum.

Patients receive a phosphate enema the morning of surgery. Prophylactic antibiotics are not routinely used. The operation is performed under general or regional anesthesia, often aided by a perianal block. The patient is positioned in the lithotomy or prone position, depending on the location of the tumor. A large operating proctoscope with a built-in suction channel to eliminate the smoke is commonly used. Coagulation can be applied in a variety of ways. Salvati and associates use bipolar electrocautery with a large ball tip to coagulate the tumor surface.[96] Madden combs away the tumor with a wire loop connected to a low-intensity cutting current.[97] Crile and Turnbull claim to achieve greater heat penetration and better tactile discrimination with a needlepoint electrode connected to an electrocautery unit having a spark-gap generator.[98] The coagulated tissue is removed with uterine curettes and tissue forceps until normal tissue is exposed. Postoperative fever is common. Patients can usually be discharged within 48 hours of the operation, tolerating regular diet and with minimal discomfort. Complications include bleeding, stricture, urinary retention, electrical burns, perianal abscess, and perforation.

Close follow-up with monthly proctoscopic examination is recommended during the first year. Any indurated area should be biopsied. Repeated electrocoagulation is indicated for recurrences localized to the bowel wall. Recurrences that involve the perirectal fat or perirectal lymph nodes should be treated by radical excision.

The 5-year survival rate after electrocoagulation for rectal cancer varies between 47% and 67%, but comparisons between these series and other forms of local therapy are limited by differences in selection criteria.[95]

Conclusion

The aim of local treatment of rectal cancer is to decrease the morbidity and the functional sequelae associated with radical surgery without compromising local tumor control and long-term survival. Selecting the optimal therapy for an individual patient with rectal cancer requires consideration of both the tumor and patient characteristics. Endorectal ultrasonography is essential for the accurate assessment of rectal wall invasion and nodal metastasis. The tumor should be removed by full-thickness local excision with an adequate normal margin for pathologic evaluation. Only patients with well-differentiated or moderately well-differentiated T1 tumors without blood vessel or lymphatic vessel invasion, and without production of mucin, are candidates for curative local excision as the only form of treatment. Tumors penetrating the muscularis propria should not be treated by local excision alone. The addition of postoperative chemoradiation therapy may improve the results of local excision in T2 tumors. Endocavitary radiation therapy and electrocoagulation result in similar tumor control as that observed after local excision. However, these ablative techniques do not provide a surgical specimen to confirm stage and tumor histology. Close follow-up is critical for early diagnosis of local recurrences, as many of them may be surgically salvaged by radical resection. Local treatment can also be used for palliation of patients with histologically unfavorable or advanced tumors and patients medically unfit for radical surgery.

References

1. Miles WE. A method of performing abdominoperineal excision for carcinoma of the rectum and of the terminal portion of the pelvic colon. Lancet 1908;2: 1812–1813.
2. Lavery IC, Lopez-Kostner F, Fazio VW, et al. Chances of cure are not compromised with sphincter-saving procedures for cancer of the lower third of the rectum. Surgery 1997;122:779–785.

3. Rothenberger DA, Wong WD. Abdominoperineal resection for adenocarcinoma of the low rectum. World J Surg 1992;16:478–485.

4. Williams JT, Slack WW. A prospective study of sexual function after major colorectal surgery. Br J Surg 1980;67:772–774.

5. Neal DE, Williams NS, Johnston D. A prospective study of bladder function before and after sphincter-saving resections for low carcinoma of the rectum. Br J Urol 1981;53:558–564.

6. Havenga K, Enker WE, McDermott K, et al. Male and female sexual and urinary function after total mesorectal excision with autonomic nerve preservation for carcinoma of the rectum. J Am Coll Surg 1996;182:495–502.

7. Balslev I, Harling H. Sexual dysfunction following operation for carcinoma of the rectum. Dis Colon Rectum 1983;26:785–788.

8. Karnajia ND, Schache DJ, Heald RJ. Function of the distal rectum after low anterior resection for carcinoma. Br J Surg 1992;79:114–116.

9. Lewis WG, Holdsworth PJ, Stephenson BM, Finan PJ, Johnston D. Role of the rectum on the physiological and clinical results of coloanal and colorectal anastomosis after anterior resection for rectal carcinoma. Br J Surg 1992;79:1082–1086.

10. Biggers OR, Beart RW, Ilstrup DW. Local excision of rectal cancer. Dis Colon Rectum 1986;29:374–377.

11. Morson BC. Factors influencing the prognosis of early cancer of the rectum. Proc R Soc Med 1966;59:607–608.

12. Fisher B, Anderson S, Redmond CK, et al. Reanalysis and results after 12 years of follow-up in a randomized clinical trial comparing total mastectomy with lumpectomy with or without irradiation in the treatment of breast cancer. N Engl J Med 1995;333:1456–1461.

13. Zenni GC, Abraham K, Harford FJ, et al. Characteristics of rectal carcinomas that predict the presence of lymph node metastases: implications for patient selection for local therapy. J Surg Oncol 1998;67:99–103.

14. Brodsky JT, Richard GK, Cohen AM, Minsky BD. Variables correlated with the risk of lymph node metastasis in early rectal cancer. Cancer 1992;69:322–326.

15. Sitzler PJ, Seow-Choen F, Ho YH, Leong APK. Lymph node involvement and tumor depth in rectal cancers: an analysis of 805 patients. Dis Colon Rectum 1997;40:1472–1476.

16. York Mason A. Rectal cancer: the spectrum of selective surgery. Proc R Soc Med 1976;69:237–244.

17. Nicholls RJ, York Mason A, Morson BC, Dixon AK, Fry IK. The clinical staging of rectal cancer. Br J Surg 1982;69:404–409.

18. Whiteway J, Nicholls RJ, Morson BC. The role of surgical local excision in the treatment of rectal cancer. Br J Surg 1985;72:694–697.

19. Willet CG, Compton CC, Shellito PC, Efrid JT. Selection factors for local excision or abdominoperineal resection of early stage rectal cancer. Cancer 1994;73:2716–2720.

20. Killingback M. Local excision of carcinoma of the rectum: indications. World J Surg 1992;16:437–446.

21. Sasaki O, Atkin WS, Jass JR. Mucinous carcinoma of the rectum. Histopathology 1987;11–259–272.

22. Minsky BD, Rich T, Recht A, et al. Selection criteria for local excision with or without adjuvant therapy for rectal cancer. Cancer 1989;63:1421–1429.

23. Cohen AM, Wood WC, Gunderson LL, Shinnar M. Pathological studies in rectal cancer. Cancer 1980;45:2965–2968.

24. Madsen PM, Braendstrup O. The predictive value of diagnostic biopsies in histologic grading. Dis Colon Rectum 1985;28:676–677.

25. Phang PT, Wong WD. The use of endoluminal ultrasound for malignant and benign anorectal diseases. Current Opinion in Gastroenterology 1997;13:47–53.

26. Beynon J, Foy DMA, Roe AM, Temple LN, Mortensen NJ. Endoluminal ultrasound in the assessment of local invasion in rectal cancer. Br J Surg 1986;73:474–477.

27. Beynon J, Mortensen NJ, Foy DMA, et al. Preoperative assessment of local invasion in rectal cancer: digital examination, endoluminal sonography, or computed tomography? Br J Surg 1986;73:1015–1017.

28. Beynon J, Mortensen NJ, Foy DMA, et al. Preoperative assessment of mesorectal lymph node involvement in rectal cancer. Br J Surg 1989;76:276–279.

29. Holdsworth PJ, Johnston D, Chalmers AG, et al. Endoluminal ultrasound and computed tomography in the staging of rectal cancer. Br J Surg 1988;75:1019–1022.

30. Milsom JW, Graffner H. Intrarectal ultrasonography in rectal cancer staging and in the evaluation of pelvic disease. Ann Surg 1990;212:602–606.

31. Hinder JM, Chu J, Bokey EL, Chapuis PH, Newland RC. Use of transrectal ultrasound to evaluate direct tumour spread and lymph node status in patients with rectal cancer. Aust N Z J Surg 1990;60:19–23.

32. Lok Tio T, Coene PPLO, van Delden OM, Tytgat GNJ. Colorectal carcinoma: preoperative TNM classification with endosonography. Radiology 1991;179:165–170.

33. Herzog U, von Flue M, Tondelli P, et al. How accurate is endorectal ultrasound in the preoperative

staging of rectal cancer? Dis Colon Rectum 1993;36: 127–134.

34. Nogueras JJ. Endorectal ultrasonography: technique, image interpretation, and expanding indications in 1995. Seminars in Colon and Rectal Surgery 1995;6:70–77.

35. Kruskal JB, Kane RA, Sentovich SM, Longmaid HE. Pitfalls and sources of error in staging rectal cancer with endorectal ultrasound. RadioGraphics 1997;17:609–626.

36. Hunerbein M, Schlag PM. Three-dimensional endosonography for staging of rectal cancer. Ann Surg 1997;225:432–438.

37. Ivanov KD, Diacov CD. Three-dimensional endoluminal ultrasound. Dis Colon Rectum 1997;40:47–50.

38. Heneghan JP, Salem RR, Lange RC, Taylor KJW, Hammers LW. Transrectal sonography in staging rectal carcinoma: the role of gray-scale, color-flow, and Doppler imaging analysis. AJR Am J Roentgenol 1997;169:1247–1252.

39. Thoeni RF, Moss AA, Schnyder P, Margulis AR. Staging of primary rectal and rectosigmoid tumors by computed tomography. Radiology 1981;141:135–138.

40. Dixon AK, Fry IK, Morson BC, et al. Preoperative computed tomography of carcinoma of the rectum. Br J Radiol 1981;54:655–659.

41. Grabbe E, Lierse W, Winkler R. The perirectal fascia: morphology and use in staging of rectal carcinoma. Radiology 1983;149:241–246.

42. Adalsteinsson B, Glimelius B, Graffman S, et al. Computed tomography in staging of rectal carcinoma. Acta Radiol Diagn (Stockh) 1985;26:25–55.

43. Freeny PC, Parks WM, Ryan JA, et al. Colorectal carcinoma evaluation with CT: preoperative staging and detection of postoperative recurrence. Radiology 1986;158:347–353.

44. Thompson WM, Halvorsen RA, Foster WL Jr., et al. Preoperative and postoperative CT staging of rectosigmoid carcinoma. AJR Am J Roentgenol 1986; 146:703–710.

45. Kramann B, Hildebrandt U. Computed tomography versus endosonography in the staging of rectal carcinoma: a comparative study. Int J Colorectal Dis 1986;1:216–218.

46. Rifkin MD, Wechsler RJ. A comparison of computed tomography and endorectal ultrasound in staging rectal cancer. Int J Colorectal Dis 1986;1:219–223.

47. Waizer A, Powsner E, Russo I, et al. Prospective comparative study of magnetic resonance imaging versus transrectal ultrasound for preoperative staging and follow-up of rectal cancer. Dis Colon Rectum 1991;34:1068–1072.

48. Thaler W, Watzka S, Martin F, et al. Preoperative staging of rectal cancer by endoluminal ultrasound vs. magnetic resonance imaging. Dis Colon Rectum 1994;37:1189–1193.

49. Starck M, Bohe M, Fork F-T, et al. Endoluminal ultrasound and low-field magnetic resonance imaging are superior to clinical examination in the preoperative staging of rectal cancer. Eur J Surg 1995;161:841–845.

50. Wallengren NO, Holtas S, Andren-Sandberg A. Preoperative staging of rectal carcinoma using double-contrast MR imaging. Acta Radiol 1996;37:791–798.

51. Vogl TJ, Pegios W, Mack MG, et al. Accuracy of staging rectal tumors with contrast-enhanced transrectal MR imaging. AJR Am J Roentgenol 1997; 168:1427;1434.

52. Hadfield MB, Nicholson AA, MacDonald AW, et al. Preoperative staging of rectal carcinoma by magnetic resonance imaging with a pelvic phased-array coil. Br J Surg 1997;84:529–531.

53. Blomqvist L, Holm T, Rubio C, Hindmarsh T. Rectal tumours—MR imaging with endorectal and/or phased-array coils, and histopathological staging on giant sections. Acta Radiol 1997;38:437–444.

54. Joosten FBM, Gansen J, Joosten HJM, Rosenbusch G. Staging of rectal carcinoma using MR double surface coil, MR endorectal coil, and intrarectal ultrasound: correlation with histopathologic findings. J Comput Assist Tomogr 1995;19:752–758.

55. Meyenberger C, Huch Boni RA, Bertschinger P, et al. Endoscopic ultrasound and endorectal magnetic resonance imaging: a prospective, comparative study for preoperative staging and follow-up of rectal cancer. Endoscopy 1995;27:469–479.

56. Zagoria RJ, Schlarb CA, Ott DJ, et al. Assessment of rectal tumor infiltration utilizing endorectal MR imaging and comparison with endoscopic rectal sonography. J Surg Oncol 1997;64:312–317.

57. Kulling D, Feldman DR, Kay CL, et al. Local staging of anal and distal colorectal tumors with the magnetic resonance endoscope. Gastrointest Endosc 1998;47:172–177.

58. Kraske P. Zur extirpation hochsitzender mastdarmkrebse. Verh Dtsch Ges Chir 1885;14:464–474.

59. Bleday R, Breen E, Jessup JM, et al. Prospective evaluation of local excision for small rectal cancers. Dis Colon Rectum 1997;40:388–392.

60. Christensen J. Excision of mid-rectal by the Kraske sacral approach. Br J Surg 1980;67:651–653.

61. Bevan AD. Carcinoma of the rectum: treatment by local excision. Dis Colon Rectum 1986;29:906–910.

62. York Mason A. The place of local resection in the treatment of rectal carcinoma. Proc R Soc Med 1970;63:1259–1262.

63. Allgower M, Durig M, Hochstetter AV, Huber A. The presacral sphincter-splitting approach to the rectum. World J Surg 1982;6:539–548.

64. Buess G, Mentges B, Manncke K, et al. Technique and results of transanal endoscopic microsurgery in early rectal cancer. Am J Surg 1992;163:63–69.

65. Smith LE, Ko ST, Saclarides T, et al. Transanal endoscopic microsurgery: initial registry results. Dis Colon Rectum 1996;39:579–584.

66. Mentges B, Buess G, Effinger K, et al. Indications and results of local treatment of rectal cancer. Br J Surg 1997;84:348–351.

67. Heimann TS, Oh C, Steinhagen RM, et al. Surgical treatment of tumors of the distal rectum with sphincter preservation. Ann Surg 1992;216:432–437.

68. De Cosse JJ, Wond RJ, Quan SHQ, et al. Conservative treatment of distal rectal cancer by local excision. Cancer 1989;63:219.

69. Morson BC, Bussey HJR, Samoorian S. Policy of local excision for early rectal cancer of the colorectum. Gut 1977;18:1045–1050.

70. Lock MR, Ritchie JK, Hawley PR. Reappraisal of radical local excision for carcinoma of the rectum. Br J Surg 1993;80:928–929.

71. Read DR, Sokil S, Ruiz-Salas G. Transanal local excision of rectal cancer. Int J Colorectal Dis 1995; 10:73–76.

72. Hager TH, Gall FP, Hermanek P. Local excision of cancer of the rectum. Dis Colon Rectum 1983; 26:149–151.

73. Obrand DI, Gordon PH. Results of local excision for rectal carcinoma. Can J Surg 1996;39:463–468.

74. Garcia-Aguilar J, Mellgren A, Sivatvongs P, et al. Local excision of early rectal cancer: the Minnesota experience. Unpublished data.

75. Gastrointestinal Tumor Study Group. Prolongation of the disease-free interval in surgically treated rectal carcinoma. N Engl J Med 1985;312:1465–1472.

76. Swedish Rectal Cancer Trial. Improved survival with preoperative radiotherapy in resectable rectal cancer. N Engl J Med 1997;336:980–987.

77. Mendenhall WM, Rout WR, Vauthey JN, et al. Conservative treatment of rectal adenocarcinomas with endocavitary irradiation or wide local excision and postoperative irradiation. J Clin Oncol 1997;15:3241–3248.

78. Minsky BD, Cohen AM, Enker WE, Mies C. Sphincter preservation in rectal cancer by local excision and postoperative radiation therapy. Cancer 1991;67:908–914.

79. Rosenthal SA, Yeung RS, Weese JL, et al. Conservative management of extensive low-lying rectal carcinomas with transanal local excision and combined preoperative and postoperative radiation therapy. Cancer 1992;69:335–341.

80. Bailey HR, Huval WV, Max E, et al. Local excision of carcinoma of the rectum for cure. Surgery 1992;111:555.

81. Ota DM, Skibber J, Rich TA. MD Anderson Cancer Center experience with local excision and multimodality therapy for rectal cancer. Surg Clin North Am 1992;1:147–152.

82. Coco C, Magistrelli P, Granone P, et al. Conservative surgery for early cancer of the distal rectum. Dis Colon Rectum 1992;35:131–136.

83. Rouanet P, Saint Aubert B, Fabre JM, et al. Conservative treatment for low rectal carcinoma by local excision with or without radiotherapy. Br J Surg 1993;80:1452–1456.

84. Wong CS, Stern H, Cummings BJ. Local excision and post-operative radiation therapy for rectal carcinoma. Int J Radat Oncol 1993;25:669–675.

85. Graham RA, Atkins MB, Karp DD, et al. Local excision of rectal carcinoma: early results with combined chemoradiation therapy using 5-fluorouracil and leucovorin. Dis Colon Rectum 1994;37:308–312.

86. Minsky BD, Enker WE, Cohen AM, Lauwers G. Local excision and postoperative radiation therapy for rectal cancer. Am J Clin Oncol 1994;17:411–416.

87. Fortunato L, Ahmad NR, Yeung RS, et al. Long-term follow-up of local excision and radiation therapy for invasive rectal cancer. Dis Colon Rectum 1995;38: 1193–1199.

88. Weber TK, Petrelli NJ. Local excision for rectal cancer: an uncertain future. Oncology 1998;12:933–947.

89. Despretz J, Otmezguine Y, Grimard L, Calitchi E, Julien M. Conservative management of tumors of the rectum by radiotherapy and local excision. Dis Colon Rectum 1990;33:113–116.

90. Mohiuddin M, Marks G, Bannon J. High-dose preoperative radiation and full thickness local excision: a new option for selected T3 distal rectal cancers. Int J Radiat Oncol 1994;30:845–849.

91. Ahmad NR, Nagle DA. Preoperative radiation therapy followed by local excision. Sem Rad Oncol 1998;8:36–38.

92. Papillon J, Berard P. Endocavitary irradiation in the conservative treatment of adenocarcinoma of the low rectum. World J Surg 1992;16:451–457.

93. Sischy B. The role of endocavitary irradiation for limited lesions of the rectum. Int J Colorectal Dis 1991;6:91–94.

94. Gerard JP, Romestaing P, Ardiet JM, Mornex F. Endocavitary radiation therapy. Semin Radiat Oncol 1998;8:13–23.

95. Chinn BT, Eisenstat TE. Electrocoagulation of selected adenocarcinoma of the distal rectum. Seminars in Colon and Rectal Surgery 1996;7:233–237.

96. Salvati EP, Rubin RJ, Eisenstat TE, et al. Electrocoagulation of selected carcinoma of the rectum. Surg Gynecol Obstet 1988;166:393–396.

97. Madden JL, Kandalaft S. Clinical evaluation of electrocoagulation in the treatment of cancer of the rectum. Am J Surg 1971;122:347–352.

98. Crile G, Turnbull RB Jr. The role of electrocoagulation in the treatment of carcinoma of the rectum. Surg Gynecol Obstet 1972;135:391–396.

16

Coding and Billing for Colon and Rectal Surgery

Frank G. Opelka, M.D., F.A.C.S.

Physicians nationwide are experiencing increasing difficulty resolving medical claims. Many physician offices still process medical claims manually through the mail. This delays reimbursement for up to 4 months. The claim process is expedited by using electronic submission. Today, claims require more detailed patient information and precise data entry unique to each insurance carrier. Misinformation delays reimbursements, and insuring agents deny or delay payment of claims for increasingly petty reasons. They commonly assert that procedures were "not precertified," are "not medically necessary," or constitute "experimental treatment" or that the charges "extend beyond the reasonable and customary norms." Even more frustrating, the cost of reprocessing a denied claim is five to ten times greater than that of the original claim.

Why has the claims process become so difficult? Rising health care costs and attempts at cost reduction by insurance carriers are central to this question. National health care expenditures broke the $1.0 trillion mark in 1996, representing 13.6% of the gross domestic product.[1] Although the rate of health care growth has stabilized, the immediate future portends further increases with the aging of the "baby boomers." As this population becomes eligible for Medicare, the number of patients needing routine and emergent health care services will grow sharply. The rising costs of health care have received attention from major industries and the federal government. In an effort to stem cost increases and promote efficiencies, each has tried to impose numerous controls on health care expenditures. These controls take many forms, from fee-for-service care to fully capitated care. An effective

and early measure in cutting costs involves controlling the coding and billing systems. Despite the changing nature of the system, this chapter outlines aspects of proper coding and billing that facilitate appropriate reimbursement for health care services. Because of the large number of insurance companies and the inconsistency among policies, it is impossible to provide detailed guidance for each carrier. Therefore, the primary discussion concentrates on Medicare and Health Care Finance Administration policies, which influence over 45% of the health care dollars and serve as the template for most other insurance carriers.

Medical Economics

Medical economics has matured during the past 10 years. This has created integrated systems for various aspects of capitated health care. Evidence-based medicine (disease management) uses treatment plans as a reproducible management instrument and, ideally, promotes innovation to improve care with maximal quality and minimal cost. The three major components competing for health care revenues today are the insuring agents, the providers, and the health care facilities. The insuring agents continue to develop new strategies for patients that begin with indemnity plans and extend through complex levels of capitation to a fully capitated system.

The provider format has changed from the previously ubiquitous individual physician practices to groups of physicians concentrating in either specialty or multispecialty groups. Each physician group works to capture more market share. The word *provider* now encompasses physician assistants, nurse practitioners, nurses, pharmacists, dietitians, physical therapists, and social workers.

Hospitals continue to shift from predominantly inpatient facilities to providing more outpatient services. In order to compete, hospitals are compelled to seek contractual or physical integration with insurers and providers within their market. New concepts of profit and risk sharing permeate the markets.

All these economic pressures are bringing changes to the entire health care system. Patients seek care in an educated and efficient fashion, and market-driven health care is gaining importance. As a result, outpatient surgery has quickly become a significant opportunity for improved and efficient care. Within these fiscal challenges, providers are forced to accurately document, code, and bill for the services rendered. In addition, appropriate coding and billing are critical legal documents that protect physicians in fraud and abuse investigations from auditors working for the Health Care Financing Administration (HCFA), the Office of the Inspector General of Health and Human Services, or the U.S. Justice Department.

The Proper Code

Most insurance carriers use the American Medical Association's coding nomenclature called the Physician's Current Procedural Terminology (CPT),[2] making it the industry standard. CPT codes are developed through a process that has extensive physician input and control. Codes exist to describe virtually every accepted medical and surgical procedure. New codes and revised codes are added annually in an attempt to stay abreast of medical advances and changing technology. Each section of the CPT manual contains generic codes to cover procedures that the CPT manual does not fully describe. Finally, the CPT coding system is set up so that *any* provider can use *any* code to describe the service delivered. For example, either gynecologists or other providers may use gynecological procedure codes.

Once the CPT code is chosen, physician services are coded in combination with the appropriate diagnosis code using the *International Classification of Diseases, 9th Revision* (ICD-9).[3] Together, these codes define the actual treatment delivered and whether or not it is a covered service. Hospital services are billed separately from physician services and rely on diagnosis-related groups (DRGs). When used in concert, these three elements describe the physician service (CPT) provided within a group of coded diagnoses (DRG) for a specific diagnosis (ICD-9).

Choosing the proper codes refers to finding a CPT code that best describes the procedure or service the patient receives in concert with the appropriate ICD-9 code. Despite the existence of over 9000 CPT codes, not all procedures are accurately described in the CPT manual. The CPT text is divided into several sections. Anesthesia has a set of codes, the evaluation and management services have a section, and surgery has the single largest section. Within each section is the primary code descriptor. For example, 44140 is a code with the descriptor "Colectomy, partial; with anastomosis." The primary descriptor is the language to the left of the semicolon. The comments to the right of the semicolon describe additional elements of the primary descriptor. The subsequent codes in CPT (ranging from 44141 to 44147) are formatted with an indentation. This indicates that these codes use the same primary descriptor as 44140, "Colectomy, partial." These subsequent codes substitute their descriptors to the right of the semicolon. For example, the descriptor for code 44141 is "with skin level cecostomy or colostomy." It is understood from CPT nomenclature that, using the first portion of Code 44140, this translates to "Colectomy partial; with skin level cecostomy or colostomy" (Table 16.1). In addition to the primary code descriptors, each section has a group of "modifiers." The modifiers clarify the codes used and enhance reimbursement.

TABLE 16.1. Current Procedural Terminology (CPT) codes for colorectal surgery.

44140	Colectomy, partial; with anastomosis
44141	with skin level cecostomy or colostomy
44143	with end colostomy and closure of distal segment (Hartmann type procedure)
44144	with resection, with colostomy or ileostomy and creation of mucofistula
44145	with coloproctostomy (low pelvic anastomosis)
44146	with coloproctostomy (low pelvic anastomosis), with colostomy
44147	abdominal and transanal approach

Use of Modifiers

The modifiers are the most commonly underused aspects of coding. The purpose of modifiers is to precisely define the specifics of each code and the treatment rendered. The reason modifiers are so underemployed is multifactorial. Providers and practice managers often will fail to use modifiers because of the possibility of triggering manual review and audit by the insurance carrier. Carriers do not readily recognize modifiers and thus tend to deny the claim. If used properly, and recognized appropriately by the carrier, modifiers enhance the entire patient care database and appropriately increase provider reimbursement.

Modifiers and associated nomenclature emanate from two different sources:

- *Physician's Current Procedural Terminology (CPT)* is used for the definition of CPT-4 numeric modifiers.
- The Health Care Financing Administration's Common Procedure Coding System (HCFA-PCS) alpha modifiers were developed by the HCFA for the Medicare program.

For the purposes of this text on ambulatory anorectal surgery, the primary modifiers of concern are the numeric modifiers related to surgical procedures. These modifiers define the procedure more clearly and also describe the subsequent care that occurs within the global surgical period. Surgical procedures have a defined global period that varies with each procedure. The global period generally corresponds to the surgical procedure and the attendant postoperative care required until complete recovery. Three global periods are recognized by the HCFA and are generally accepted by other insurers. They are 0 days, 10 days, and 90 days. All related services delivered during the global period are covered in the corresponding procedural fees. Surgical modifiers define the other elements of provider services rendered in the 90-day global period. Listed below are some modifiers that are frequently misused. It is beyond the scope of this text to comprehensively review every modifier.

Several modifiers are used to indicate a billed service that is not part of a global surgical package, and therefore is eligible for separate reimbursement. **Modifier 24** is "Unrelated Evaluation and Management Service by the Same Physician During a Postoperative Period." The modifier indicates that an evaluation/management (E/M) service was performed during the postoperative period for a reason unrelated to the original procedure. This circumstance is reported by adding the modifier 24 to the appropriate level of E/M service. For example, a patient undergoes a colectomy and is discharged from the hospital. The CPT code reported is 44140. The postoperative global period for this code is 90 days. The patient subsequently returns to the office within a week and is treated for hemorrhoidal irritation. These two episodes of care have unrelated ICD-9 diagnostic codes and represent separate diseases. The physician should report the appropriate evaluation and management code followed by the 24 modifier, e.g., 9921224. In order for the E/M service to be payable in the postoperative period with the 24 modifier, the diagnosis code supporting the service must be different from the diagnosis code reported for the previously performed surgery. Modifier 24 should not be used for the medical management of a patient by the surgeon after surgery.

Modifier 25 is "Significant, Separately Identifiable Evaluation and Management (E/M) Service by the Same Physician on the Day of a Procedure." For example, a patient returns for a visit to complain about an incisional hernia. The appropriate evaluation and management service is provided. During the course of the visit, the provider determines that the patient should receive a screening flexible endoscopy. Since these two episodes of care carry different diagnoses, each is separately billable.

Modifier 50 is used for "Bilateral Procedures." Bilateral procedures performed at the same operative session should be identified by first coding one procedure. The second procedure is coded with the addition of a modifier 50. Some procedures are exempt from this modifier because the procedure represents a bilateral operation, such as a hemorrhoidectomy.

Modifier 51 is used for "Multiple Procedures," other than evaluation and management services, performed on the same day or at the same session by the same provider. The primary procedure or service is coded as usual, and the additional procedure is reported with the modifier 51. Providers should be careful not to use this modifier for add-on procedures. Appending the procedure with a modifier 51 requests separate reimbursement for the additional procedure. That reimbursement is reduced to represent the services provided in the operating room. Add-on procedures have already been reduced. By adding the 51 modifier to an add-on code, the reduced service will be further restricted.

Modifier 53 is used for a "Discontinued Procedure." Due to extenuating circumstances or those that threaten the well-being of the patient, the physician may elect to terminate a surgical or diagnostic procedure. It is then necessary to indicate that a surgical or diagnostic procedure was started but discontinued. This circumstance is reported by adding the modifier 53 to the code for the discontinued procedure. Documentation describing the circumstances requiring the discontinuation should be provided with the claim submission. This modifier is not used to report the elective cancellation of a procedure before the patient's anesthesia induction and/or surgical preparation in the operating suite. This modifier is effective for services rendered on or after January 1, 1997. It should be used with procedure code 45378 when billing for failed colonoscopies (those that do not pass the splenic flexure) performed on or after January 1, 1997.

Modifier 54 is "Surgical Care Only." When a patient receives surgical care only and then is transferred to the care of another specialty or surgical group, the procedure is reported using the appropriate code and modifier 54. This usually results in a significant reduction in fees and varies with each procedure.

Modifier 55 is "Postoperative Management Only." This modifier applies when a patient receives surgical care elsewhere and a new physician or group provides the postoperative care. The group providing the postoperative care uses the operative code with the modifier 55. This permits reimbursement for the portion of the surgical fee set aside for postoperative care.

Modifier 57 is "Decision for Surgery." Adding modifier 57 to the appropriate level of E/M service identifies an evaluation and management service that results in the initial decision to perform the surgery. E/M services on the day before or on the day of major surgery (90-day global period) that result in the initial decision to perform the surgery are not included in the global surgery payment. These

E/M services may be billed separately and identified with the 57 modifier. This modifier should not be used for visits during the global period of minor procedures (0- or 10-day global period) unless the purpose of the visit is a decision for major surgery. This modifier is not used with minor surgeries, because the global period for minor surgeries does not include the day before the surgery. When the decision to perform the minor procedure is typically done immediately before the service, it is considered a routine preoperative service and a visit or consultation is not billed in addition to the procedure.

Modifier 58 is "Staged Procedure or Service by the Same Physician During the Postoperative Period." The physician may need to indicate that the performance of a procedure during the postoperative global period represents a planned return to the operating room. Examples include a planned "second look" for ischemic bowel or intraabdominal abscess. It is best to identify the planned second procedure in the documentation for the first procedure.

Modifier 59 is "Distinct Procedural Service." Under certain circumstances, a provider may need to indicate that a procedure or service was independent from other services performed on the same day. This modifier developed from the Correct Coding Initiative. The modifier defines an episode of care or a procedure that is separate and distinct from another episode of care. For example, a patient undergoes a large intestine resection, CPT code 44140. During the course of surgery, the segment of bowel involved was densely adherent to the splenic flexure of the colon. Thus the entire splenic flexure required mobilization, CPT code 44139. Proper coding requires a modifier 59 for the splenic flexure mobilization code to pass. The carrier's computer would not allow for the CPT code 44139 without the modifier. In a different sense, the CPT code 44139 is considered a component of a low anterior resection, CPT code 44145. In this case, the modifier does not recognize reimbursement for both CPT 44145 and 44139.

Modifier 62 is "Two Surgeons." For some procedures, two surgeons are required because of differing skills. For example, during a pelvic exenteration, the services of a urologist and a colorectal surgeon may be required for the operation. In this instance, the total reimbursement is 125% of the original fee. Each surgeon should document his or her individual aspects of the procedure. This modifier is distinctly different than an assistant at surgery.

Modifier 66, "Surgical Team," is more rare than a procedure requiring two surgeons. An example might be a pelvic exenteration with a partial sacrectomy. The surgeons involved could be a team composed of a colorectal surgeon, a urologist, a neurosurgeon, and possibly a gynecologist. Each physician must provide proper documentation of his or her role in the operative and postoperative management. The HCFA prices these cases by individual report.

Modifier 78 is "Return to the Operating Room for a Related Procedure During the Postoperative Period." This most commonly represents a complication of a previous procedure. An example would be an anastomotic leak following a colon resection. The subsequent operations to treat this complication would be coded with the modifier 78 added to the appropriate procedure code.

Modifier 79 is "Unrelated Procedure by the Same Physician During the Postoperative Period." The physician may need to indicate that the performance of a procedure or service during the postoperative period was unrelated to the original procedure. This circumstance may be reported by using the modifier 79. For example, a repair of an incisional hernia (49565) is performed. The postoperative period designation for this procedure code is 90 days. Within 2 weeks, the same physician performs a cholecystectomy, CPT code 47600. The physician should report the cholecystectomy as 4760079.

Modifier 80 is "Assistant Surgeon," and **Modifier 82** is "Assistant Surgeon (when qualified resident surgeon not available)." Assistants at surgery are subject to review and approval by HCFA each year. The American College of Surgeons vigorously defends the right of the patient to have assistants at surgery with appropriate reimbursement. Modifier 80 is used in a nonteaching environment, or 82 is used when residents are documented as being unavailable. The operative report must clearly reflect that the assistant surgeon was required because of the complex nature of the procedure. The HCFA reserves the right to determine eligibility for this modifier.

Claim Forms

Numerous claim forms exist, and each insurance carrier has a specific form. The standard form for Medicare serves as the prototype and will be briefly reviewed. The HCFA form 1500 is familiar to almost every medical practice. The form is designed to reveal the patient's insurance coverage and individual demographics. The form also identifies additional insurance coverage called Medigap coverage. This is a health insurance policy or other health benefit plan offered by private entities to patients who are entitled to Medicare benefits. Medigap coverage is specifically designed to supplement Medicare benefits. The 1500 form also identifies the referring physician and the ordering physician. The date, location of service, type of care, and diagnoses are all entered on the form.

Incomplete or invalid information often leads to claim denials. In 1996, the HCFA began disallowing all appeals for incomplete or invalid information. The billing records are returned to the billing agent marked "return as unprocessable." Preventing a claim appeal was introduced by HCFA to be a cost and time saving measure for the appeal process. A denied claim can still be resubmitted within 6 months with the needed corrections.

Appeals and Hearings

For the Medicare population, the appeal process starts with "post payment review." In a post payment review, the claim receives an independent review. The actual filing of a request for review can occur in writing, by fax or telephone, or electronically. The appeal begins from the date noted on the reconciliation voucher (Explanation of Medicare Benefits [EOMB]). It may be necessary to provide supporting documents, including anesthesia records, laboratory or pathology reports, computed tomographic scans, and more. A Medicare insurance claim review request must be completed for each claim. If the post payment review proves unsatisfactory and if the amount in dispute exceeds $100, a "fair hearing" may be requested. In addition to written documentation, the hearings may be conducted in person, over the telephone, or solely in written format. The carrier is required to respond to the hearing in 45 to 120 days. If the hearing officer denies the claim, further appeal involves an administrative law judge. The action must involve a $500 minimum and must be filed within 60 days of the fair hearing. Unfortunately, other insurance agencies do not provide the same organization and due process as Medicare.

Each insurance company varies its billing and reimbursement practices. Nearly all agencies have computerized the processing of claims. The vendors that provide the software have provided the carriers with numerous options to implement payment policies. The software that determines payment is easily adjusted and is often inconsistent with accepted norms for procedures, coding, and billing. This allows an insurance company to constantly change its payment policies by simply altering the software through built-in "switches." For example, the carrier can decide to stop paying for all preoperative evaluation and management services that include a decision to operate. By simply adjusting the computer program, all such claims are denied. For the provider to be reimbursed for the service provided, each denied claim requires an appeal. Some evidence suggests that carriers and payment vendors promote payment policy changes to increase claims denials. To reverse such carrier and vendor practice requires extensive legislative efforts. Unpublicized rules and policies further complicate the claims process for each clinical practice.

Conclusion

New technologies and improved treatments are increasing the quality of health care. Although new technologies offer potential cost savings to society as a whole, the opportunities for savings and more efficient care are rarely appreciated by the insurance carriers. Often, technological advances extend health care services to new frontiers with unimaginable quality. Initially, however, the costs only escalate. For example, laparoscopic surgery has decreased hospital length of stay and reduced recovery periods with early patient return to work.

But the increased cost of laparoscopic procedures has not been fully reimbursed by the third-party payers, particularly the federal government. Additionally, more patients are undergoing surgery than before because the new technology offers improved outcomes. If the present health care system is to survive, similar cost-saving measures and greater efficiency must be developed.

Understanding coding, documentation, and billing improves office efficiency and health care delivery systems. During the past 5 years the reduction in available health care dollars has encouraged insurers to exert influence over coding and billing. It is imperative that individual practices improve coding to be able to provide quality and efficient care. Accurate coding benefits the entire system by improving reimbursement and by providing an accurate model for predicting future health care needs.

Finally, the nation should develop a physician-sponsored national health care coding policy. Such a policy would serve as a benchmark to evaluate and grade the various insurance carriers nationwide. The national health care coding policy, with the endorsement of the HCFA, would ensure that federal and nonfederal insurance agencies follow national standards. Such an effort to standardize payments, prevent unwarranted denials, and limit senseless delays in care would create health care policies rather than insurance policies. Standards would limit fraud and abuse, improve correct coding, shift emphasis toward proper care, and improve the overall quality of the coding database.

References

1. Highlights: National Health Expenditures, 1997. Available at: http://www.HCFA.gov/stats/nhe-oact/hilites.htm. Accessed March 16, 1999.
2. American Medical Association. Physician's Current Procedural Terminology (CPT), 4th edition. Chicago: American Medical Association, 1998.
3. World Health Organization. International Statistical Classification of Diseases and Related Health Problems, 9th Revision (ICD-9). Geneva: World Health Organization, 1989.

17

Ambulatory Anorectal Surgery in Australia

Ian G. Faragher, M.B., B.S., F.R.A.C.S., F.R.C.S.(Ed.)

The Australian Health Care System

Ambulatory surgical services are less common in Australia than in the United States. The reasons for this are multifactorial and are predominantly due to different economic incentives and public attitudes in the two countries. In Australia medical care in public institutions is funded by the federal government and is available without additional charges. About 70% of the population receives its medical care through this system. This system includes the university teaching hospitals and the vast majority of undergraduate and postgraduate medical education. The remaining 30% of the population have health insurance and may elect to receive their health care within the private health care system.

Ambulatory surgery is performed in both the private and public sectors. The federal government and the private insurers in Australia have not demanded a move from inpatient to outpatient procedures to the same extent as have the managed care organizations in the United States. Despite a recent trend for health insurance companies to move from the nonprofit to the commercial domain, there are currently no requirements for pretreatment authorization or limitations on length of stay. In addition, there has not been a strong stimulus promoting ambulatory surgery within the public sector. Limiting the growth of health care costs within the public system has been accomplished by rationing health care. Patients are stratified by need and are placed on waiting lists for elective procedures. Less emphasis is placed on either decreasing the length of stay for inpatient surgery or performing more ambulatory surgery. The public appears to tolerate the

increased time both waiting for surgery and remaining hospitalized postoperatively.

Despite these generalizations, there is a true desire to increase the role of ambulatory surgery in Australia. Until recently, outpatient procedures were scheduled in the same surgical suites as inpatient procedures. Many hospitals now are developing specific outpatient surgery units. Although there are still far fewer freestanding ambulatory facilities in Australia than in the United States, such facilities are slowly gaining acceptance.

Method

The number and corresponding length of stay of four anorectal operations (selected by International Classification of Diseases, Ninth Revision [ICD-9] codes) were retrieved by electronic searches of local and national databases for the most recent financial year (July 1 to June 30). Hospital 1 has a dedicated day surgery facility, and hospital 2 does not. The Australian Institute for Health and Welfare (Canberra, Australia) supplied the national figures for Australia. The data from the United States were retrieved from the U.S. Department of Health and Human Services[1] via the Internet. These data are summarized in Table 17.1.

Results

Only 11% of hemorrhoidectomies in Australia in 1996–1997 were performed as outpatient procedures, compared with 74% of such operations in the

TABLE 17.1. Ambulatory and inpatient anorectal operations in Australia and the United States.

		Number of operations			
	ICD-9 code	Ambulatory	Inpatients	Average stay (days)	Ambulatory cases (%)
Hospital 1 (1997–98)					
Incision perianal abscess	49.01	31	29	5.5	52
Anal fistulotomy	49.11	18	12	7.3	60
Hemorrhoidectomy	49.46	40	58	2.7	41
Excision pilonidal sinus	86.21	37	16	3.2	70
Subtotals		126	115		52
Hospital 2 (1997–98)					
Incision perianal abscess	49.01	3	31	8.4	9
Anal fistulotomy	49.11	13	18	2.9	42
Hemorrhoidectomy	49.46	11	74	2	13
Excision pilonidal sinus	86.21	11	31	1.7	26
Subtotals		38	154		20
Australia (1996–97)					
Incision perianal abscess	49.01	354	3,469	3	9
Anal fistulotomy	49.11	576	1,611	2.8	26
Hemorrhoidectomy	49.43/4/6	1,240	9,780	3.6	11
Incision pilonidal sinus	86.03	164	1,045	2.8	14
Subtotals		2,334	15,905		13
United States (1994)					
Hemorrhoidectomy	49.43–6	80,000	28,000		74

United States during 1994. Anal fistulotomy is the most common ambulatory anorectal operation performed in Australia. Comparing the data between the two Australian hospitals demonstrates a wide variation in local practice. The rates of ambulatory procedures were generally higher in hospital 1, which has a dedicated day surgery unit, than in hospital 2.

The national length-of-stay data for Australia reveal that patients admitted for these procedures spend an average of 2 nights in the hospital. Again, there is substantial local variation between institutions.

Discussion

The Royal Australasian College of Surgeons created a committee on outpatient surgery in 1980. This committee developed into the Australian Day Surgery Council. It currently determines the standards and clinical indicators for accreditation of ambulatory surgery centers. The council now realizes that increasing the utilization of ambulatory surgery will provide significant benefits for patients as well as economic and institutional advantages.[2] Despite our understanding the advantages of ambulatory surgery in general, anorectal operations in Australia are usually performed on inpatients,

whereas in the United States the majority are ambulatory procedures. Although no data exist to explain this difference, my personal opinion attributes the lower rate of ambulatory anorectal surgery in Australia to a combination of historical, economic, and regulatory issues. It is unlikely that Australian patients have higher comorbid conditions mandating inpatient treatment.

Historically, patients were admitted to the hospital on the day before surgery. Patients were kept in hospital until the first bowel movement, which often occurred on the fifth postoperative day. Many surgeons still justify an overnight stay for possible problems with analgesia, urinary retention, or constipation.

Increasing the amount of ambulatory surgery performed in Australia requires acceptance by the surgical staff and paramedical personnel as well as by the general community. Once a commitment to outpatient surgery is made, the surgeon may adopt a range of techniques that facilitate this method of care.

In anorectal surgery, these techniques include preoperative use of a high-fiber product with or without an enema; infiltration of long-acting local anesthetic around the anal canal at surgery; restriction of intravenous fluids during anesthesia to minimize the risk of postoperative urinary retention;

continuing the fiber product postoperatively; adequate regular oral analgesia; liberal use of sitz baths; and the availability of 24-hour telephone support. Patient education, consisting of verbal and written information covering the events on the day of surgery and possible problems in the postoperative period, is invaluable in facilitating recovery and compliance. Of note is the fact that the prescription of medications by telephone is not allowed in Australia.

Institutional services may also assist in increasing ambulatory surgery. For example, a nursing service can convert a patient from oral coumarin to low–molecular weight heparin injections while at home, then supervise the return to oral anticoagulation. This is invaluable and avoids inpatient perioperative heparin infusions. A visiting nurse may also perform wound care and change dressings, if required.

Despite many benefits for patients, practitioners, and institutions, the rate of ambulatory surgery remains low in Australia. In the current environment, in which change is directed more by accountants than by clinicians, the aim is often to do the same for less, rather than to do more in an efficient manner. Increasing the rate of ambulatory surgery will meet both of these objectives. However, the "same for less" policy prevents the investment of enthusiasm and resources required to effect more rapid change. Until recently, the funding formula for Australian public hospitals was biased toward inpatient procedures. If true economic incentives existed, I am sure the rate of ambulatory anorectal surgery would rise in Australia to approximate levels in the United States, as the underlying biological problems are identical.

References

1. Pokras R, Kozak LJ, McCarthy E. Ambulatory and inpatient procedures in the United States, 1994. Vital Health Stat 13 1997;Dec(132):1–113.
2. Royal Australasian College of Surgeons. Report and Recommendations on Day Surgery. Melbourne: Royal Australasian College of Surgeons, 1997.
3. Day Surgery. Report and recommendations of the Royal Australasian College of Surgeons, Australian and New Zealand College of Anaethetists, and the Australian Society of Anaethetists. Revised edition 1997. (Published) Royal Australasian College of Surgeons, Melbourne Australia.

Index

ISBN 0-387-98603-0

9 780387 986036 >